ALMOST HOME:
REFORMING HOME AND COMMUNITY CARE IN ONTARIO

Almost Home is a rich and comprehensive study of the policy questions underlying the shift in medical care from hospitals to homes and communities, a change that is reshaping Canadian health care policy and politics. Using document analysis and interviews with government officials and other key stakeholders in the policy community, the authors analyse the policy content and process of five different attempts to reform home and community care in Ontario between 1985 and 1996, as introduced by Liberal, New Democratic, and Conservative governments.

As this study demonstrates, the ongoing shift from the Medicare 'mainstream' of physician and hospital care to the Medicare 'margins' entails not only a shift in the site of care but an erosion of the post-war state's role in health care. While Medicare continues to resist political and ideological forces aimed at shrinking the state's role, cost constraints, demographic pressures, and technological advancements are increasing pressure on home and community care.

The authors have made a significant contribution to research on policy development and change. Their rigorously analytical approach fills a major gap in book-length literature on long-term health care in Canada.

PATRICIA M. BARANEK has an adjunct position in the Department of Health Policy, Management, and Evaluation at the University of Toronto.

RAISA B. DEBER is a professor in the Department of Health Policy, Management, and Evaluation at the University of Toronto.

A. PAUL WILLIAMS is an associate professor in the Department of Health Policy, Management, and Evaluation at the University of Toronto.

Almost Home

Reforming Home and Community Care in Ontario

PATRICIA M. BARANEK
RAISA B. DEBER
A. PAUL WILLIAMS

UNIVERSITY OF TORONTO PRESS
Toronto Buffalo London

© University of Toronto Press Incorporated 2004
Toronto Buffalo London
Printed in Canada

ISBN: 0-8020-8965-8 (cloth)
ISBN: 0-8020-8639-X (paper)

Printed on acid-free paper

National Library of Canada Cataloguing in Publication

Baranek, Patricia M., 1946–
   Almost home : reforming home and community care in
   Ontario / Patricia M. Baranek, Raisa B. Deber, A. Paul Williams.

   Includes bibliographical references and index.
   ISBN 0-8020-8965-8 (bound)   ISBN 0-8020-8639-X (pbk.)

   1. Home care services – Government policy – Ontario – History –
   20th century.   2. Long-term care of the sick – Government policy –
   Ontario – History – 20th century.   3. Home care services – Government
   policy – Ontario.   4. Long-term care of the sick – Government policy –
   Ontario.   I. Deber, Raisa B., 1949–   II. Williams, A. Paul (Alan Paul),
   1951–   II. Title.

   RA645.37.C3B37 2004   362.1' 4' 0971309049   C2004-900723-8

University of Toronto Press acknowledges the financial assistance to its
publishing program of the Canada Council for the Arts and the Ontario
Arts Council.

University of Toronto Press acknowledges the financial support for its
publishing activities of the Government of Canada through the Book
Publishing Industry Development Program (BPIDP).

To Frank and Gemma Baranek

Contents

Acknowledgments

Almost Home: Reforming Home and Community Care in Ontario is based on Patricia Baranek's doctoral thesis. In that work successive attempts by three Ontario governments to reform home and community care were analysed, and it was noted that policy agreement remains elusive. Since then, both the Romanow Commission and the Kirby Committee have recommended adding a limited range of home and community care, primarily targeted at individuals with short-term needs who have been discharged from hospitals. The issue of how best to deal with the other populations who might benefit from home and community care, however, remains unsettled. The original thesis has been extended and put into this wider context.

A number of individuals were key to the successful completion of the doctoral research. We would like particularly to recognize the contribution of Professor Ronald Manzer, a member of the thesis committee, for his thorough and constructive questioning and suggestions. We are grateful to the Ontario Ministry of Health who gave generous access to information. The comprehensiveness and the richness of the data are also due to the generosity of all those who participated in interviews and provided further documentation. We would especially like to thank those individuals, who encompass public servants, politicians, and representatives from consumer and labour groups, provider organizations, and associations, who provided their time and insights. However, we bear responsibility for the interpretation of their input. Our appreciation is extended to the anonymous reviewers from the University of Toronto Press and the Social Science Federation of Canada for their insightful comments. Considerable administrative and research assistance was provided throughout by Ann Pendleton, Scott McDonald, and Cathy Bezic in the Department of Health Policy, Management and Evaluation.

We would like to acknowledge the financial support of the University of Toronto Open Fellowship, the National Health Research Development Doctoral Fellowship, the National Health Research Development Program, the M-THAC (From Medicare to Home and Community) Research Unit, funded by the Canadian Institutes for Health Research, and the Department of Health Policy, Management and Evaluation.

Our thanks to Virgil Duff, the executive editor at the University of Toronto Press, for his encouragement and support. We are indebted to Frances Mundy, editor, for overseeing the manuscript to completion and to Catherine Frost, copy editor, for her meticulous readings and revisions to the text.

This book is the product of many minds and hearts. However, the wisdom and support of those listed above were supplemented with the encouragement, respect, and constancy of family. Our appreciation and love go to Tony and Joshua Doob, Liba Nicholls and Denise Ballentine, Charles and Jonathan Deber, Abraham and the late Norda Berlin, and Janet Lum.

Abbreviations

ACE	Advocacy Centre for the Elderly
ADM	Assistant deputy minister
AMO	Association of Municipalities of Ontario
CAP	Canada Assistance Plan
CCAC	Community Care Access Centre
CCCO	Comprehensive Community Care Organization
CCHO	Council of Chronic Hospitals of Ontario
CHA	Canada Health Act
CHO	Community Health Organization
CHST	Canada Health and Social Transfer
CMSO	Comprehensive Multi-Service Organization
COTA	Community Occupational Therapist Associates
CPC	Canadian Pensioners Concerned
CRCS	Canadian Red Cross Society
CUPE	Canadian Union of Public Employees
CWL	Catholic Women's League of Canada
DHC	District Health Council
ED	Executive director
EPF	Established Programs Financing
FP	For profit
GDP	Gross Domestic Product
GNP	Gross National Product
HSTAP	Health Sector Training and Adjustment Program
HTAB	Hospital Training and Adjustment Board
IHP	Integrated Homemaker Program
LTC	Long-term care
MC	Ministry of Citizenship

MCRR	Ministry of Citizenship, Culture and Recreation
MCSS	Ministry of Community and Social Services
MOH	Ministry of Health
MPP	Member of Provincial Parliament
MSA	Multi-Service Agency
NDP	New Democratic Party
NFP	Not for profit
OCSA	Ontario Community Support Association
OCSCO	Ontario Coalition of Senior Citizens' Organizations
ODP	Office for Disabled Persons
OECD	Organisation for Economic Cooperation and Development
OFHN	Ontario Family Health Network
OHA	Ontario Hospital Association
OHCPA	Ontario Home Care Programs Association
OHHCPA	Ontario Home Health Care Providers' Association
OHIP	Ontario Health Insurance Plan
OMA	Ontario Medical Association
ONA	Ontario Nurses' Association
ONHA	Ontario Nursing Home Association
OPSEU	Ontario Public Sector Employees Union
OSCA	Office for Senior Citizens' Affairs
PC	Progressive Conservative Party
PHC	Primary Health Care
RFP	Request for Proposal
RPN	Registered Practical Nurses
St Eliz.	Saint Elizabeth Visiting Nurses' Association of Ontario
SAO	Service Access Organization
SCA	Service Coordination Agency
SCCA	Senior Citizens' Consumer Alliance
USCO	United Senior Citizens of Ontario
VON	Victorian Order of Nurses
WCB	Workers' Compensation Board
WHO	World Health Organization

ALMOST HOME:
REFORMING HOME AND COMMUNITY CARE IN ONTARIO

CHAPTER ONE

Introduction and Overview

1.1 From Hospital to Home and Community

Hospitals are changing; care is increasingly occurring outside hospital walls in outpatient clinics, offices, and even in people's homes (Canadian Home Care Association, 1998; Canadian Institute for Health Information, 2000; Hospital Report Research Collaborative, 2001; Shamian and Lightstone, 1997; Sheps et al., 2000). The Federal-Provincial-Territorial Advisory Committee on Health Services Working Group on Continuing Care has defined home care as 'an array of services which enables clients, incapacitated in whole or in part, to live at home, often with the effect of preventing, delaying, or substituting for long-term care or acute care alternatives' (Dumont-Lemasson et al., 1999).

But the home is a location; it is not a coherent service. Home and community services can substitute for *acute* care in hospitals and/or provide services to *post-acute* patients who have been discharged from a hospital. They can substitute for long-term care in *nursing homes*. They also can represent an appropriate way of *maintaining* health and allowing clients to remain independent for a longer period of time, thus avoiding or delaying the need for institutional care. Finally, they can *prevent* deterioration through additional services and monitoring. The mix of clients, services, and providers varies accordingly.

The shift of care out of hospitals has been enabled by technology. An increasing range of services, some of remarkable complexity, now can be delivered safely in the home. Yet the fact that something *can* be done does not tell us why policy makers *wish* it to happen. They have adopted two primary justifications for encouraging this shift. The first reason is tied to *costs*, driven in large part by assumptions that many services provided in hospitals and other health care institutions can be provided less expensively in the community or, at the very least, that expenditures can be contained more easily through 'capped' funding arrangements (Chappell, 1994; Coyte and Young, 1997a,b; Hollander, 1994; Jackson, 1994; Jacobs et al., 1995). The second is tied to *quality*, driven by the belief that services provided 'closer to home' respond to consumer preferences and can enhance consumer choice, independence, and quality of life, positively affecting health and well-being (B.C. Royal Commission on Health Care and Costs, 1991; Shapiro, 1992). It should be noted that the policy shift occurred before there was systematic evidence that the ongoing shift from hospital to home and community would produce more favourable outcomes in terms of health costs, quality, or improved health status. The results of recent evaluations are somewhat equivocal; some find improved outcomes (Hollander, 2001; Hollander and Tessaro, 2001; Hollander et al., 2002), while others do not (Fassbender, 2001; Jacobs, 2001; Saskatchewan HSURC, 2000a).

As we argue in this book, the shift from hospital to home and community is fundamentally reshaping Canadian health care policy and politics – both the way in which health care services are funded and delivered and the dynamics of health care policy making. This is because the move out of hospitals does more than simply change the *site* of care; it results in an increasing proportion of care moving beyond the collective 'logic' and institutionalized boundaries of the 'Medicare mainstream,' which consists of publicly funded, 'medically necessary' services delivered in hospital or by physicians. Within this mainstream the costs of illness are shared across society and access to services is based on need. Outside, the more individualistic 'logic' of private competitive markets, where care is not an entitlement and where access to services is more likely to be a function of the ability to pay, places the costs of illness on the ill. Within the mainstream of Canadian Medicare there is sustained public and political support for the principles of universal access to medically necessary care, buttressed by the concentrated power of the organized medical profession. Outside, even in proximate fields like home- and community-based care, there is a relative legislative vacuum at the national level, there is little agreement on principles, and policy communities are highly fragmented. In these less visible, less politically mobilized and highly fragmented terrains, governments are largely free to act as they see fit either to extend the public logic of universal coverage or to move to the private logic of competitive markets. Thus, while the hospital and physician 'mainstream,' not only in Canada but in other industrialized countries, has proved relatively resistant to political change, particularly when compared with other components of the post-war state (such as welfare, education, or housing), change outside the mainstream is politically less constrained.

In this book we concentrate on two sets of issues by examining home and community care reform in Ontario between 1985 and 1996. At the level of policy *content*, we delineate the different policy choices considered by successive governments concerning the appropriate boundaries between the roles and responsibilities of public governments and private markets – the 'public-private mix.' As we discuss in more detail in following chapters, three dimensions of this mix can be distinguished: *financing* (who pays for which services and for whom); *delivery* (how services are organized and operated); and *allocation* (the mechanisms and incentive structures inherent in how resources flow from those financing care to those delivering it). At the level of policy *process*, we analyse why policy within the home and community care sector has swung wildly across policy choices, whereas policy within the adjacent sectors of physician services has remained relatively static. We argue that one key reason is the difference in the structures and institutions surrounding decision making in these adjacent arenas, which in turn are strongly influenced by the policy legacies associated with the development of Canadian Medicare or the lack thereof.

1.1.1 The Medicare Mainstream

Canadian Medicare evolved gradually, shaped by the realities of 'fiscal federalism.' Constitutionally, health care is a responsibility of provincial governments. Yet provinces vary considerably in their fiscal capacity. In the early days of the nation, medical science was limited in its ability to treat and heal, and its purchase was left to the individual patient. Over time, as medical knowledge has expanded, governments in all countries have come under increased public pressure to ensure that all residents have access to a basic level of services. In Canada, it was clear that richer provinces (of which Ontario was among the richest) would be able afford a far higher level of services than their poorer counterparts. This disparity translated into a series of cost-sharing agreements, whereby the federal government redistributed resources to help pay for the most expensive parts of health care delivery, leaving the other, admittedly important, services to markets and/or charity. To respect provincial jurisdiction, these arrangements provided federal money to provincial governments, initially in the form of direct grants for purposes such as

hospital construction, public health, and the training of health professionals. In 1957 the Hospital Insurance and Diagnostic Services Act provided for the federal government's sharing approximately half the cost
of provincial hospital insurance plans as long as the provinces complied
with a set of national terms and conditions. (Because it was more difficult for poor provinces to find the matching funds, the funding formula
was not precisely 50-50, but was based on a combination of provincial
and national average expenditures for hospital services. This in turn
meant that poor provinces would receive a higher proportion of their
expenditures for hospital services from federal sources, whereas richer
provinces would receive a higher per capita grant, thus allowing all provinces to feel aggrieved.) A similar plan, the 1966 Medical Care Act
extended cost sharing to insurance for physician services. By 1971 every
Canadian province had in place provincially run insurance plans that
reimbursed private providers of hospital and physician services. Other
services were not included in the cost-sharing formula, although provincial governments could (and did) pay for them with provincial
resources. Mental health, for example, was delivered largely within provincially run psychiatric hospitals and, as such, did not attract federal
cost sharing. Neither did public health, which was traditionally paid for
and delivered by combinations of provincial and local governments.

The vision of health care in Canada was thus solidly based upon how
medicine was practised in 1957. At that time, sickness was largely treated
on an in-patient basis. The definition of hospital services included everything seen as required, including nursing, diagnostic tests, physiotherapy, pharmaceuticals administered to in-patients, and so on. Little
thought was given to what might happen if such services could be delivered outside the hospital to very sick people.

It was soon realized that the cost-sharing formula was overly rigid and
discouraged innovations in delivery. Care given inside a hospital or by a
physician would attract '50 cent dollars' (more or less) from the federal
government. Care given in the community – for example, by a nurse
practitioner – would have to be paid for from provincial resources only.
Both levels of government accordingly agreed to shift the funding formula to a per capita entitlement – intended to increase with growth in
the Gross Domestic Product – made up of a combination of 'tax points'
and residual cash. The federal government agreed to reduce its tax rate
for individuals and business by a specified amount, allowing provinces
to increase their own taxes with no net cost to taxpayers. After 1977, with
the passage of Established Programs Financing (EPF), the cost-sharing

for hospital insurance, medical (physician) insurance, and post-secondary education (colleges and universities) was replaced by this new formula. Federal control was reduced; the new money became part of provincial general revenues. Provinces had only to comply with the (rather general) national terms and conditions for health care; no conditions whatsoever were attached to the post-secondary education funding. Neither were any restrictions attached to the additional per capita grant labelled as being for 'extended health services,' in order that provinces could experiment with different ways of delivering care in the home and community should they wish to do so. After 1977 provincial governments were free to set their own priorities and to innovate with delivery mechanisms.

In 1984 the Canada Health Act (CHA) (Government of Canada, 1984) clarified the terms and conditions. Provincial plans would have to meet the following five conditions: *universal* coverage (everyone eligible for coverage would be part of the plan); *public administration* of the insurance plan in a way that maintained accountability for the use of public money(although widely misunderstood, this condition did not require public delivery; indeed, almost all care was delivered by private physicians and private not-for-profit hospitals); *comprehensive* coverage of all medically necessary hospital and physician services (without defining what was meant by medically necessary); *portability* across provincial boundaries for insured services to insured persons; and reasonable *access* to insured services by insured persons, unimpeded by financial or other barriers. The last provision included a prohibition against user fees to insured persons for insured services. Provincial governments did not have to adhere to the CHA terms and conditions; health care remained under their constitutional authority. If they did not do so, however, the federal government was empowered to impose fiscal penalties, including dollar for dollar withholding of the amount charged in user fees from the federal contribution.

These definitions erected a barrier around the set of services protected by the terms of the Canada Health Act. Within the CHA, services had to be provided universally, on the basis of need, without co-payments or user charges. Outside the barrier, however, provincial governments retained autonomy to decide who to cover, for what, and under what circumstances. Although section 6 of the Canada Health Act allows for the provision of extended health care services, these services were not made subject to the five principles of the act. CHA services accordingly became the 'mainstream' of Medicare. As Tuohy (1999a,b) and Maioni (1998) have noted, the CHA thus served to insulate these services from the cost-cutting pressures evident on other components of the welfare state.

The economically difficult times in the 1980s and 1990s initially were met by deficit financing. As national debt exploded, however, governments were forced to take severe steps to bring their finances under control. In Canada, the federal government unilaterally changed the funding formula; the per capita entitlement for EPF payments no longer grew at the same rate as inflation. Since tax revenue did keep pace, the cash contribution shrank dramatically, to the point where it was in danger of disappearing altogether. Although formally there was no longer a federal contribution for health care – and there had not been since 1977 (Auditor General of Canada, 1999; Deber, 2000a) – this was a complex case to make. Instead, provincial governments were successful in convincing the public both that the transferred tax points should not be counted as part of the federal contribution and that the federal government was no longer paying 'its share' of health care costs. This campaign was accompanied by considerable fear that, in the absence of a sizeable federal cash contribution, there would be few levers with which to enforce compliance with CHA terms and conditions. However, the federal government was reluctant to hand its revenues over to provincial general revenues or to threaten its hard-won fiscal flexibility.

A sleight-of-hand solution was found. In 1996 the EPF programs (hospital insurance, medical insurance, post-secondary education) were combined with the last major cost-sharing program, the 1966 Canada Assistance Plan (CAP), which covered both income assistance to the poor and a series of means-tested social service programs to assist the elderly and disabled populations. The new transfer, again a mixture of cash and tax points, was renamed the Canada Health and Social Transfer (CHST). The federal government was able to cut its transfer (by approximately the amount of the former CAP payments), while introducing a 'cash floor' below which payments would not fall.

This shift had considerable impact on home- and community-based programs, many of which had formerly been funded under CAP. Indeed, because the CHA terms and conditions continued to apply only to those services delivered by doctors and by hospitals, although there was no longer dedicated funding for those social programs formerly covered under CAP, the demise of CAP reinforced the protection of those programs in the 'mainstream' while clarifying that decisions about whether or not to provide or fund other programs would be fully under the control of provincial decision makers.

On one level, Medicare has been an enormous success. Indeed, the concept of universal health care insurance remains the top policy priority and top-ranked national symbol for Canadians (Donelan et al., 1999; Ekos Research Associates Inc., 1998, 2001; Mendelsohn, 2002). Although Medicare is (perennially) under stress, the single-payer public system has been relatively successful in constraining expenditures for hospital and physician services – indeed, perhaps too successful. All Canadians have access to medically necessary hospital and doctor services without regard to their economic means. Indeed, Medicare has been one of the most successful progressive income distribution programs; access to care is based on need rather than on ability to pay. The subsidy and transfer dimension of public health care in Canada shows the progressive pattern of taxation and health care benefits. Those in the highest income brackets on average pay the most taxes and consume the least health care dollars, while those in the lowest income brackets derive the greatest benefit from Medicare (Ross et al., 2000). However, the limitations of the Canada Health Act's definition of comprehensiveness have become more evident as attention shifts to the needs of those with chronic illness and as technology allows care to shift from hospital into home and community. One recurring issue has been the role of community-based care for those with long-term needs for services.

1.1.2 Outside the Mainstream: Community-Based Long-Term Care

'Community-based long-term care' (LTC) traditionally has referred to the network of personal care, support, and health services required on a periodic or ongoing basis by people who, because of physical disability or ageing, need assistance to function as independently as possible. This network can be distinguished from the care given in long-term care *facilities*, such as chronic care hospitals, nursing homes, and homes for the aged (Ontario Ministry of Community and Social Services [MCSS], Ministry of Health [MOH] and Ministry of Citizenship [MC], 1991) and the supports falling outside the health care system (e.g., housing, income support), which nonetheless may be essential if people are to be able to function. In this book we concentrate only on the community-based LTC services.

It is important to note that nomenclature for community-based LTC is not standardized across Canada – some provinces refer to 'continuing care,' others to 'home care,' and still others to 'community care' (Hollander and Baranek, 1997). This system comprises services, programs, and facilities funded by and accountable to a mix of private organizations and governments. The formal system (which represents about 20 per cent of the services provided) includes both health and social services. The informal system involves the support given by family, friends, and volunteers, which represents over 80 per cent of help provided (MCSS et al., 1990). Although a considerable amount of care is provided in the community by providers falling within the medical mainstream (e.g., physician offices, ambulatory clinics, laboratory tests), neither government LTC programs nor this book will include these fully insured ambulatory services within the definition of community LTC.

Community-based LTC services in turn can be roughly broken down into (1) *in-home services* provided in people's homes by paid workers, further subdivided into *professional care* (e.g., nursing, physiotherapy), *personal supports* (e.g., assistance with bathing and toileting), *homemaking* (e.g., laundry, cleaning, meal preparation), and *respite* services to family caregivers; and (2) *community support services*, provided primarily by volunteers, largely but not entirely in people's homes (e.g., meals-on-wheels, transportation, security checks, friendly visiting), or in community centres (e.g., adult day programs, Alzheimer community programs) (MCSS et al., 1991).

As noted above, these services could be aimed at a number of different target populations. *Acute* and *post-acute* clients require the kinds of professional services, such as nursing and rehabilitation, which otherwise might have been provided within a hospital, but should be needed only for a limited period of time; 'cure' and discharge from the program are reasonable goals. The *chronic* clients, on the other hand, might need services for the foreseeable future, but would have a greater reliance upon homemaking and other support services to allow them to manage in their own homes. At one extreme, an oxygen-dependent individual might need skilled nursing. At the other extreme, a frail elderly person might need help only with cleaning and shopping.

Community-based LTC services, as organized in Ontario, accordingly could be dichotomized as falling either into the health sector or into the social service sector, a fact that has significance both historically and in terms of reform. Each set of services evolved. For example, Ontario first offered an Acute Home Care Program as a demonstration project in 1958; by 1974 it had been implemented through the province as an insured service under the Ontario Health Insurance Plan (OHIP) (Deber, 1992). The Acute Home Care Program was designed to facilitate early discharge of patients from acute-care hospitals by fully insuring in-home services for those clients requiring at least three professional services (among physiotherapy, occupational therapy, speech therapy, registered nursing, or social work) per month; because the program was intended for acutely ill rather than chronically ill clients, a time limit was placed upon eligibility for services. The plan also covered a range of support services, particularly some homemaking, but only for those also receiving the professional services. Coverage was implemented under the Ontario Health Insurance Act (Government of Ontario, 1990a), which defined how medically necessary physicians' services would be paid for. As such, this home care would be fully financed by government. In the terms later used, the client groups being targeted by the Acute Home Care Program were only the *acute* or the *post-acute* populations, rather than those needing either *chronic* or *preventive/maintenance* care. The program fell under the auspices of the Ministry of Health and adopted a medical model of care.

In contrast, the community support services included what is commonly referred to as the 'soft' services, such as meals on wheels, home maintenance, friendly visiting, transportation, security checks, adult day programs, elderly persons centres, and senior volunteer services. These services came under the jurisdiction of the Ministry of Community and Social Services (MCSS) and the Ministry of Community and Social Services Act (Government of Ontario, 1990b). The Ministry of Community and Social Services was colloquially referred to as 'Com Soc' at the beginning of the research period; subsequently, it became known as MCSS. We will refer to the ministry as MCSS throughout the book, except when an interviewee uses Com Soc in a response. In contrast to services falling under the auspices of the Ministry of Health (MOH), MCSS programs were not fully insured; patients were means tested and required to pay a portion of the costs if they were able to do so, while local governments were also expected to contribute. Accordingly, MCSS programs were not uniformly available across the province. Instead, they were provided by grass roots organizations driven by a large number of volunteers and funded by different levels of government and a variety of private sources, which included private insurance, charitable giving, and out-of-pocket expenditures. In practice, the actual services provided by the various programs overlapped; clients might receive home nursing or homemaking from either program. However, there were clear differences in how such services would be paid for. The clear 'cultural' differences between the MOH and MCSS were evident in these program models (Deber, 1992). These differences between a universal/medical/entitlement model and a local/social/means-tested user fee approach would recur throughout the discussions about LTC reform.

However, both the MOH and the MCSS programs fell outside what we are terming the mainstream of medicine; as such, federal legislation placed no constraints on the freedom of provincial governments to redesign this sector, should they wish to do so.

1.1.3 Policy Content: Financing, Delivery, and Allocation

With respect to *financing*, the Canada Health Act requires that to qualify for federal funding, provincial health care plans must comply with five national conditions (universality, comprehensiveness, accessibility, portability, and public administration); however, the definition of comprehensiveness does not require coverage of even medically necessary care once care shifts outside hospitals to providers other than physicians. On the one hand, this flexibility gives provinces considerable freedom to restructure health systems in innovative ways, to integrate services, and to shift funding away from acute care towards goals such as health promotion and population health. However, these innovations may not always represent improved efficiency. Instead, they frequently involve the shifting of responsibilities (and costs) to local/regional levels of government and even outside the public sector altogether. In the process, non-'mainstream' health care services (e.g., rehabilitation, drugs, home nursing, and personal support) may become fragmented (eroding the extent to which standards are national) and subject to the logic of commercial, increasingly globalized markets. For example, in our case study of Ontario, detailed in following chapters, a combination of hospital restructuring and long-term care reform shifted more and more care into the community and outside the purview of the CHA, but it also removed acute home care as a universal entitlement. Individuals are now guaranteed only that they will be assessed for publicly funded services, not that they will receive them. Thus, those who previously would have received some or all of their care in hospitals may now receive them from publicly funded Community Care Access Centres (CCACs), or they may be forced by capped budgets, restricted eligibility criteria, and service maximums, to seek care in private markets from both not-for-profit (NFP) and for-profit (FP) providers.

With respect to *delivery*, a potential expansion of the role of corporate FP providers (in comparison with historically predominant but relatively small NFP community-based agencies) raises important additional questions about service costs, quality, and professional power, which can be particularly problematic in areas such as home care and rehabilitation, in which there are few established standards and outcome measures and little systematic evaluation of costs or effectiveness. In contrast to other markets in which consumer choice and discretion may provide sufficient incentives to ensure an optimal balance of cost and quality, 'necessary' health care is often not discretionary, and many consumers may not be able to judge quality, to 'voice' concerns about poor quality, or to 'exit' from services or providers that do not meet their needs (Hirschman, 1970). Anecdotal evidence suggests that in Ontario there has already been a province-wide decline in the number and capacity of established NFP providers, who have experienced difficulty competing with larger FP competitors.

Further, the complexity of the community-based sector makes it inherently difficult to define and measure service quality. Community-based services are paid for by a mix of public (including local governments) and private sources (including private insurance, out-of pocket payments, and charities). Services are delivered by for-profit and not-for profit organizations and by an assortment of professionals, volunteers, and family caregivers. They are received by consumers with diverse characteristics and needs, ranging from home-based substitutes for acute-care hospital services to assistance with activities of daily living. In community-based LTC many consumers are not ill in a clinical sense; in addition to maintaining functional capacity and avoiding or delaying institutionalization, LTC aims for the attainment of more subjective and difficult-to-quantify goals, such as 'wellness,' 'independence,' 'empowerment,' and 'quality of life' (Béland and Arweiler, 1996a,b; Havens, 1995). Services are provided in geographically dispersed settings, including the consumer's home, where direct supervision and peer scrutiny may not be possible and where poor quality of care may be more difficult to detect than it would be within conventional health services organizations (Federal, Provincial and Territorial Working Group on Home Care, 1990).

The third dimension, *allocation*, refers to the mechanism by which finances flow to providers, who may be individuals or organizations in public or private sectors. Allocation includes resource allocation (how a resource envelope is determined and the mechanism for transferring funds to providers) and reimbursement (the formula for determining how much is to be paid to a provider for a service). A key question here is the extent to which the state intervenes to control the flow of funding or, conversely, the extent to which it allows other mechanisms, such as competitive market forces, to dominate.

Within the mainstream of Canadian Medicare, for instance, the terms and conditions required for federal funding have ensured that public funding has flowed to hospitals and doctors with relatively few strings attached. Hospitals have been given global budgets within which they were expected to provide a specified range of services, and individual physicians were reimbursed by provincial health care insurance plans on a fee-for-service basis for virtually every service they deemed to be medically necessary. This reflects both a greater emphasis on stability of health care providers and the field as a whole and caution about experimenting with different allocation approaches. As a result, major providers of care have not experienced any marked degree of direct competition with each other. In the field of home and community care, however, there has been a greater willingness to rely more on allocation through competitive market mechanisms. Such mechanisms usually involve a specified format for negotiating and administering contracts usually based on cost and price, and they encourage both experimentation in delivering services and competition among a pool of providers. As we will see in the case of Ontario, successive initiatives aimed at reforming home and community care used different allocation mechanisms, ranging from central command and control to market competition.

1.2 The Case of Ontario's Reform of Community-Based Long-Term Care

A series of initiatives by four successive governments in Ontario, over the period 1985 to 1996, to reform community-based long-term care provides an excellent case study for examining such issues. None of the three provincial governments (Liberal, NDP, and Progressive Conservative) that held office over that time period disputed the need for change, just as all stakeholders appear to have agreed that home care was a priority for reform. Nonetheless, each government found it difficult to develop and implement a policy that did not spark intense debate and was not immediately reversed by the next government. In this section we describe the range of services that constitute community-based LTC, a range that goes well beyond the hospital and doctor mainstream of Medicare and thus locates much of the field outside Medicare's institutional framework; and we identify factors that 'pushed' successive governments of different political stripes to attempt major reforms in this field.

1.2.1 Factors Pushing towards Reform

Multiple factors pushed governments toward reform of community-based LTC. Some were related to demand, such as the projected increases in the population of elderly and disabled individuals living in

Ontario. Others were related to supply. Within the hospital sector, downsizing had pulled beds and resources from the system; hospitals no longer were willing or able to provide care that in theory could be provided in 'alternative levels of care.' Some were related to a more educated and demanding clientele no longer willing to deal with the existing fragmented 'non-system' and the fact that comparable levels of service were not available across the province. There was a proliferation of 'one-off' services with varying eligibility criteria. There was little integration across the two ministries involved: MOH services in general employed a medical model (with universal entitlements and no co-payments) and MCSS a social model. At the level of the client, there was confusion. Individuals often had difficulty accessing care. Providers were frustrated. Projections implied that it was unlikely that the current hospital-focused system could be affordably extended to the population that would require such services. Reform was clearly indicated, and policy makers felt that a win-win situation was possible – reform might both improve quality and lower costs. As usual, the devil was in the details.

The demand projections seemed sobering. Ontario was a young population, but Canada had been highly affected by the baby boom (Foot and Stoffman, 1998, 2000). In 1980, 10 per cent of Ontario was over the age of sixty-five. At the time the reform process began, this proportion was predicted to double by the year 2021. Of more concern was the growth of the frail elderly, a high proportion of whom were single women. Between 1970 and 1980, although the elderly population increased by 34 per cent, government spending on services for this age group increased by 600 per cent. However, the dramatic increase in utilization of services was more a reflection of the newness of most of the programs. By 2001 it was estimated that the number of elderly between the ages of sixty-five and seventy-four would increase by about 38 per cent, the number between seventy-five and eighty-four by 75 per cent, and the number over age eighty-five by 110 per cent. The major impact of the demographic change was expected to be felt in health and social services (Van Horne, 1986). Because of the dramatic increase in utilization of acute health care by the frail elderly, the development of lower-cost alternatives was seen as crucial. While income support for the elderly was viewed as an important concern, the fact that the federal government had the largest responsibility in this area made it a less pressing issue for the province. In addition, over the decade the income of the elderly had increased by approximately 20 per cent, and approximately 86 per cent lived independently in the community, two-thirds of them in their own homes, most of which were mortgage free (Ontario Task Force on Aging, 1981).

The fear of cost escalation was not unwarranted. In the last two decades home care expenditures in Canada have grown at an average annual rate of 21.3 per cent and were predicted to reach almost $3 billion in 1998. This growth in spending is almost double the average annual rate of growth in other health expenditures and more than triple the inflation rate. In Ontario, government funding for home care grew from $132.6 million in 1984–5 to an estimated $1,040.0 million in 1998–9, representing a 668 per cent increase (Schlesinger, 1998). By 2003 it was anticipated that the number of home-based clients would grow by approximately 50 per cent to almost 1 million, or 9 per cent of the population of Ontario (Health Services Restructuring Commission, 1997).

The proliferation of one-off service programs, with no efforts at coordination and integration and the split in jurisdictional responsibility between MOH and MCSS, made this 'system' extremely difficult to access and navigate. As both sets of programs grew, increasingly they were serving the same clients, albeit, with different eligibility criteria, funding mixes, and requirements. These factors, along with geographic inequities in program availability across the province, resulted in unnecessary institutionalization or underservicing.

1.2.2 Models for Reform

While there was broad agreement on the need for reform, different governments took distinctive and often contradictory approaches to reform. Three basic types of model were recommended over the reform period. One type was the 'brokerage' model: a coordinating agency would be given a budget with which to purchase services from existing providers through a variety of informal methods. This model represented an incremental reform in terms of the divergence from the existing system. Two versions of the brokerage model were proposed by the Liberals (One-Stop Shopping/Access and Services Access Organization (SAO)), and another by the NDP (Service Coordination Agency (SCA)). The second type of model, subsequently proposed by the NDP, was a quasi-public delivery system, to be created through the amalgamation of existing and new services; almost all service providers would become employees of this new agency. The NDP's version would be called a Multi-Service Agency (MSA). To encourage the trend to unified delivery, there would be a limit on how many services could be purchased outside the MSA. This model represented both an almost total restructuring of the system and a movement in terms of government involvement/encroachment in service provision that ran contrary to mounting popular sentiments for smaller government. Finally, the third type of model, proposed and implemented by the Conservatives, was a managed competition model, where publicly funded services were purchased through a formal competitive contract process based in theory on price and quality, although to this day quality remains difficult to define. Although this model in terms of delivery decisions may have been consistent with notions of smaller government, it did not imply less centralized control by government, a point that will be highlighted in chapter 7.

On the financing side of the LTC reforms, all three governments, while maintaining the full funding of home care services (professional health and homemaking services), recommended its removal from the Health Insurance Act to a global capped budget. As a result, home care moved from its former status in Ontario as a fully funded entitlement (albeit an entitlement not required under the terms of the Canada Health Act or its precursor legislation), to one in which availability of publicly funded services could be constrained by budget pressures.

With respect to the delivery of services, the three successive governments shifted from a design that maintained the status quo of a mix of NFP and FP providers, to a preference for NFP providers, to a quasi-public delivery monopoly, and finally to a design that in its impact favours FP providers.

On the allocation dimension, the government model shifted from an informal, cooperative, brokerage-type model with a purchaser/provider split to a more centrally planned model, where the purchaser and provider of services were the same, and finally to a formal, competitive, market-type model with a purchaser/provider split.

1.3 Looking Ahead: The Making and Meaning of LTC Reform in Ontario

In the remaining chapters of this book we will tell the story of these series of attempted reforms and draw lessons for future efforts to reform the system. In chapter 2 we present a conceptual framework within which we analyse 'design decisions' and the implications for the ability of the state to bring about reform. In chapter 3 we outline the methods employed in the conduct of this research, the data collected, and the analytic tools employed. We begin the story in chapter 4, starting with the status quo before 1985 and then describing the interplay of ideas, interests, and institutions during the years of Liberal government between 1985 and 1990, when the One-Stop Shopping (and the One-Stop Access pilot projects that emanated from it) and the SAO models were proposed. In chapter 5 we move on to the New Democratic Party years between 1990 and 1993 and the development and rejection of the SCA model. In chapter 6 we depict the development of, and reaction to, the NDP's MSA model between 1994 and 1995. In chapter 7 we provide an analysis of the first six months of the Progressive Conservative government in 1995, during which the CCAC model was developed. In chapter 8 we provide an overall analysis of the design decisions inherent in the five models and an analysis of the dynamics within the policy community that underlay these changes in decision. We conclude by suggesting the implications of these attempts to reform LTC both for the future of health care in Canada and, more broadly, for the ability to change programs.

CHAPTER TWO

Conceptual Framework

2.1 Introduction

From the 'brokerage' proposals of the politically moderate Peterson Liberals, to the centralized 'command and control' approach of the socialist-leaning New Democratic Party (NDP) under Bob Rae, to the 'managed competition' reform of the market-oriented Mike Harris Progressive Conservative (PC) Party, the series of reform initiatives analysed in this book involved substantially different and often contradictory decisions about how community-based long-term care (LTC) services should be funded and delivered. Two sets of questions arise.

From the perspective of the policy analyst trying to develop optimal models for financing and delivering services and mechanisms for allocating resources, it is important to understand the implications of different approaches to the *policy content* on the performance of the resulting system. Answering these questions requires clarification of (1) the different 'design decisions' inherent in the different potential models; (2) the evaluation criteria which might be used to prefer one set of options to another; and (3) the relationship between responses on each of these design decisions and performance on the evaluation criteria, in full recognition that they may vary for different stakeholders. Insight about these matters is critical to anyone setting up a program, as well as to those providing and receiving services. In the case of community-based LTC, at some point most Canadians are likely to require such services, either for themselves or for members of their families. Health care is also an expensive program, a reality that affects us as taxpayers and citizens. Most of us, then, have a stake in reaching wise policy conclusions in this arena.

Political scientists, however, also are interested in a broader set of questions relating to *policy process*, particularly with respect to the capacity of 'the state' to react to policy demands. Answers to these questions extend well beyond issues of financing or delivering particular services, to focus on change and the ability to adapt to changing times. Key questions arise: What accounts for such volatility in this policy field? What can the dynamics of policy change in the case of community-based long-term care in Ontario reveal about the dynamics of change or stasis in other proximate policy fields?

We argue that answers to these questions need to go beyond simple description of the historical course of policy initiatives to analyse the complex interplay of ideas, institutions, and interests that characterized the 'policy community' in this field. All theories of policy making must deal with the interplay between 'the state' and society. In that sense, the state refers to the distinct set of political institutions within a defined geographic territory that are concerned with 'the organization of domination, in the name of the common interest' within that territory (McLean, 1996). The state enjoys sovereignty over its members and possesses a formal apparatus of authoritative roles and law norms through which that sovereignty is exercised. The state thus extends beyond a particular government, or even a particular political system. In contrast, 'society' refers to the individuals and groups living in that territory and includes individuals, families, interests, and interest groups. Theories vary on the relative importance of and power balance between 'state' and 'society' in policy making.

The 'historical institutional' or 'neo-institutional' theory we draw upon goes some way towards redressing a tendency in the policy literature to explain policy simplistically as a function only of societal interests and interest group politics, with the state as a relatively minor actor; or, equally simplistically, to explain them as only a function of the internal dynamics and structures of the state, with societal interests as a mere backdrop. Neo-institutionalism requires that the state be understood within its historical/societal context and that the state, its institutions, and the ideas that it promotes play a key role in shaping that context.

An ongoing issue in the analysis of changes in health policy is the extent to which the state can act autonomously, as opposed to the extent to which it is a prisoner of vested interests and global forces. Indeed, Tuohy (1999a,b) has argued that the Canadian health care system has remained relatively static because powerful interests, particularly physicians, have impeded the capacity to introduce reforms. Maioni (1997,

1998) has similarly attributed the inability of the United States to introduce universal health insurance to the rigidities inherent in the American political system and the extent to which the medical profession has
been able to take advantage of this to block policies it opposes.

In contrast, an examination of Ontario's attempts to reform the LTC
sector illustrates the power of the state. Rather than being neutral
bystanders or arbiters, the provincial governments took a lead role in
shaping not only policy options, but the internal dynamics of the policy
community. The state was able to take such a 'strong' role, we suggest,
for a number of reasons. First, each of the three governments examined
here was new to power (two with clear majorities) and was characterized
by relatively untempered ideological and political commitments. The
most extreme contrast was between the Rae (NDP) and the Harris (PC)
governments: while the former favoured an extended state role in
health and social care and saw itself as the champion of labour rights,
the latter aggressively asserted a greater role for competitive markets
and viewed organized labour as a 'special interest' and an impediment
to business.

Second, all governments faced a relatively weak and fragmented policy
community. In contrast to the 'mainstream' of health care characterized
by strong, organized interests, including the Ontario Hospital Association (OHA) and the Ontario Medical Association (OMA), by strong public and political support for the principle of universal public coverage,
and by the robust institution of Medicare itself, the LTC policy community was characterized by relatively small and difficult-to-mobilize consumer and provider groups, by little ideological agreement on the role
and responsibilities of public governments and private interests in the
provision of home and community care, and by minimal legislative constraints. This allowed the state to make major changes in policy without
much effective resistance. Indeed, as we discuss later, one of the actions
of the Rae government was to enact legislation (Bill 173) that removed
home care from the Ontario Health Insurance Plan (OHIP), thus also
removing it from the universal entitlements of the Canada Health Act
(CHA). For its part, the Harris government contended at different
points that community-based care and the Community Care Access Centres (CCACs) it established to manage such care were created not as a
matter of legislation, but as a matter of government policy outside legislation. Indeed, even within the NDP's Bill 173, there was nothing that
stopped an erosion of access to publicly funded services; one of the main
features of the bill was to centralize authority to identify intermediary

agencies and to set their budgets in the hands of the minister of health. Given such degrees of freedom, the provincial state encountered few major obstacles to the expression of its authority, and when governments changed (e.g., Liberal to NDP to PC) or when governments changed their minds (e.g., the NDP shift from a brokerage model to a centralized command-and-control approach to service delivery), change reverberated not simply in the formulation of policy, but throughout the web of relationships constituting the policy community.

The conceptual framework we employ to understand these dynamics is based on the concepts of policy communities, ideas, interests, and institutions. In this chapter, we give a brief introduction to these concepts. We then return to policy content, decomposing policy into a number of key 'design decisions' related to the financing and delivery of community-based LTC services and to the mechanisms for allocating resources to providers. We then bring the pieces together to outline how our conceptual framework will be applied throughout the course of following chapters to an analysis of the case of Ontario's successive community-based long-term care reform initiatives between 1985 and 1996.

2.2 Neo-institutionalism and Policy Communities

Neo-institutionalism may be described as an analytic perspective that emphasizes the impact of formal and informal institutions on policy outcomes (Brooks, 2000). As Coleman and Skogstad note, 'the preferences and values of policy actors are shaped fundamentally by their structural position. Institutions are conceived as structuring political reality and as defining the terms and nature of political discourse' (1990b, 2). A recognition of the importance of institutions is neither new nor surprising, being well established within sociological theories on organizations and political science analyses of constitutional and legal-legislative frameworks. Neo-institutionalism goes further, however, to examine the broader social and political dynamics that shape institutions at key historical junctures (often referred to as 'critical junctures') and the ways in which institutions then create their own historical pathways, thus shaping future events (given the shorthand description 'path dependence'). Neo-institutionalism presents an important qualification and corrective to theories of policy that either focus too narrowly on the characteristics and agency of the state without taking into account the broader societal context in which the state exists or focus too narrowly on factors outside the state, (e.g., organized interests, pressure groups, voter constituencies and social classes) without considering the independent capacity of the state to make policy – sometimes even in opposition to powerful societal interests, pressure groups, constituencies, and social classes. Indeed, neo-institutionalism draws attention precisely to the relative capacity or autonomy of the state and state actors to make policy decisions that do not simply respond to or mediate the demands of dominant societal interest, such as business, the capitalist class, or, in the case of health care, the medical profession, but that reflect the state's own structural interests and internal logic, including the political and ideological predispositions of governing parties at key historical junctures.

Of course, and this point must be emphasized, the capacity and relative autonomy of the state are not static: they waxes and wane. The key theoretical question addressed by neo-institutional theories is therefore: Under what conditions does the state have relatively more or less capacity to assert its own internal logic and shape the broader context in which it exists rather than being shaped by this context?

In this connection, it is equally important to observe that the state's context is also not static. Not all elements and features of the broader societal context are equally important or relevant at all times in all policy fields. For instance, with respect to organized interests, while the major oil and gas companies are likely to have vested interests, actively involve themselves in, and have major influence on issues of energy, environmental policy and global trade, they have had little involvement in issues of community-based LTC.

In this connection, Coleman and Skogstad's conceptualization of 'policy community' is particularly useful. A policy community is that part of a political system that, by virtue of its functional responsibilities, its vested interests, and its specialized knowledge, acquires a dominant voice in determining government decisions in a specific field of public activity. It is populated by government agencies, pressure groups, media organizations, and individuals who have an interest in a policy field and attempt to influence it (Coleman and Skogstad, 1990a; Pross, 1992). The constituent parts of this community will vary from policy field to policy field and from time to time. Of major theoretical interest, therefore, is the composition of a policy field at a particular historical juncture and the extent of the state's capacity, vis-à-vis the other main constituents of a policy community, to assert its authority.

According to Coleman and Skogstad, state capacity is a function of multiple factors. Within the state, they include the presence of professional bureaucracies able to generate their own information, backed by legal mandates and unambiguous regulations, and able to coordinate and concentrate decision making through a single agency or interdepartmental committees. But such factors, even when they are present, are balanced by the internal dynamics and relative capacity of the policy community external to the state. They use the term 'policy networks' to refer to the set of relationships that form around an issue of importance to the policy community; these networks can be characterized in terms of the relative strength, autonomy, and capacity of both state and societal groups. A strong, cohesive group of societal actors with shared interests provides less opportunity for state actors to promote their interests than a loosely organized, uncoordinated set of societal actors (Coleman and Skogstad, 1990b).

Even within a policy community such as health care, the power of specific groups and interests will change over time; for instance, the relative power of the organized medical profession vis-à-vis the state and factors influencing that power have been major topics of interest for medical sociologists in both the United States (Starr, 1982) and Canada (Naylor, 1986; Taylor, 1987; Tuohy, 1999a; Williams et al., 1995). Indeed, organized groups that should, on the face of it, figure as central players in a given policy field or policy community may consciously choose not to play an active role. For example, as we will discuss later, the Ontario Medical Association, a latecomer to the policy discussions, chose to absent itself from the field of community-based long-term care at the end of the NDP period, abandoning its alliances with other groups and interests opposed to the NDP's reform, thus removing an additional potential constraint on the Harris government as it embarked on its reforms. In stark contrast to the relative inertia in the health-related fields relating to physician services (Tuohy, 1999a), we find that, in the field of community-based long-term care, the provincial state proved to have few external constraints on its actions. One key reason, we argue, is because it faced a policy community that can be characterized as a loosely organized and uncoordinated set of societal actors.

Clearly, analysis of policy communities and the relative capacity of the state requires careful attention to the institutions of the state as well as the characteristics of the organized and the diffused societal interests confronted by the state in any given policy field. However, institutional factors do not fully explain policy dynamics. Like the neo-institutionalists, we suggest that, in addition to these two main conceptual dimensions of institutions and interests, a third dimension must be distinguished: ideas. Particularly in the field of Canadian health care, ideas have played and continue to play a crucial role, in many ways independent of changes in institutions and interests, but intimately related to them. Canada's health care system is the only one in the industrialized world based on explicit principles: universality, comprehensiveness, accessibility, public adminis-tration, and portability. While these principles are institutionalized in the Canada Health Act and continue to enjoy strong popular and political support, they nonetheless define an important terrain for political strug-gle. Indeed, these ideas demarcate a political landscape that is important not only for what it includes, but for what it *does not* include. This is because the dominant idea of health care consolidated under the CHA is focused on hospital and physician care; competing definitions that go further to include care outside hospitals and care provided by health pro-fessions other than doctors are beyond the boundaries of this idea. Thus, ideas play a major role not only in defining the nature of illness, health, and health care, but in identifying the role of the state, the rights and responsibilities of individuals, and a hierarchy of interests. As such, they 'constrain' the actions of both governments and societal interests. Out-side the Medicare mainstream, however, as is the case for community-based long-term care, there is a greater diversity of ideas and less consen-sus on which ideas should prevail. The extent to which ideas focus the policy agenda and policy action thus is a key consideration.

In the following subsections we elaborate these three key concepts of ideas, institutions, and interests that underpin our analysis of Ontario's series of community-based LTC reform initiatives in subsequent chapters.

2.2.1 Ideas

There is broad consensus in the literature about the role that ideas play in policy making. As Manzer (1994) states, public policies are made within frameworks of political ideas that structure thinking about what constitutes a public problem, what means are available to deal with it, and what evaluations are made retrospectively. This definition is part of understanding ideas as policy determinants, used not simply strategi-cally but instrumentally to understand problems and actions. He argues that political ideas can be examined as determinants of policies or as meanings of policy. As determinants, ideas are used strategically to mobilize, persuade, and manipulate other interests in support of one's own. As such, ideas are instruments of political power. Manzer main-tains that understanding participants' political ideas helps to explain their actions in a particular policy debate.

This line of argumentation can be seen in Schattschneider's (1964) early recognition that conflict is at the root of politics. He places partic-ular emphasis on the 'scope of the conflict' (how the issue is defined, which in turn affects who participates in decision making and the rules by which decisions are made). As a result, he views the definition of alternatives as the supreme instrument of power. The way in which a policy problem is framed will determine who gets involved, the degree of conflict, and the possible solutions. Similarly, Simeon (1976) argues that ideas are very closely connected to power and must be linked to the group whose interests they promote.

Stone (1997) sees ideas as both a medium of exchange and a mode of influence, as both object and subject. Shared meanings motivate people to action and coalesce individual desires into collective action. However, information is interpretive, incomplete, unequally available, and strategically withheld. Because politics is driven by how people interpret information, much activity is devoted to controlling interpretations. She views policy making as a constant struggle over the criteria for classification, the boundaries of categories, and the definition of ideals that guide the way people behave. Boundaries are constantly contested either because they are ambiguous or because their positioning differentially allocates benefits and costs.

Public policy is usually about the distribution of concentrated or diffuse benefits and costs. The distribution of costs and benefits of any program, whether they fall in a concentrated or diffused way, influences the type of political contest that follows. As a result, participants strategically represent programs as contests between different types of costs and benefits. The description of the problem one way or the other mobilizes different groups into actions. In such ways, ideas have a direct influence on political interests as well as on institutional arrangements.

Operationally, however, there are diverse approaches to conceptualizing and empirically measuring ideas. Apart from analysing the content of ideas, some political scientists distinguish between levels of ideas on the basis of how well organized the ideas are and how overarching are the concepts they attempt to explain. For example, Doern and Phidd define ideas as 'the desired end states, the sense of public purposefulness, that individuals and groups seek to obtain through state action, or often through preventing the state from acting' (1992, xv). Recognizing that the lines can be fuzzy, they distinguish between four levels of ideas: ideologies, dominant ideas, paradigms, and objectives.

2.2.1.1 Ideologies
Ideologies are 'explicit, detailed, and politically focused ideas, which explain the political world, provide a framework for interpreting particular events, and offer a recommendation and prescriptions for future

action' (Simeon, 1976, 570) In his study of educational policy, Manzer (1994) distinguishes among three ideological traditions in Canada: liberalism and both conservative and radical communitarianism. In liberalism, the focus is on the individual and the efficiency of the market. The role of the state should be limited to facilitating fairness in competition in order to allow for individuals to achieve their potential. Emphasis is on the fairness of process, even if it results in inequalities.

In contrast, Manzer sees communitarian ideologies as centred on communities and humans as social beings. The difference between conservative and radical communitarianism lies in their views of the political community. To the former, the community is a hierarchical order in which individuals are unequal, governed by obedience to a legitimate authority. To the latter, the community is composed of equal individuals governed by cooperation and consensus.

In Canada, the distinctions across traditional political ideologies have been less clear as parties adopt aspects of each other's ideologies. As a result, Deber (1991) argues, in the health sector it is more helpful to speak of reforms from the right versus reforms from the left. Although there may be overlap in these concepts and in reality they more closely represent the extremes of a continuum, it is helpful to look at the overall cluster of ideas distinguishing the two positions.

Reform from the left within the health sector would include the following collection of ideas and beliefs: a belief in public administration to ensure social goals of equity; the need for a redistribution of goods and services by the state; universal coverage of programs; entitlement to services; security as a motivating force; and a shift to healthy public policy (specific public policy initiatives required to improve the health of residents and beyond the traditional jurisdiction of the formal health care system).

Reform from the right would include: a diminished belief in the capacity and ability of the state to perform certain functions; a need to limit the responsibilities of the state and reduce spending; the importance of individual liberty; the reduction of coverage of necessary services to a minimum; a greater belief and reliance on the private and informal (families) sector in the financing and provision of care; targeting of social programs based on need and ability to pay; the debilitating impact of the welfare state on individual initiative; the importance of need as a motivating force; and a continued belief in the medical model of care.

As will be documented in the later chapters, the second LTC model (Multi-Service Agency) legislated by the NDP government is a prime

example of 'reform from the left,' while the model (CCAC) introduced
by the Harris Conservatives represents 'reform from the right.' The two
Liberal models (One-Stop Shopping/Access and Service Access Organization) and the first NDP model (Service Coordination Agency) lie
between.

2.2.1.2 Dominant Ideas

Dominant ideas, according to Doern and Phidd (1992), are a second-
order construct that provides shape to a particular policy issue. They are
derived from broader ideologies, and it is often conceptually difficult to
separate the two. Although the same dominant ideas tend to be used in
public policy debates, the interpretation or spin put on the idea
depends on the wider beliefs and interests of the participants. Some of
the dominant ideas that underlie public policies are equity (sometimes
viewed as justice), which deals with equity or fairness in the distribution
of public benefits and burdens (Manzer, 1994); security; liberty (often
synonymous with choice or freedom from state interference); efficiency;
and effectiveness.

Stone (1997) sees equity involving distributions, which are regarded
as fair even though they may contain both equalities and inequalities.
Distributions are at the heart of most public policy debates, especially
those involving the goal of equity. In any distribution there are three
possible dimensions: the recipient (who is included and excluded in the
distribution); the item being distributed (definition of the boundaries
and the value of the item being distributed); and the process for making
the distribution (fairness with which the item is being distributed). In
LTC policy, financing decisions often deal with equity issues, that is, the
scope of services, who is eligible for service, and the determination of
user fees.

Liberty embraces various notions ranging from economic freedom to
freedom of expression. The concept of liberty is usually applied to individuals, not to social groups. Restriction of individual action most often
is justified by a reduction of harm to others. To define a simple criterion
of harm that tells which activities are or should be forbidden is problematic, however, because liberty, according to Stone, is constructed in political life. She sees it as a matter of cultural history and political choice as
to what kinds of harm are privileged and which are punished. From the
consumer's perspective, liberty often refers to the freedom to choose a
service or a service provider. From a provider's perspective, liberty often
refers to autonomy and freedom from government regulation. In LTC
reform, the allocation method chosen had different implications for

consumer choice, while delivery decisions had ramifications for for-profit economic participation in this sector.

The idea of security usually implies the satisfaction of needs. It often involves conflicts over the kinds of security government should provide, the kinds of needs it should meet, and the way in which burdens making security a collective responsibility should be distributed. The idea that security can be reduced to objective and countable needs is politically problematic. The definition of security, like other policy goals, is an exercise in political claims making. In LTC, financing decisions that dealt with service availability and quality as well as with the amount and determination of user fees were security issues from a consumer perspective. Delivery and allocation decisions had security implications for workers (job security, compensation, and working conditions) and for providers (viability).

Efficiency, for Stone, is a comparative idea. It has come to mean the ratio between input and output, efforts and results, expenditure and revenue, or cost and benefit. Efficiency is always a contestable concept, and the measures used in any analysis of efficiency can also be viewed as political claims. As Stone points out, one person's efficiency can be seen as another person's waste. By offering different assumptions, sides in a conflict can portray their preferred outcomes as being the most efficient. According to Stone, conflicts over efficiency arise over three questions: Who gets the benefits and who bears the burdens of a policy? How should we measure the benefits and costs of a policy? What mode of organizing activity is likely to yield the most efficient results? As Manzer argues, 'concepts of effectiveness and efficiency are embedded in politically contested concepts of public purpose, norms of legitimacy and justice, and theories of policy intervention' (1994, 12). The evaluation of efficiency or effectiveness of public policies is part of the ideological context. In LTC reform, efficiency permeated the debate of all three design decisions: the efficiency of public funding versus mixed financing models, the efficiency of for-profit (FP) versus not-for-profit (NFP) provision, the efficiency of competition versus cooperation.

Ideas rarely stand alone, but often they conflict. Equality and efficiency are often thought to be in a zero-sum relationship. Equality, it is claimed, eliminates the differential rewards necessary to motivate people to be productive, interferes with individual choices curbing experimentation and innovation, or is not productive because a large administrative machinery is required to maintain it. Security and liberty often conflict: the redistribution of benefits to increase the security of disadvantaged individuals usually results in infringement on the ability of more affluent individuals to dispose of their assets as they choose, as well as adversely affecting efficiency by removing the motivating force of need. In the reform of the LTC sector, there were many trade-offs as will be argued in chapter 8, below.

2.2.1.3 Paradigms

'In technically complex fields of policy ... decision-makers are often guided by an overarching set of ideas that specify how the problems facing them are to be perceived, which goals might be attained through policy and what sorts of techniques can be used to reach those goals. Ideas about each of these matters interlock to form a relatively coherent whole that might be described as a policy paradigm. Like a gestalt, it structures the very way in which policy makers see the world and their role in it' (Hall, 1992, 92). Paradigms act as prisms through which certain policy options pass easily while others do not. Shifts in policy paradigms often account for policy innovation.

In the LTC sector in Ontario, two policy paradigms were in evidence: (1) the medical model and (2) the broader determinants of health model. The medical model (Lomas and Contandriopoulos, 1994) favours the primacy of the physician, is reactive, focuses on cure as opposed to health promotion and disease prevention, centres on the individual rather than whole populations, and views health narrowly as an absence of disease rather than a state of complete physical, mental, and social well-being (definition of health according to the World Health Organization).

The broader determinants of health model was informed and developed over the years by a number of national and international reports. It sees the scope of health and health care as being broader than illness/disease and physician/hospital care. The 1974 publication of the internationally acclaimed Lalonde report, *A New Perspective on the Health of Canadians* (Lalonde, 1974), represented an important milestone in the evolving concept of health. In this document the Health Field Concept is outlined, which emphasizes that health is influenced by four areas: lifestyle, human biology, environment, and the organization of health care. Later, the (Ontario) Premier's Council on Health Strategy adopted the World Health Organization's (WHO) definition of health: 'Health is the extent to which an individual or group is able, on the one hand, to realize aspirations and satisfy needs; and, on the other hand, to change or cope with the environment. Health is therefore seen as a resource for every day life, not the objective of living; it is a positive concept emphasizing social and personal resources, as well as physical capacity' (Premier's Council, 1989a, Introduction, n.p.).

This broader approach is focused on health promotion and disease prevention rather than on cure, where health promotion has been defined as 'the process of enabling people to increase control over, and to improve, their health' (WHO, 1978, n.p.). At the World Health Assembly in 1977 WHO resolved that 'a main social target of governments, international organizations and the whole world community in the coming decades should be the attainment by all peoples of the world by the year 2000 of a level of health that will permit them to lead a socially and economically productive life' (WHO, 1978, n.p.). The endorsement of this resolution and the subsequent birth of the Health for All by the Year 2000 movement (HFA 2000) were significant developments for health promotion. In 1978 at the International Health Conference on Primary Health Care (PHC) in Alma-Ata, USSR, it was further declared that the Health for All goal was to be attained through PHC. The major features of PHC were defined as health education, health promotion, community participation and intersectoral cooperation (WHO, 1978).

LTC reform took place in an environment that was informed by the above national and international events and reports. Many of the efforts in LTC reform concerned realigning the sector away from a medical model to a broader determinants of health approach. Among the themes we examine in this book are the use of ideology, dominant ideas, and paradigms as a way of framing issues to influence who participates in or stays out of the debate, who forms alliances, how interests are represented, why certain institutions are established, and in understanding the policy outcome itself.

2.2.2 Institutions

Institutions include both formal organizations and informal rules and procedures that structure conduct (Thelen and Steinmo, 1992). In neo-institutionalism, institutions are never the sole determinant of policy outcomes. Nevertheless, they consolidate the power and influence of certain ideas and interests over others, and they structure political struggle around policy issues. Change in institutions modifies the constraints under which actors make strategic choices, and it can reshape the goals and ideas that stimulate political action.

A critique of traditional institutional analysis has been its tendency towards static and sometimes deterministic accounts, better able to explain continuity and permanence rather than change. Thelen and Steinmo (1992) outline a number of sources of institutional dynamism. First, broad changes in the socio-economic or political context can produce a situation in which previously latent institutions suddenly become salient, or in which old institutions are used in the service of different ends, which in turn introduce new actors. Second, external changes can produce a shift in the goals or strategies being pursued within existing institutions. Lastly, changes occur when political actors adjust their strategies to accommodate changes in the institutions themselves, that is, acting on openings provided by the different context in order to defend or further their positions.

Considerable evidence in international contexts demonstrates the influence of institutions in policy making. Immergut (1992) shows how the difference in institutional factors (constitutional rules that create different veto points, political parties and party discipline, and electoral results) accounted for the differences in national health schemes introduced in France, Switzerland, and Sweden, rather than differences in ideas or in preferences and the organization of interest groups. She concludes that no view of politics can rely exclusively on either institutions or interests. Both are necessary.

Hall, (1992), in his study of the way in which Britain moved from Keynesianism to monetarist policies, shows how institutions interact with interests and ideas. For him, the following institutional factors influenced the policy outcome: capital relations of production and democratic electoral institutions; a party system characterized by intense, two-party competition, which gave the Conservatives strong incentives to seek a clear alternative to Labour policies; the centralization of power in the cabinet and the prime minister, which gave the Conservatives the capacity to institute radical change; and the routines and procedures of the British Treasury, which acted as filters to new incoming ideas. Institutions emerge from his analysis as a critical mediating variable, however, not as a substitute for interests and ideas.

As discussed in subsequent chapters, institutional factors such as legislation (and lack of legislation) and government structures influenced the shape and power of ideas, the authority of societal interests, and policy outcomes.

2.2.3 Interests

Individuals with common goals often come together into what are variously termed 'interest groups,' 'pressure groups,' or 'special interest groups.' Pross defines them as 'organizations whose members act together to influence public policy in order to promote their common interest. (1975, 2). The key dimension is organization: rather than being a haphazard collection of people, interest groups require at least a modicum of institutional or formal structure.

Interests, as distinct from interest group structures, refer to the policy preferences, motives, or objectives of state and societal actors in a policy field or policy issue (Manzer, 1994). Interests may be either explicit or implicit, openly declared or hidden. Not only do groups promote their own interests, but also they shape the reception of opposing interests by their public interpretations of them.

Interest groups might be considered a form of institution, in that they are formal organizations that structure relationships and outcomes within a policy community. However, they are not part of government. Nonetheless, it can often (although not always) be convenient for government to have an organized contact through which it can consult and deal with key stakeholders, particularly if successful policy implementation will require their cooperation. The ability of interest groups to promote their interests thus will depend not only upon their own institutional characteristics, or even the institutional characteristics of the state, but also upon the network of relationships among interest groups and the relevant components of the state. These networks are usually found within a specific policy community. For example, the interests of the labour movement are mediated through organized unions and their institutional set of rules and procedures, and the successful promotion of these interests is dependent on the particular network of relationships the movement has with other societal interests, such as provider associations, and with the state. As Schattschneider has pointed out, policy debates are often determined by the 'scope of conflict' – that is, who participates, and under what ground rules (Schattschneider, 1964; Kellow, 1988).

According to Pross (1992). interest groups perform a number of functions within a policy community, including interest promotion, communication, legitimation, regulation, and administration. They transmit demands and information from sectoral communities to public authorities and information and demands from the authorities to their members; they build public support for programs and policies; they administer some public programs; and they engage in regulatory activity. An understanding of the reciprocal benefits provided by the state and interest groups offers some insight into why some groups have more influence than others.

To achieve their goals, public officials must generate support in the relevant policy community (or at least overcome dissent). If interest groups do not exist, state agencies often encourage their formation. At times, governments try to break up old policy communities to create new ones. In this way, governments can try to control the agenda and to frame the scope of conflict. Schattschneider indicates that the development of cleavages is the prime instrument of power: 'Every change in the direction and location of the line of cleavage produces a new majority and a new allocation of power' (1964, 63). In addition, without the support of well-organized interest groups, state agencies may find their agendas usurped by central agencies or other departments. At times, ministers use groups as a source of policy countervail to departmental advice.

To perform the above functions, interest groups must possess the attributes of organization: a formal structure, a clear definition of roles, a system for generating and allocating resources, rules governing behaviour, and procedures for reaching and implementing decisions. Pross categorizes interest groups along a continuum ranging from institutional groups to issue-oriented groups. Institutional groups possess organizational continuity and cohesion; have extensive knowledge of the sector and enjoy an ease in communications within the sector; have a stable membership; have concrete and immediate goals; and organizational imperatives are generally more important than any particular objective.

Issue-oriented groups are at the other end of the continuum and possess characteristics opposite to those possessed by institutional groups. They allow their concern with one or two issues to dominate both their internal affairs and their relations with government. Their weak base, however, does not make them ineffective. They can achieve their objectives through techniques normally shunned by institutional groups, such as demonstrations, media events, and inflammatory rhetoric. Their chief advantage lies in their flexibility. They can disrupt a policy field, breaking down and challenging its consensus.

Within the LTC sector, most groups were issue oriented, and some tended more towards the definition of institutional groups. The composition of societal groups and the fragmented network they formed accounts in large part for the dominance of the state in the LTC policy sector and for the volatility in alliance formation and dissolution.

Interest-group power or influence is not a property possessed by groups solely by virtue of their organizational characteristics, their number of members, or their budgets, however, as some interest group theorists would contend. Understanding interest group influence in terms of social, economic, or organizational resources is not enough. According to Immergut (1992), political influence comprises the relationship of these groups to the political system, and one therefore needs to understand the receptivity of political institutions to political pressures. Institutional mechanisms structure the process and provide interest groups with different opportunities for influencing decisions. As well, new ideas, as stated above, change the boundaries of a debate and realign interests.

In LTC reform there were a number of policy interests that can readily be identified. The government had an interest in constraining costs by shifting publicly financed care to the private sector by transferring care to less costly providers and agencies; in strengthening and regaining its political support base; in improving access to care; in reducing or increasing the involvement of the FP sector in care; and in extending consumer participation in program decisions. Consumer interest included ease of access, broadening the types of care provided, rights, and choice of providers. Unions were interested in successor rights, job protection, and promotion, while provider groups were interested in income protection and autonomy.

2.3 Policy Outcomes: Design Decisions

The outcome of Ontario's series of attempts to reform community-based long-term care was the establishment by the Mike Harris Progressive Conservatives of a provincial network of Community Care Access Centres. CCACs were mandated to assess the needs of individuals residing within their geographic catchment areas, and to purchase necessary services through a process termed 'managed competition.' This process, which pitted traditional NFP community service agencies against a growing number of FP agencies, was touted as achieving 'best quality' at the 'lowest cost.' In limiting CCACs to the purchase rather than the direct provision of services, and in relying on market forces as a means of driving down costs, this reform differed in key respects from reforms proposed by the earlier Liberal and NDP governments. Such differences may best be understood by 'decomposing' both the final and proposed policies into different component parts or 'design decisions.' As detailed below, the first overarching decision concerns the appropriate role of the state in the provision of services. Additional decisions address: the specific role of the state in funding of services; appropriate mechanisms for 'flowing' funding between government and service providers either directly or through mediating institutions such as CCACs; and the extent of state responsibility for actual service delivery.

2.3.1 The Public/Private Mix

To understand the policy decisions available to and taken by the provincial governments, it is necessary to summarize the arguments justifying the role of the state versus the private sector in the provision of goods and services, what is meant by 'public' and 'private,' and how we discern shifts in direction from public to private.

The debate about public versus private operationalizes deep views about values. What is the boundary between the responsibilities of the state and the responsibilities of members of society either individually or in non-governmental collectives? When do personal tragedies – such as ill health or unemployment – become the concern of others? Which issues should be 'socialized,' and which remain the responsibilities of individuals and their families?

A number of justifications have been offered for the intervention of governments and the superiority of state or collective provision over private market provision of goods and services (Deber, 1991; Pal, 1992). The first rationale is that of public or collective goods. The benefits of these types of good cannot be rationed and are susceptible to the 'free-rider' problem – the refusal by rational individuals to pay for such goods while benefits are guaranteed. The resolution is for governments to compel the provision and financing of such goods and services. A second rationale for government provision is externalities: even in the case of private goods, there are often positive or negative consequences as a result of their consumption. Governments intervene in these instances to ensure standards are met in the provision of such services or goods. A third rationale is that of market failure. Governments can improve efficiency by becoming monopoly providers or by regulating private monopolies. The provision of order, a fourth rationale, is ensured by the state's monopoly of force and its sovereign authority. Lastly, the promotion of social justice through government redistribution is often a correction to unjust or unfair market outcomes.

On the other hand, the questioning of government's capacity in social welfare provision is linked to calls for deficit/debt reductions and arguments of efficiency. Distrust and loss of faith in the public sector, in terms of both motives and competence, seem to be increasing (Bendick, 1989). Critics of government provision advocate the introduction of more market-like mechanisms in public services – mechanisms such as consumer choice, competition, and performance measurements based as much as possible on profit considerations. Calls for greater privatization and minimal public provision are other suggestions (Deber, 1991; Kamerman and Kahn, 1989; Saltman and von Otter, 1992b). The guiding beacon for social policy reform is no longer 'market failure' but 'government failure' (Williams, Deber, et al., 2001).

As a countermovement to the growth of government, privatization emerges as the most serious conservative effort to pose an alternative. The most notable efforts have occurred in New Zealand, Australia, Britain, and the United States (Osborne and Gaebler, 1992). According to Kamerman and Kahn, (1989) the privatization proponents argue that reliance on the private sector results in greater efficiency, responsiveness to clients, scope for innovation and specialization, and improved management. Despite the popularity of the movement, precision in the definitions of public and private is lacking.

Paul Starr (1989), in his essay on the meanings of privatization, states that public and private are usually paired to describe a number of related oppositions in our thought – public is to private as open is to closed or as the whole is to the part. Public often means governmental or official. Private often characterizes what lies beyond the state's boundaries, that is, in the market or in the family. Saltman (Saltman and von Otter, 1995) states that 'public' can refer to branches of government or to semi-autonomous agencies, which are publicly capitalized but autonomously managed and are accountable to public officials for long-term outcomes. On the other hand, 'private' is less precise, sometimes, but not always, including NFP organizations with commercial ones, which may range from small owner-operated firms to large stock-issuing corporations. The distinction between FP and NFP is also less precise, sometimes separated by whether an excess of revenues to expenditures is called 'profit' or 'surplus.' One has to look not only at the ownership structure but also at the framework of incentives that determine the behaviour of these institutions. Deber et al. (1998), in their definition of public and private, divide public into four levels of government (nation, province/state, region, and local) and private into five sectors (corporate FP, small business / entrepreneurial, charitable/NFP run by paid employees, charitable/NFP run by volunteers, and family/personal).

Privatization generally means the withdrawal from variously conceived public spheres: a shift of individual involvement from the whole to the part; an appropriation by an individual or a group of some good formerly available to all; or a withdrawal from the state of assets and functions. Public policy is concerned with privatization at the latter level.

Starr (1989) cautions that public and private do not have consistent meanings in different institutional settings and that it is risky to generalize about the merits of privatization as public policy beyond a particular institutional or national context. As a result, he argues, privatization reflects a direction of change and does not denote a specific origin or destination. Critical to this change is movement from open to closed (as in access to information) or from the whole to the part (particularly in the distribution of benefits).

There are four types of government policy that can bring about a public/private shift:

- the cessation of public programs and the disengagement of government from specific kinds of responsibilities (implicit privatization), or the restriction of publicly produced services in volume, availability, or quality, leading to a shift by consumers towards privately produced and purchased substitutions (privatization by attrition);
- the transfer of public assets to private ownership;
- the financing of private service (contracting out or vouchers) instead of direct government service production; and
- the deregulation of entry by private firms into activities that were previously treated as public monopoly.

Bendick (1989) defines privatization as a shift into non-governmental hands, of some or all roles formerly involved in publicly producing a good or service. He differentiates between 'governmental load-shedding' and the 'empowerment of mediating institutions.' For Bendick, 'load-shedding' refers to arrangements where both the means of financing and the means of delivery are divorced from government, for example, budget reductions, the introduction of user fees, and increased use of volunteers. Many of the policies of both the Thatcher and the Reagan governments were examples of 'load-shedding.' The empowerment of mediating institutions involves arrangements where government delegates production and delivery of services while retaining some or all responsibility for financing, for example, the use of vouchers, contracting out services, or public/private partnerships.

The normative theories justifying privatization as a possible direction for public policy emanate from different visions of a good society. Laissez-faire individualism that accepts inequality in resources as natural and free market economics that promises greater efficiency, a smaller government, and more individual choice are most influential. Another vision is grounded in a return of power to communities through a greater reliance on families, churches, and NFP institutions for social provision. In another view, privatization is a political strategy for diverting demands away from the state, thereby reducing government overload. Starr (1989) argues that some advocates of privatization draw on all three.

Saltman (1995) cautions that we not confuse privatization and competition. While privatization refers to the private ownership of capital resources and the private objective for which these resources are deployed, competition is a particular methodology for allocating resources. Competition uses a variety of mechanisms (consumer choice, open bidding, negotiated contracts, etc.) to compare the performance of multiple players. As monopolies can exist with private ownership, competition can exist within public ownership and administration. The concept of competition will be discussed below under 'Allocation' (subsect. 2.3.4).

LTC reform illustrates the attempts by government to move both the financing and the delivery of services along this public-private continuum. As will be documented in later chapters, the NDP shifted delivery away from FP provision. This policy was later reversed by the Harris Conservative government. In financing all three governments either intended to or did put in place structures that have the potential to increase the private component of LTC funding. It will be argued that this act has broader implications for health care in general.

2.3.2 Financing

At root, the debate about financing is a debate about who should bear which costs. It is often argued in terms of the 'basket of services' and what should be 'in' or 'out.' In Canada, there is general consensus that 'core services' – including 'medically necessary' hospital and physician services – should be paid for publicly. (Commission on the Future of Health Care in Canada, 2002; Standing Senate Committee on Social Affairs, Science and Technology, 2002). However, community-based LTC is not so simple to deal with. The wide range of services and clients compounds the policy dilemma. At one extreme, community-based LTC involves services that clearly would be paid for collectively if offered in hospitals: palliative care for a terminally ill patient who wishes to die at home, wound care for a post-surgical patient who has been discharged soon after an operation, and so on. At the other extreme, it involves services that are readily open to exploitation by those who could pay for them: house cleaning or assistance with lawn maintenance. Other services might otherwise be offered by family members or volunteers: meal preparation, friendly visiting, or transportation for shopping. There are strong economic and moral arguments for universal coverage for services in the mainstream of medicare; few individuals would wish an unnecessary appendectomy, and few citizens would be willing to let individuals die simply because they were unable to pay the costs for such life-saving therapy. These arguments become increasingly attenuated as one moves towards the social end of programs. On the other hand, such services are often essential – arguably more essential than medical care to keep the frail elderly living in the community (Hollander and Prince, 2002). The debate about which services should be publicly financed, and for which populations, proved to be a contentious element within the successive reforms (Deber and Williams, 1995).

A number of participants may be involved in the financing of health and social services. The public sector can take responsibility for funding some services or some portion of the population. Private sources of funding can come from private insurance, out-of-pocket spending, or charitable giving. When financing of health care is reviewed internationally, evidence indicates that the public share in total health care financing, on average, has increased in the industrialized nations from about 60 per cent in 1960 to 80 per cent at the beginning of the 1980s (Poullier, 1986). Many publicly funded systems include not only hospital and physician services, as is the case in Canada, but also drugs, dental care, and long-term care services (Organisation for Economic Co-operation and Development (OECD), 2000; Poullier, 1986; Schieber and Poullier, 1991). At the international level, a greater share of public financing is available for hospitals and other institutional care than for ambulatory care and medical goods; home care and social services are even less likely to receive public financing.

In addition to more equitable access to care, another argument for public financing is based on the evidence that single-payer systems tend to have lower costs than public-private systems, as is true in the United States (Culyer and Jönsson, 1986; OECD 1987, 1990). Mixed funding sources give rise to two policy problems: first, cost control measures can be achieved through cost shifting, that is, moving costs from government to the private sector or from one level of government to another, rather than through actual efficiencies; and second, monopsony bargaining power over providers is harder to achieve with multiple payers. (Deber, 2000a)

Despite the evidence of the merits of public financing of health care and its increasing use, there are continued attempts to introduce increased private funding of health care through user fees or co-payments, as a solution to increase revenues and reduce costs to the public system and to prevent abuse of the system. Robert Evans refers to these attempts as 'zombies', ideas that are intellectually dead but nevertheless keep returning from the grave (Evans et al., 1993a,b). Evidence shows that user fees for services deemed 'medically necessary' will generate more revenue for providers; will increase, not decrease, the total cost of health care; and will redistribute the benefits to the healthy and wealthy and the costs to the sick and the poor (Evans et al., 1994a; Stoddart and Labelle, 1985). Private health insurance for such services has been shown to have similar negative effects (Evans, 1984). However, these arguments do not address the core issue: which community-based LTC services could be classified as medically necessary and which, although important, were not as obviously candidates for full public payment. Boundaries must be drawn; the issue of where to do so, and for which target groups, would become a major focus of the reform debate.

In redesigning the financing side of the LTC system, governments were dealing not only with health services, but also with social support services, most of which are traditionally not considered part of government's responsibility, such as housekeeping and the provision of meals. Government intervention in these areas has traditionally been based on financial need. Governments have had to untangle the effects of these social needs on health, however, to the extent that their lack contributed to deterioration in health of the client. With respect to traditional professional health services in community-based LTC, provincial policy at the time fully funded them, but there was no legal requirement to do so. As a result, governments were free to privatize them. In other LTC services, there was already an ongoing practice of charging user fees.

Because of developments in technology and pharmaceuticals, acute care traditionally provided by physicians or in hospitals increasingly was being performed in the community. In 1995–6 it was estimated that 46 per cent of Home Care cases was acute care (Health Services Restructuring Commission, 1998). As a result, publicly funded care was being shifted to a sector of care that no longer fell under the protection of the CHA and therefore was no longer mandated to be publicly insured. Reform of LTC services thus has wider implications for the future of Canadian health care.

In redesigning the financing dimension of community-based LTC, governments, although aware of the research evidence supporting public financing, were also conscious of the rising demand in care due to an ageing population, decreasing fiscal transfers from the federal government, rising provincial debts and deficits, and the need to control and cut costs. These factors would play a part in the shifts in the public/private mix.

2.3.3 Delivery

In exploring the delivery dimension we consider who should provide the service. Possibilities include the public sector (that is, the state) or the private sector (either NFP or FP providers). In Canada, there has been relatively little public delivery, and the debate instead revolves around the relative merits of NFP versus FP organizations. In turn, FP can be divided into FP/s (small businesses) and FP/c (investor-owned corporations) (Deber, 2002). Within the medicare mainstream, most hospitals are NFP, whereas most practising physicians are FP/s entrepreneurs. FP/c firms provide significant services, however, including clinical items such as pharmaceuticals, laboratory tests, and medical devices, as well as a range of non-clinical services (e.g., telecommunications, cleaning, meals).

The issue of delivery has evoked heated political discussion. Clearly, the *CHA* does not prohibit the commercial delivery of services; indeed, as noted above, a considerable amount of public money already goes to FP organizations. However, many argue that FP has no place in dealing with health care. Others have attempted to move the debate to the relative efficiencies of various delivery formats and the degree of choice available for 'consumers.'

Both the academic literature and the policy advocacy community accordingly have been engaged in an avid, ongoing debate about the relative merits of public, private NFP, and private FP delivery. Some argue that better incentives and competition make FP organizations more nimble and flexible than 'complacent' NFPs (Crowley, Zitner, and Faraday-Smith, 2002; McFetridge, 1997; Ontario Home Health Care Providers' Association, 2001; Osborne and Gaebler, 1992; Preker, Harding, and

Travis, 2000; Premier's Advisory Council on Health for Alberta, 2001; Zelder, 2001). Others maintain that the profit motive encourages inferior care (Armstrong and Armstrong, 2003; Armstrong, 2000; Browne, 2000; Canadian Council for Policy Alternatives (CCPA) et al., 2000; Fuller, 1998; Himmelstein, Woolhandler, and Hellander, 2001; Himmelstein et al., 1999; Rachlis, 2000; Rachlis et al., 2001; Relman, 1992; Shapiro, 1997; Sutherland, 2001; Vogel, 2000) and may even result in high mortality rates (Devereaux et al., 2002). The debate is complicated by the fact that these organizations often prove to provide different services and to serve different populations; comparisons frequently are those of 'apples with oranges.' For example, Martin Knapp (1986) compares the relative efficiency of public, voluntary, and private producers in the provision of publicly financed residential childcare in the United Kingdom. After controlling for technologies of care and characteristics of clients, he draws the tentative conclusion that in the privatization of production, the private and voluntary sectors are more cost effective than the public sector. The study was not able to take into account the final output, however, particularly the long-term effects of care on children and their families. He suggests that tax concessions, low wages, long hours, and charitable giving were possible reasons for cheaper care in the private and voluntary sectors.

Bendick (1989) examines the efficacy of the privatization of publicly delivered services within a framework of public financing. He concludes that FP privatization tends to be more efficient in services where goals are measurable, easily monitored, and evaluated, for example, garbage collection. Where problems are complex, such as health and social welfare programs, and processes are not well understood, he argues that the FP sector does no better or worse than the public sector. As an alternative strategy, he recommends the privatizing of programs with complex goals to the NFP sector over the FP sector, which he refers to as the empowerment of mediating institutions. Evidence indicates that NFP deliverers have a better record in providing services in the interest of clients beyond what is precisely specified in contracts. Bendick also argues that the empowering of mediating institutions would draw service providers into the political constituency that advances and defends public programs.

The literature on the implications of public versus private delivery has been reviewed by Deber, who examined case studies of diverse services such as privatization of local government activities; public-private partnerships for capital development (e.g., the Private Finance Initiative);

and comparisons among public, NFP, and FP delivery for sectors such as acute-care general hospitals, nursing homes, managed care companies, social services / residential care, ambulatory clinics, laboratory services, and home care (Deber, 2002). Although some researchers find differences in outcomes, others do not, particularly when services are professionally controlled. Nonetheless, it is obvious that FP providers are in business to make profits; the literature is clear that one of the major ways in which they achieve 'efficiencies' proves to be through controlling the wages paid to their employees. FP providers often employ a different skill mix (usually hiring lower-paid workers) and/or pay less in wages and benefits. It is not surprising that unions were opposed to the idea of allowing FP provision, while payers had some interest in 'union busting.'

Even with services and programs for which goals and costs are easily monitored and evaluated, savings from FP delivery have often not materialized. By 31 March 1999, under the alternative service delivery strategy, the Ontario Ministry of Transportation had entered into a number of contracts with the private sector to provide road maintenance services for approximately 6,800 kilometres, or 30 per cent of the provincial road system. The Ontario auditor in his 1999 report (Office of the Provincial Auditor General of Ontario, 1999) found that the ministry had not achieved the target savings of 5 per cent on the four outsourcing contracts reviewed, which covered about 20 per cent of the province's highway system. In health care and social support services, where services are harder to predict, monitor, and evaluate, provincial auditors have found that delivery by FP organizations has often been even more problematic (MacDonnell, 2001; Office of the Auditor General of New Brunswick, 1998; Office of the Auditor General of Nova Scotia, 1997, 1998, 1999; Office of the Provincial Auditor General of Ontario, 1998a,b, 2000). Unions accordingly have been highly resistant to issues around FP delivery. As a result, however, they have often blurred the important distinctions between small businesses (which tend to be less susceptible to incentives to 'cut corners' but also are unlikely to achieve economies of scale) and investor-owned corporations (which generate most of the problematic events cited in the anti-FP literature).

The Ontario government had a number of delivery options: by the public sector, where workers would be government employees; by the NFP private sector, using paid workers (e.g., Ontario public hospitals); by the NFP sector, relying on volunteers (e.g., most agencies delivering meals on wheels); by individuals and their families; and/or by the FP private sector (e.g., many homemaker agencies). As indicated above, one key issue in this design decision is the determination of the appropriate balance among paid workers, volunteers, and 'informal care givers' (families and friends). In Ontario, another issue that surfaced in the reforms was the extent to which governments encouraged the unionization of the sector and promoted the rights of unionized workers over those of their non-unionized counterparts.

In redesigning the delivery side of the sector, governments therefore had the option of retaining the status quo of largely NFP providers with some FP groups providing homemaking services; shifting the NFP/FP balance of providers to one or the other end of the continuum; assuming responsibility for publicly delivering some or all services; or shifting more of the responsibility for care outside formalized care systems to individuals and their families.

2.3.4 Allocation

Allocation refers to the method/mechanism by which finances are flowed to providers, who may be individuals or organizations. Allocation includes resource allocation (how a resource envelope is determined and the mechanism for transferring funds to providers) and reimbursement (the formula for determining how much is to be paid to a provider for a service) (Hollander, Deber, and Jacobs, 1998). None of the models, with the exception of the CCAC, was developed to the stage of making micro-allocation decisions concerning formulae for reimbursements of services. As a result, this aspect of allocation will not be further considered.

Most models of health care contain a number of components between the funders of the system and the care deliverers. They can include third-party payers (government, private insurers) as well as intermediary provider organizations. Allocation is not so much a public/private issue as it is one of control of finances and incentives for reimbursement. Although it is not a public/private issue, certain forms of allocation lend themselves better to particular forms of financing and delivery (Deber et al., 1998).

Hollander et al. (1998) distinguish between partnership models and market models of funding services. In the former, government takes a more flexible approach in the development, negotiation, and administration of contracts. They are more concerned about the stability of the industry and more cautious about experimenting with different service

FIGURE 2.1
Allocation Models for Publicly Financed Services

Client follows money		Money follows client	
Centrally planned	Regionally planned	Managed competition / public competition	Market

delivery approaches. Providers of care, because they are not in direct competition with each other, are more cooperative, exchanging 'best practices.' Market models, on the other hand, develop criteria for measuring efficiency and effectiveness; have a specified format for negotiating and administering contracts, usually based on cost and prices; and encourage experimentation in delivering services and competition among a pool of providers.

Figure 2.1 illustrates Saltman and von Otter's (1992a) continuum of allocation mechanisms, which apply to both publicly and privately financed sources. They range from centrally planned models (associated with command and control models), in which money is assigned to providers and patients must follow the money, to market models, in which resources follow the clients. A range of mixed models, termed 'managed competition' or 'public competition', attempts to blend the merits of both approaches.

Market allocation models are not to be confused with market-based financing, since the allocation mechanisms being discussed in this book apply to *publicly* financed services. Another distinction that can be made about allocation methods is whether the client follows the money or the money follows the client. At the centrally planned end, clients follow the money, that is, the planner decides where services will be provided, a global budget is allocated to the particular provider organization, and the client goes to that organization for service. Choice of provider for the patient is considerably reduced. The British National Health Services represents a model closer to the planned end. In market allocation models, money follows the client, that is, the client chooses the provider and the provider is reimbursed for services provided to that client. An example of this model is fee-for-service reimbursement of physicians in Ontario, where the physician's income is largely determined by the number of patient visits and patients choose their physician. The models that fall between attempt to create a compromise between central planning and markets.

During the 1980s and 1990s there was considerable experimentation on allocation mechanisms within publicly financed health systems in the United States, Britain, and Europe. In their work on the publicly operated health systems of northern Europe, Saltman and von Otter (1992a,b) developed a conceptual framework of 'planned markets' as an option that could strongly influence reform efforts in such systems. The authors suggested that structural problems with the 'command-and-control' public delivery model were at the root of the search for alternative models. Pressures to constrain spending, for publicly operated systems to be more responsive to patient concerns, and for more employee participation in decision making have forced these societies to experiment with new organizational frameworks that rely more upon market mechanisms.

The other distinction in allocation mechanisms is the purchaser/provider split. As Hollander, Deber, and Jacobs (1998) indicate, a purchaser/provider split can technically occur in only one of two circumstances; (1) the client is the sole purchaser of services (there are no third-party payers, such as governments or insurance companies); and (2) the client has delegated his/her decision on where to receive services to a purchasing agent (e.g., government or private insurer). In the first condition clients are threatened by catastrophic risk. In the second condition client choice is diminished. It is argued that splitting the purchaser function from that of the provision of care can increase efficiency and removes conflicts of interest inherent in situations where the functions are combined.

In the case of publicly financed services governments can flow funds either directly to their own employees (e.g., Ontario psychiatric hospitals); directly to individual private service delivers (e.g., most Canadian physicians); directly to private FP or NFP provider organizations (e.g., most Ontario hospitals or nursing homes); indirectly through a mediating agency, such as Ontario Home Care Programs; or directly to individuals who purchase their own services. There is no purchaser/provider split in the first example. The funders and deliverers of services are part of the same organization, the provincial government. In the other four instances there is a purchaser/provider split in that the purchasing function is undertaken by government, but the delivery of care is provided by non-governmental employees. For mediating agencies and direct funding to individuals, there is an additional purchaser/provider split when the agency or individual then purchases services external to the organization.

In LTC reform in Ontario, recommended allocation mechanisms swung from one end of the continuum to the other. Allocation methods varied from a very informal brokerage model close to the planned end of the continuum to a much more centrally planned model, then to a managed competition model closer to the market end of the continuum. All three governments also introduced pilot projects that allowed persons with disabilities to purchase their own services directly.

2.4 Summary and Conclusions: Policy Legacy

We posed two key analytic questions in our introductory comments to this chapter. The first question concerns policy content and provides a framework for examining the design decisions in each of the reforms. The second question deals with policy process and examines the interplay of ideas, institutions, and interests that explains the shape that reform takes. In particular, the latter question also tries to account for the volatility of this policy field. Finally, we try to show what an understanding of the dynamics of policy change in the case of community-based long-term care in Ontario can reveal about the dynamics of change or stasis in other proximate policy fields.

We suggest that answers to these questions must consider the relative autonomy or capacity of the state to assert its authority in a given policy field. Such capacity, we argue, waxes and wanes at different historical junctures. It does so not only because of change in the internal characteristics, interests, and logic of the state, including the ideological predilections of the party in power, but because of the changing characteristics and dynamics of the broader policy community in which the state is situated.

In the following chapters, we trace the different responses made by successive provincial governments to the reform of community-based LTC services in Ontario. These reforms differed in content and process. The content of the various reforms showed both similarities and differences in 'design decisions' about how best to finance, deliver, and allocate resources in the sector. The process of reform reflected different balances of ideas, institutions, and interests. In the next chapter, we clarify our methods of data collection and analysis before moving to the details.

CHAPTER THREE

Research Methodology: The Case Study Approach

3.1 Qualitative Research and Case Studies

Data-gathering techniques cannot be divorced from theoretical orientations (Berg, 1998). Certain problems lend themselves to certain forms of enquiry; in turn, the sort of data collected influences the sort of questions that can be asked. In this study we examined the influence of ideas, institutions, and interests on LTC reform. The purpose was to understand more clearly the reasons for the shifts in 'design decisions' about financing, delivery, and allocation reflected in the successive reform proposals and how they related to the ideas and interests that were expressed by stakeholders regarding reform. To do so, we employed a particular qualitative analysis approach: the case study design.

The case-study design is recognized (Johnson and Joslyn, 1995) as a distinctive form of empirical enquiry directed towards understanding the development of public policies, developing explanations, and testing theories. It represents a guided empirical enquiry in which a contemporary phenomenon is investigated within its real-life context, when the boundaries between phenomenon and context are not clearly evident and in which multiple sources of evidence are used (Yin, 1989). The case study is used in research where in-depth understanding is the goal and in situations where the researcher is unable to assign subjects, manipulate variables, or control the context of the study. The design allows for in-depth understanding of processes, explanatory theories, and hypothesis generation (see Johnson and Joslyn, 1995). Case studies are useful for answering 'how' and 'why' questions and for generating hypotheses for future research. For example, the results of this research should prove useful for understanding the nature of policy communities in general, the influence and interrelationship of various forces on policy, and the different dynamics in other policy communities in adjacent sectors. In case studies, typically a number of data collection methods are used, such as interviews, document analysis, and personal observations.

3.2 Data Sources

The period of time covered in this research is May 1985 to January 1996, which spans the mandates of the successive Liberal, New Democratic (NDP), and early Progressive Conservative (PC) governments. There were two primary sources of data documents and interviews, each of which was used to supplement the limitations in the other.

Analysis of the written word affords certain advantages. It is a permanent record that permits retrospective analysis; it is non-reactive; it promotes ease of access; and despite the possible intentional bias in the presentations, it is the public representations of participants' views, perhaps strategically advanced, to promote their interests. The usual disadvantage of document analysis – that records may not be accessible – is not an issue. All the documents in this research form part of the public record, accessible through Freedom of Information legislation.

Because of the span of time covered in the study, availability of records inevitably was uneven. Documentation from the Liberal period at the time of data collection either had been destroyed or was lodged in archives; at best, it was incomplete. Although records from the PC period were fresh, the government was relatively new during the period when the research data was being gathered. As a result, the data that inform this analysis are much more extensive from the NDP period. This in no way is meant to convey a hierarchy of importance in reform periods but rather is seen as a flaw inherent in research that is dependent to some extent on the record keeping of others. Nevertheless, these gaps form a limitation on the research.

Interviews allowed us to fill in gaps in data in the written documents and allowed for further exploration of our respondents' interpretations of the relative influences of ideas, interests, and institutions and the potential outcome of policies. It is important to recognize that memories of past events are shaped by subsequent history. In addition, people move in and out of positions and forget details. We therefore emphasized more recent events in the interviews and sought to cross-check interview data against other sources and against published material, where available.

While implicit theoretical assumptions and limitations exist with each data source, each represents 'a different line of sight directed toward the same point' (Berg, 1998, 4). The use of multiple sight lines or triangulation allows a richer understanding and a means of verifying insights. The triangulation of the data is not merely a combination of different kinds of data but an attempt to relate them.

3.2.1 Documents

The following documents were collected and used to inform analysis and provide support for interpretations.

1. Published government reports from the Liberal, NDP, and PC periods outlining reform models. They include Liberal – One-Stop Shopping model: *A New Agenda*, 1986 (Van Horne, 1986); Liberal – Service Access Organization (SAO) model: *Strategies for Change*, 1990 (Ontario Ministry of Community and Social Services (MCSS), Ontario Ministry of Health (MOH), Ontario Office for Senior Citizens' Affairs (OSCA), and Ontario Office for Disabled Persons (ODP), 1990); NDP – Service Coordination Agency (SCA) model: *Redirection of LTC*, 1991 (MCSS, MOH, and Ministry of Citizenship (MC), 1991); NDP – Multi-Service Agency (MSA) model: the multi-coloured reports on the MSA, 1993 (MOH, MCSS, and MC, 1993a,b,c,d) and Bill 173 An Act respecting Long-Term Care, 1994 (MOH, 1994); PC – Community Care Access Centre (CCAC) model: *Alternatives to the MSA: A Summary of Discussion with Key Groups Representing LTC Consumers, Providers, and Workers*, 1996 (Government of Ontario, 2001; MOH, 1996a,b,c,d; Wilson, 1996).
2. *Hansard* from the Legislative Assembly for the research period, and the Standing Committee on Social Development reviewing Bill 173, media releases, and speaking notes from ministerial addresses.
3. Written submissions from a sample of societal interests plus government-type agencies to the Standing Committee on Social Development reviewing Bill 173. Other written material from these groups on earlier reforms was also reviewed, but it was not as systematically organized or available.
4. Annual reports and other reports from societal interest groups, where available.
5. Newspaper stories and press releases were also employed, although this material also was not as systematically available.

3.2.2 Interviews

Questions for a semi-structured, open-ended interview schedule were developed based on material gathered from preliminary interviews with key informants and on the need for information required to test out the influence of the theoretical constructs. This schedule was pre-tested and modified accordingly. Face-to-face interviews, with the exception of one- and a half interviews that were done by telephone, were conducted with thirty-eight key informants. They included informants from twenty-three societal organizations and fifteen government informants (seventeen were approached). The latter group included government ministers and members of the opposition parties, ministry officials from government bureaucracies, and other types of government agencies. Key informants from societal organizations typically were the head of the organization in smaller organizations or in larger organizations the policy manager/analyst most involved with the reform.

Although it is the organization, its interests, and its influence that are of interest, one cannot interview organizations per se. Our assumption in the research, while we recognized its precariousness, was that the answers of individuals represent the organizational or institutional perspective. Because the research period encompasses eleven years, key informants were not always involved with their organization for the entire period. While it would have been optimal, given infinite resources, to track down and interview all the key informants for each organization over the entire time period, resources and time did not permit such an approach. As a result, some interviewees new to their organization had to infer the answers to questions pertaining to earlier periods.

Only two individuals from the 'government' category refused an interview. Interviews ranged from one to four hours in length. With permission from the interviewees, the interviews were tape-recorded and later transcribed.

3.3 Determination of the Policy Community

An early task in data collection was the determination of the make-up of the policy community in the community-based long-term care (LTC) sector, accomplished through an examination of government LTC files during the Liberal, NDP, and PC periods; government consultation documents; and information gathered from preliminary interviews with key informants.

The government institutional structures most closely associated with reform (in chronological order) included OSCA, MOH, MCSS, ODP, and MC, which combined OSCA and ODP during the NDP mandate. The Standing Committee on Social Development, the Premier's Council on Health Strategy, and later the Premier's Council on Health, Well-Being, and Social Justice, other government agencies, and local government also had key roles in the reform at specific times.

The societal interest groups in the community-based LTC sector numbered in the thousands, as evidenced by the claim of the NDP government to having included 75,000 participants during the consultation process (MOH, MCSS, and MC, 1993d). Clearly, not all groups had equal input. Given the limitations on time and resources and our intent to undertake in-depth analysis of reform during this period, it was essential that we focus the research on the key influential groups. During our review of government files, certain groups tended to surface more than others. From this preliminary review, it was clear that groups that had a provincial mandate were more influential than those whose mandate was local. This view was further substantiated by the fact that during the NDP consultation the central LTC Division, which was developing the policies, conducted the meetings with provincial associations, while the fourteen Area Offices undertook the consultations with local groups and forwarded only summaries (rather than transcripts) of their discussions to the central Division. As a result, the policy-making ear in government received a distillate, prepared by the Area Offices, of the input from local groups.

It was decided, therefore, to focus on organizations with a provincial mandate. However, they numbered in the hundreds. To ensure the inclusion of the different and influential interests in reform, a purposive sample was chosen, using a snowball sampling technique from the following category of groups: consumers (seniors, disability, and ethno-cultural), providers (for-profit [FP], not-for-profit [NFP], professional services, support services, professional associations, unions), and other (e.g., charitable organizations). In total, twenty-three organizations were included in the final sample: five consumer groups, seventeen provider groups, and one other type of organization. One 'local' provider organization deemed important by key informants was included as a surrogate for a set of interests that had no provincial association. Because the numbers in each category are small, a further breakdown cannot be done for reasons of confidentiality.

Within the government category, the fifteen key informants included government ministers, members of the official opposition, political staff, members of the bureaucracy from deputy ministers to policy analysts, and representatives from municipal government and government-type agencies.

3.4 The Community-Based LTC Policy Community

A description of the policy community involved in community-based LTC services when the Liberals came to form the government will help to set the stage for an analysis of the events that unfolded over the period in question. Government agencies included the MOH and the MCSS. Societal interests included the Home Care Programs, which were NFP agencies fully funded by the MOH, provider groups (health and social support agencies that were both commercial and NFP and funded by both MCSS and MOH), volunteer agencies, and consumer groups (seniors, disability groups, multicultural groups, and religious groups). Over time, the relative influence of these groups would change, shifting the balance of interests. Similarly, government proposals for reform would often change the scope of policy, awakening otherwise dormant interests or bringing disparate interests into alliances with some commonality to support or oppose the reform.

The health provider organizations were largely NFP agencies providing nursing or rehabilitation therapy services. While these organizations had been in existence for some time, in terms of resources and access to government, they did not rival the more 'institutionalized groups' (Pross, 1992) in health care, such as the medical or hospital organizations. The diverse nursing and therapy provider agencies, while having their own provincial organizations (e.g., the Victorian Order of Nurses [VON] agencies belonged to VON Ontario), did not form either a nursing coalition or a health provider coalition at the provincial level.

Although powerful medical associations like the Ontario Medical Association (OMA) existed, they were not, on the whole, involved with LTC reform. They had other issues to fight that were more important to them, such as extra-billing. In 1984 the Canada Health Act came into effect, banning extra-billing but giving provinces a three-year grace period to comply with the act. Negotiations between provinces and physicians proceeded relatively smoothly in all provinces except Ontario (Heiber and Deber, 1987). In 1986 the new Liberal government was embroiled in a bitter doctors' strike during which they brought in the ban on extra-billing practices (Tuohy, 1992). Similarly, hospital administrations and their professional groups, such as the Ontario Hospital

Association (OHA), did not engage in the reforms with much vigour. In the mid-1980s the reform of this policy sector was viewed primarily as involving community services and residential care and therefore not the concern of the OHA. Approaching 1990, these organizations would also be distracted by other pivotal issues such as hospital cutbacks and restructuring.

The social and personal support service organizations provided services such as attendant care, homemaking, food preparation, meal delivery, and security checks. They were mostly single, one-off, NFP agencies, whose services were provided by largely low-paid workers or volunteers. Organizational resources included a small, paid administrative staff. At the provincial level, the NFP agencies, which provided similar types of care, had associations; for example, homemaking agencies belonged to the Visiting Homemakers' Association, or meals on wheels agencies belonged to Meals on Wheels of Ontario. There were a few FP agencies such as Extendicare and Dynacare. The support services sector as a whole, however, was not unified at the provincial level. Without a uniform voice, this set of organizations was not effective during the Liberal reform period. In addition, government found it challenging to consult support service agencies.

In the mid-1980s consumer groups consisted of various seniors' groups (pensioners' or consumer advocacy groups); disability groups, which broke down into largely disease-focused groups; diverse ethnocultural groups separated by their ethnicity; and religious groups. During the Liberal reform period these groups, although somewhat vocal, were not forceful.

In the context of this analysis, we adopt the term 'consumer' to refer to seniors, persons with disabilities, children, and other potential recipients of community-based LTC services. Alternative terms have been suggested, such as recipient of care, client, or patient. Clearly, none of these terms is politically neutral. 'Consumer' and 'client' have meanings that pertain to private markets, that is, a completely informed person guided by individual preferences who exercises choice among options. Many 'clients' in the LTC sector are the frail elderly or the cognitively impaired, for whom the concept of informed choice is not meaningful. On the other hand, the term 'patient' is often associated with a medical model, that is, the authority of the physician and a narrow focus on cure and on health as being the absence of disease. 'Recipient of care,' other than being cumbersome, has an undertone of passivity. While the latter two terms, 'patient' and 'recipient of care,' are appropriate for a patient who, after an acute episode of illness is discharged early from a hospital, they are forcefully rejected by non-ill seniors (commonly referred to as well-seniors) and persons living with physical disabilities. The latter two groups lobbied heavily during the reforms for autonomy in decision making and for empowerment in designing not only their program of care but also the LTC system. As will be argued, well-seniors and persons with physical disabilities were more vocal and became more organized than other recipients. These two groups favoured the market moniker 'consumer' precisely because it implied the kind of recognition and power they were seeking. While adopting the term 'consumer,' we recognize that it has a narrow meaning and is not appropriate for all groups receiving LTC services.

In the following chapters, respondents are identified by a letter designating the type of group to which they belong. (The letter 'I' indicates a comment or query by the interviewer.) The letters designating the types of group are as follows:

C – Consumer organizations (including seniors,' disability, and ethno-cultural organizations)
P – Provider organizations (including all provider groups, both professional and support services, FP and NFP, professional associations, as well as organized labour)
G – Government officials (including members of the bureaucracy, members of the political arm of government, members of the official opposition, and members of other types of government agency)
O – other types of organizations, such as volunteer organizations

Although it would provide greater clarity to the analysis if the subcategories in which respondents belong were further identified, ethical considerations prevent such a strategy. Clearly, knowing whether it is a government minister or a member of the bureaucracy, whether it is a respondent from an NFP or an FP provider organization who is speaking in interview excerpts would make the analysis stronger. Because the numbers of interviewees in each subcategory are small, however, respondents could be readily identified, which would negate the assurances of anonymity and confidentiality given to them in return for their participation.

3.5 Analytical Strategies

There were three types of analyses undertaken: historical review, policy analysis, and content analysis.

3.5.1 Historical Review

Documents were used to construct a historical account of the events, process, and environment around the reform over the research period. The historical account of events and decisions is included in chapters 4–7.

3.5.2 Policy Analysis

Government policy documents also were used to compare and evaluate each recommended model in terms of the decisions made regarding the three design dimensions of financing, allocation, and delivery. Specifically, the shifts in the public/private mix in financing and delivery and the allocative mechanisms across the models were analysed. The implications of the design decisions in each model were analysed in terms of the role of the state in this sector and in terms of meeting traditional policy goals of access to services, quality of services, efficiency, choice, and availability of services. This analysis for each of the five models is undertaken in chapters 4–7.

3.5.3 Content Analysis

A content analysis was done using the Qualitative Solutions and Research non-numerical unstructured data indexing searching and theorizing (QSR NUD*IST) qualitative analysis software (Qualitative Solutions and Research, 1997). The interview transcripts and the written submissions to the Standing Committee on Social Development on Bill 173 were systematically analysed using this software. The purpose of this analysis was to develop an understanding of the development of each reform model using the framework of ideas, interests, and institutions; to answer questions of who, how, what, when, and why. The other documentation outlined above was used to inform and supplement these analyses.

QSR NUD*IST is a computer package designed to aid users in handling non-numerical and unstructured data in qualitative analysis. QSR NUD*IST manages data documents, explores documents through the creation of categories and coding of the text, manages and explores ideas, searches for patterns in coding, and allows for the exploration of theories about the data. This software replaces earlier cumbersome and time-consuming methods of undertaking qualitative analysis and permits a more in-depth, faster, and flexible exploration of the data.

Interviews were transcribed and documents (reports and submissions) were optically scanned into Text Format and imported into NUD*IST. The selection of categories for coding the documents was an iterative process. Reliability and validity checks for the coding were conducted.

Analyses of both the content and the process of reform are presented in chapters 4–7.

CHAPTER FOUR

Long-Term Care Reform in the Liberal Period, 1985–1990

4.1 Long-Term Care Reform under the Liberal Governments

In 1985 the formation of the Liberal government of David Peterson ended forty consecutive years of Progressive Conservative (PC) rule. The 2 May election had given the PCs, under the relatively conservative leadership of Frank Miller, a plurality of 52 seats in the 125-seat Legislature; 48 seats went to the Liberals, and 25 to the social democratic New Democratic Party (NDP) under Bob Rae. Although the Liberals received fewer seats than the PCs, the NDP was unwilling to support Miller. Instead, it formed an 'accord' with the Liberals, promising support for at least the limited future as long as its policy priorities were dealt with. On 4 June Miller delivered his throne speech; his government was promptly defeated on a non-confidence vote. Rather than calling a new election on the heels of the previous one, the province's lieutenant governor agreed to respect the accord and allowed the Liberals to form the government. Although no NDP members entered cabinet, Peterson agreed to a number of key NDP policy priorities. Long-term care (LTC) reform was not on this list.

It is noteworthy that, despite the low priority accorded to LTC reform by the politicians, senior bureaucrats continued to push for action. As noted in earlier chapters, this perceived urgency was driven by both external and internal forces. On the demand side, an ageing population and the technological ability to shift care into the community increased the pressure on available services, while an orientation towards health as well-being rather than as sickness care led to an increased recognition of the advantages of community-based treatments. From a policy viewpoint, decisions to lower hospital budgets and bed numbers reduced the availability of institutional care and left more (and sicker) people needing care within the community.

The first Liberal mandate (1985–7) was conducted under the constant threat that NDP support might be withdrawn, which muted reform in those areas not on the agreed-upon priority list. The resulting policy proposal for LTC reform, One-Stop Shopping (later known as One-Stop Access) could be seen as representing little more than the gathering of information, although in hindsight, some suggestion of what future reform might look like could be discerned.

In 1987 the accord ended. Peterson went to the polls and won a majority. During this mandate, the Liberals had more freedom to innovate; the proposal for Service Access Organizations represented a more comprehensive attempt at LTC reform, but one firmly rooted in managerial imperatives, with policy development left clearly under bureaucratic control. Not surprisingly, their proposal was incremental, leaving the delivery side of LTC largely unchanged. The main policy goals were the introduction of better coordination of the system, more accountability in the way home care organizations contracted their services, and more control over future costs. Nonetheless, the Liberals did begin to advance the agenda of shifting thinking (and power) within health care. Conventional wisdom among most health policy analysts inside and outside government appeared to be that the LTC system should be reoriented away from the medical model by promoting services that would keep seniors healthy in their own homes for as long as possible. In turn, this would require efforts to reduce the power of physicians and hospitals and shift resources into home and community care.

The Liberals began modestly, with a relatively inexpensive 'exhortation' policy instrument; they reformed the institutional structures by setting up new advisory bodies. These in turn had the potential of changing the 'scope of conflict' by changing which participants were at the decision-making table. One high-profile example was the Premier's Council on Health Strategy, which was composed of elite representatives from the health and social services arena plus senior members of the bureaucracy in a wide variety of health-related departments. Although advisory, its members could be in a position to champion most changes recommended by the council (e.g., powerful deans of Ontario medical schools could take forward suggested changes in medical education). The Premier's Council was both symbolic – embracing the popular ideas of public participation – but also practical; it diluted the power of physicians and hospitals by including influential voices from nursing, social services, and the business community, and it helped to shift emphasis from the medically dominant view towards a population health orientation.

The Liberal government attempted to create a similar focus for seniors' issues within government through the advocacy ministry of the Office for Senior Citizens' Affairs (OSCA). This initiative again served a symbolic function: it gave voice to a growing constituency who were demanding more independence in living. However, it also served the practical function of wresting responsibility for reform of the LTC sector away from the two dominant ministries that currently had the responsibility for providing the majority of LTC community services, namely, the ministries of Health (MOH) and Community and Social Services(MCSS). The Liberals hoped to be able to develop policy without its being paralysed by dissension between these two conflicting organizational cultures.

As we will note, the reform of the LTC policy field was aided by the nature of the policy community, which consisted of many small independent agencies largely working on their own. No single group dominated. As further evidence of the incremental nature of the Liberal reform proposals, there was no attempt to mount concerted, coordinated action.

4.2 Liberal Minority Government, 1985–1987: One-Stop Shopping

4.2.1 Institutional Changes and Underlying Government Interests

One of the Liberals' first acts was to set up the Office for Senior Citizens' Affairs, and appoint Ron Van Horne as its minister; he was given responsibility for guiding the development of a system of services for the elderly. It was believed to be the first time in Canadian history that a minister had been appointed solely to deal with seniors' issues (Nickoloff et al., 1994). Seniors were not only a growing demographic group who were living longer and therefore would be requiring more services, but they were also a much more affluent and vocal group than earlier generations had been. They were becoming a constituency that governments could not ignore. They had been lobbying for some time to have a spokesperson within cabinet to represent their interests. Without a focal point within government, seniors' groups had been forced to approach separately each of the several ministries (including, but not restricted to, MOH, MCSS, Housing, Municipal Affairs, and Finance) that provided programs for them. This new office provided an institutionalized mechanism for concentrating access to government for seniors and thereby, it was hoped, both strengthening their voice and assuaging organized groups of seniors. OSCA was given neither the mandate nor the budget to deliver programs and services to seniors, however, and accordingly, as would become apparent as time went on, it did not have the clout to deliver reform.

Van Horne moved quickly; on 12 July 1985 he announced that OSCA would conduct a public consultation to gather information for its review of programs and services for seniors. Although little information on the process is available in the Ontario Archives, the consultations appeared to have been a classic example of a 'Casablanca consultation' – it rounded up the 'usual suspects.' The process began with a round-table discussion attended by representatives of fourteen provincial senior citizens' organizations. OSCA then travelled to fourteen communities to hear the views of seniors and providers in a series of open meetings. At each of these meetings the government endeavoured to have representation from planning groups (e.g., district health councils and municipalities), health care providers, community service providers (home care and home support services), the housing sector, and LTC institutions (nursing homes, homes for the aged, and retirement homes). Approximately sixty site visits were paid to institutional programs and community service organizations serving seniors. Major interest groups also were invited to submit written submissions (OSCA, 1985).

While there was no clear-cut agreement on solutions, a consensus on the problems emerged from these consultations. Organizations made frequent mention of lack of coordination among the MOH, MCSS, and the Ministry of Housing; there was an almost unanimous belief that better coordination should begin at the provincial government level. Furthermore, they wanted a single access point or 'problem-solving centre' in each community to provide information and referral to all services for the elderly. Regarding policy content, seniors indicated that they preferred to remain in their homes for as long as possible; they endorsed further development of community services and less reliance on institutional care. Major gaps in homemaker services were highlighted; those consulted argued for both expansion of community supports and making them available without a physician's referral (OSCA, 1985). Based on OSCA's first round of consultations, it was determined that health and social services, being the largest provincial expenditures on services for the elderly, would be the first programs selected for review.

Although the review was now narrowed to health and social services,

OSCA continued to act as the 'lead agency' for reform. The prospect of intra-governmental dispute was evident; MCSS funded the social services, which received relatively few public funds but provided approximately 80 per cent of all community-based services to seniors, while the MOH-funded Home Care Program comprised 80 per cent of all expenditures on services to seniors. A government official indicated that making OSCA the lead agency for reform fitted in with the Liberal government's thinking on the need for both vertical and horizontal lines in cross-cutting policy development. The Liberals had established a number of 'advocacy' ministries whose mandate was to speak on behalf of targeted populations and their specific needs and to provide some coherence and coordination in policy analysis and development across government. This attempt to set up 'cross-cutting' ministries was also extended into particular departments. For example, the MOH, during the later Liberal period, introduced a number of 'coordinator' positions within the ministry to advocate on behalf of client groups (aboriginal coordinator), provider groups (nursing coordinator), or disease groups (cancer coordinator). These experiments tended to be described, in the language of organizational theory, as 'matrix structures.' Because such 'horizontal' structures had only moral authority (control over resources remaining within the 'vertical' structures to which budget lines were given), the experiment did not prove particularly effective.

The government's decision to have OSCA take the lead also was greeted with enthusiasm by many outside government in the policy community. It was viewed as a way of ensuring an impartial mediation of interests or ideas, as well as a potential mechanism for allowing the voice of consumers to be heard.

P: Well, because of the constant wrangling between the two ministries [MOH, MCSS] as to who should be in charge. And the view was that the Office for Seniors was more independent, was a new kid on the block, maybe more able to communicate directly with consumers, and other interested parties, wouldn't be so influenced by one or another set of provider agencies, and that it could do a better job of coordinating with the other two ministries.

There was considerable disagreement as to the net effect of having appointed OSCA as the lead ministry. Some stressed its independence and agreed that setting up such an office signaled that the government had placed a high priority on seniors' issues.

G: Oh, I think that by doing that and appointing a minister without portfolio responsible for this-that-and-the-other-thing is a very clear way for a government to signal, it hopes, that this is now a priority and is going to have special attention.

Those applauding the role of OSCA also felt that this institutional response would help to breach the schism between Health and Social Services and reflect the shift in thinking away from a medical model towards a stronger focus on prevention (e.g., P, G). These observers argued that there was no logical position within either the MOH or the MCSS that could bridge the diverse programs and assume responsibility for reform. The MOH had been concerned largely with the Home Care Program and, more particularly, with nursing homes as its primary LTC function. MCSS was seen as too soft and fractured in its approach for the more medically oriented or health-oriented elements of the needs of seniors (G).

Others were less sanguine and stressed that the absence of a line ministry with a budget and authority for programs meant that LTC reform was not a government priority.

P: If reform is in an Office, it isn't as strong as when it's entrenched within a ministerial mandate, and the minister is a member of the Priorities and Planning. It just has a stronger thrust to it ... I didn't really think the Liberal agenda was long-term care.

4.2.2 A New Agenda

On 2 June 1986, the minister for senior citizens' affairs marked Senior Citizens' Month by tabling his proposal for LTC reform in the legislature. Its title embedded a typographical pun – *A New Agenda: Health and Social Service Strategies for Ontario's Seniors* (Van Horne, 1986). The document was intended to be the first of a series of papers on services to seniors; it was stated that this was the first time an Ontario government had released a strategic plan for health and social services for seniors. The central theme of the document was enabling seniors to live active and independent lives in their own communities and in doing so to prevent unnecessary and inappropriate institutionalization. Five strategies were proposed, which represented an outline for policy and program development for health and social services over the next fifteen years, a further indication that reform was to be gradual and measured. The five strategies were:

1. to improve the health and functional status of seniors through emphasis on health promotion and illness prevention and on improvements in education and research;
2. to assist the elderly to live independently in the community by improving access to, and delivery of, community support services through the introduction of a 'one-stop-shopping' approach; and by providing a broader range of community support services;
3. to enhance the capacity of hospitals to meet the needs of the frail elderly through improvements in specialized outreach and inpatient services;
4. to provide high-quality institutional care for those elderly who are unable to live independently in the community; and
5. to introduce comprehensive planning and management at both the provincial and the local level.

The report did not represent a break with the past; its themes of prevention through community support services, functional independence, coordination of services, and the introduction of local planning had been identified under the previous Conservative government. The report reinforced both the growing awareness that the curative side of health care was not only expensive but had little effect on improving the health status of populations and the increasing hope that disease prevention and health promotion might prove both less expensive and more effective than the more traditional emphasis upon a medical model of Home Care.

One striking difference between *A New Agenda* and most proposals for health care reform was its emphasis on client groups rather than on programs. Conventionally, health reform was based on program areas, usually those associated with identifiable budgets. Accordingly, government might seek to restructure hospitals, reform primary care, or modify a drug program, with responsibility for policy development resting primarily with the branch of government running that program. In contrast, OSCA focused upon services for its client group of seniors. An immediate policy dilemma was created, since similar services could be used by other groups who were not the target of this reform. For example, persons with disabilities or people discharged from hospitals might also require nursing or rehabilitation services. As a short range solution, the government believed that it could develop a system to deal with the complete needs of the elderly (from community care to chronic and institutional care) while leaving persons with disabilities within the existing system (they would continue to be eligible for home care and support services). This approach decreased the scope of conflict and ensured that the very strong advocacy groups for the disabled would not participate in this set of discussions. (Later reforms would in turn widen the definition of affected populations and bring disability groups back into the debate.)

G: Some argued that it made much more sense to take a 'care group' approach than a 'care level' approach. The government has tended to divide the health system up on the basis of care levels, not care groups. There has never been a pure model, because there have been care group entities within government, the Office of Aboriginal Affairs ... But by and large the powerful parts of the ministry have been the care level parts ... And the concern of others, including me, was that people often use multiple levels of care and unless you create a grouping, you run the risk of losing the focus on people. You can become obsessed with care levels.

As indicated earlier, at the time there was some awareness in the policy community that the needs of the disability community were different from those of seniors, as were some of the services they relied upon. In addition, the vocal members of the disability community tended to be fairly independent adults with physical rather than cognitive disabilities; many were also associated with the Independent Living movement (G).

In *A New Agenda* the need to improve access to services and to provide a more comprehensive approach to the delivery of community health and social services was stressed (OSCA, 1987c). This strategy included several components. First, funding was enriched. In January 1986 the government had allocated an additional $11 million to community services for the elderly and for increased support for volunteers who assist in many of these services. Priority was to be given to relieving current maldistribution; services were to be expanded in northern, underserviced, rural, and remote areas. In addition, special attention was to be given to programs responding to ethnocultural needs (e.g., ethno-specific diets) of seniors. The government also increased the maximum provincial share for home support services to 60 per cent of agency costs, which would rise to 70 per cent in 1987. In addition to increasing funding for current programs, the January 1986 announcement introduced the Integrated Homemaker Program (IHP), to be delivered in conjunction with the professional services currently provided by the Home Care Program. The IHP would subsidize non-professional services needed to

assist families to care for its members by offering homemaking, shopping, meal preparation, cleaning, laundry, ironing, mending, and personal care. Although the IHP was administered by the MOH through the
Home Care Program, it was funded by the MCSS (Stewart and Lund,
1990). The government announced its hope that this strategy would
begin to bring about a functional integration of the more medically oriented services with the support services and to shift services towards prevention rather than cure. Indeed, it made it clear that its priority was to
expand support and volunteer services rather than services by health
professionals; in the document it argued the need to avoid 'excessive
professionalization' of programs (OSCA, 1987c).

In short, this reform proposal was intended to leave largely untouched
the existing system of service delivery by both formal and informal providers and the balance of public and private responsibility in the financing and delivery of these services. The increased funding was intended to
enhance and supplement, not to replace, existing or potential family
and volunteer support services. Accordingly, the reform did not move
this group of services into the public arena; individuals and their families, along with charities, would still be held responsible for meeting
these needs. The new funding was targeted at the narrower goals of
improving geographic equity, addressing cultural needs, and securing
the viability of informal and social supports.

The fifth strategy outlined in *A New Agenda* was designed to address
one of the structural barriers to an integrated and coordinated system
of care for the elderly. OSCA, working with MOH and MCSS, had concluded that the various programs delivering health and social services
for seniors should be considered components of a broad system. Service
coordination was hampered, however, because these programs were
divided among different ministerial jurisdictions, which had different
philosophies, legislative requirements, eligibility requirements, and
funding formulas. Home Care and Placement Coordination Services
were universal programs residing within the MOH, while Homemaker
and Nurses' Services, IHP, Home Support, Respite, and Attendant Care
resided within MCSS. At the local level, the thirty-eight Home Care Programs were administered by the local Health Unit (twenty-three local
boards, seven regional governments), the Victorian Order of Nurses
(VON) (four), a local hospital (three), or a special purpose body (one).
A number of interviewees talked about the conflict of interest in those
jurisdictions where Home Care Programs were run by providers who
were also eligible for contracts with the program. Others indicated that

a program run by either Public Health Units or hospitals was always the 'poor sister' to the other programs run by that agency (G). Overall, this diffusion of responsibilities made it difficult for government to plan and allocate resources comprehensively, establish priorities, and deliver health and social services on an integrated basis. The consultations leading to the report had revealed a strong consensus that these barriers to comprehensive planning and delivery should, to the extent possible, be eliminated.

How to accomplish this goal, however, was less clear. It was hoped (in retrospect rather optimistically) that at the provincial level, the placement of responsibility for planning and overall coordination of services for the elderly with the minister for senior citizens' affairs might reduce this fragmentation. At the local level, it was suggested in the Paper that a special-purpose board responsible to the province, a local government, or a provincial ministry should be created with responsibility delegated to local offices (Van Horne, 1986).

After another round of province-wide consultations with seniors, service providers, and community leaders, the minister for senior citizens' affairs announced in June 1987 the creation of five pilot projects as sites for the new 'One-Stop Shopping' approach, now called 'One-Stop Access.' One-Stop Access would offer functional assessment and take responsibility for bringing community health and social services to seniors in their own homes. All funds for service provision would come from the provincial government, but the local agency would take full responsibility for how these funds were spent (with the proviso that they could not reallocate funds from provincially designated programs without provincial approval). The local District Health Councils would oversee and provide guidance for planning, much as they did for local hospitals and public health units (OSCA, 1987c). The pilots were estimated to cost over $5 million and were to be introduced in two phases (three in 1987–8 and two in 1988–9). Local planning and management of community services and flexibility in addressing needs were highlighted. Given the government's recognition that local needs varied across the province and that a 'cookie cutter' approach was inappropriate, each of the five pilots would be free to develop its own model within the context of provincial criteria. As will be seen in later chapters, both the NDP and the Conservatives were less willing to allow local variation.

The One-Stop Access proposal represented an incremental change to the existing system, was categorized by a flexibility in approach, and was intended primarily to serve the needs of the elderly. As would become evident in future reforms, this focus had the advantage of narrowing the scope of conflict but the disadvantage of failing to deal with services offered by the same agencies to other target groups, including persons with disabilities and those discharged early from hospital. Nevertheless, to some extent, the interests of the disability community would be considered, because the initiative was to be undertaken in close cooperation with MOH, MCSS, and the Office for Disabled Persons (ODP) (OSCA, 1987a,b). In contrast, however, there was little institutional coordination between the 'long term care' branch (which was concerned with the needs of those with chronic care needs) and the activities within the 'institutional' branch (which was concerned with acute episodic care and was beginning to consider ways to reduce the demand upon 'expensive' hospitals by encouraging shorter lengths of stay and greater reliance on home- and community-based care).

4.2.3 Societal Interests and Influence on Reform

Government's freedom of action was enhanced because the policy community involved with the reform of community-based health and social services at the time had rather straightforward requests; none was calling for a major realignment of the current system.

4.2.3.1 Consumers

Although government tended to speak of 'consumers' as a unified group, these interests did not act together and did not perceive their interests as identical. The two major groups that became involved in the consultation represented seniors and the disability community. In both cases, those who became involved in the reform were relatively healthy and independent and stressed their need for social supports rather than medical care. (Those reliant upon professional services, in contrast, were rarely well enough to become involved in the consultation process.) A common theme from consumers, accordingly, was the need to disentangle access to care from existing gatekeepers – usually physicians – and to simplify 'shopping' for services.

C: What we were stressing was the one point of entry, that was the big thing; so there'd be some coordination, so we could find one place where we get what we needed, rather than have to do all of this searching for ourselves ... in many cases, consumers don't know what's available if somebody doesn't tell them. And if you're going to be possessive about your own organization, you're not necessarily going to be too helpful.

The sorts of concerns emerging from seniors' groups focused upon simplifying their ability to access care. A common complaint was that community-based services were provided by a wide variety of agencies and that no single agency was responsible for conducting comprehensive, functional (as opposed to medical) assessments of the elderly client; for coordinating the delivery of a range of services; or for monitoring changes in the individual's situation. As government officials reported:

G: Everybody was complaining. There was a lot of correspondence and groups that came forward and said, 'It's so hard to find out where to go. You get passed on from one person to the next.' And so it was just messy. It was inconvenient. Some services didn't know about other services. If somebody did manage to find out about Home Care and get through to a Home Care Program, they [Home Care] didn't necessarily mention other supports in the community that were available, and vice-versa.

G: If a client requires more than one service, then you're getting a lot of people walking in the door, and can sort of begin to feel like you're living in a train station. So that, for example, nurses want to go in and assess before they go to a client, because they want to know what they're going to come up against on a regular basis ... Homemaking agencies are going to look for completely different things and in fact not trust the assessment ... If you have more than one person [provider] you're getting a lot of different assessments, which can be very frustrating if you happen to be the person receiving all of them. And then, with three or four different agencies it means that you have three or four different agencies with completely different cultures, completely different ways of going about their business, coming in and basically invading your life.

Further fragmenting the 'consumer' voice, those in the disability community battled to be considered separately from seniors in the planning of community-based services. They saw their needs as fundamentally different from those of the elderly, noting that persons with disabilities had long been fighting to get out of the disease model of services. The more politically active parts of this community, while physically constrained, did not see themselves as ill or mentally incompetent. Their greatest need was for personal attendant services to aid in the tasks of daily living – toileting, dressing, transportation, shopping. Given the closeness of the working relationship with personal attendants, people with disabilities wanted the freedom to choose their own providers.

C: The issues at that point from the disability community side had been pretty consistent all along. One is they don't like seeing ... long-term care services as medical, and there has been a long-term fight to try to get them out. The second issue that really, I think, preoccupied the community for a long time is direct funding of attendant care services ... But up until that point I would say that the energy of the groups that were really working hardest on long-term care in the disability community were primarily focused on individualized funding and keeping disability out of [LTC reform for seniors] ... The attitude of people with disabilities is, number one, we're not seniors and there's a real difference, but more important, the real issue is the autonomy issue and the ability to choose because this is their life. I mean people think of long-term care as being illness related. But for people with disabilities it's getting out of bed in the morning and going to work, school, services like special needs.

When people with disabilities talk about consumer control they talk about people like themselves who are using wheelchairs or whatever, being involved, and that's reasonable. They're healthy people who are not deteriorating mentally. So it's not unreasonable for them to be on boards, or to be involved in advisory groups. When the seniors' community talks about consumers, what they're really talking about are family members often, because the person who's using the services is often not in any shape to be on the board.

Another set of voices came from cultural communities, who traditionally provided a considerable portion of services for the elderly. Their primary concern was to ensure that the ethno-specific services they had built over the years remained intact. Within sub-populations such as the Italian, Chinese, Greek, or Jewish communities, access and coordination were not seen as pressing issues; from their perspective, care was already coordinated and easily accessed within their own cultural groups.

C: Someone from the Italian community is quite comfortable going through COSTI or Villa Columbo, and they've got this whole circle in which they can operate reasonably effectively. Same thing with the Chinese community.

The general feeling was that during this period, reform consisted of tidying up the existing system. As such, there were no elements that would arouse consumer passion or dissent.

G: I think the consumer movement hadn't really hit a pitch at that point. There was no real series of events that would catapult a consumer movement. You know, it's doing business as usual, hearing there's some problems, saying, 'Okay, let's clean up the system. We'll get better governance; we'll try to get rid of the conflict of interest around boards; we'll strengthen the case management role; and we'll bring about one kind of phone number approach to this.' It was relatively – now when you think about it, you know – kind of a mild approach to change.

4.2.3.2 Providers
Because the suggested reforms were seen as largely incremental, most provider organizations did not feel threatened and hence tended not to become heavily involved in trying to change the direction of the reform. Similarly, unions felt no need to take an active role (P).

P: I don't think in a direct way, certainly not at the provincial level. If there was any involvement it would have been just through probably fate and circumstances at the local areas or through the Home Care Programs. But there was no government relation strategy to influence the direction.

P: Why weren't we as involved politically, as an organization, at that point? The issues weren't of a high stake. There seemed to be more balance. I guess we felt more secure, as a provider during that interval.

4.2.4 Assessment of One-Stop Access by Members of the Policy Community

The One-Stop Access approach and *A New Agenda* were not radical changes to the way business traditionally had been conducted in the sector. As such, these reforms did not upset the boundaries of the policy sector and therefore did not galvanize societal interests into action. In answer to 'Who was most influential in this period?' most respondents named the existing Home Care Programs and those already involved in delivering such services. In effect, the scope of conflict was a narrow one, and there was little disagreement about fundamental principles. In retrospect, many believed that this first reform model was a good beginning and a step in the right direction, but that more was needed.

G: I think it was a taking of what existed, and I suspect a commitment to create where there were no services, similar kinds of services, and then a commitment to making sure that you put in another layer which coordinated those services, which is probably the simplest thing that one would do.

P: As far as it went, I thought it was all right. But it was only a first step ... towards more intensive integration. But certainly the idea went a long way towards dealing with the just enormous fragmentation that still exists.

Despite the incremental nature of reform, some groups did have concerns. These concerns fell into two broad categories. First, a number of groups feared that moving decision making into a new organization would represent a change in power arrangements. This was often expressed in terms of 'inclusion/exclusion.' For example, although government believed that this reform represented a step from a provider focus to a consumer focus (G), a number of consumer and provider groups believed that One-Stop Access either cut them out of the sector or didn't do enough to bring them into the sector. Some ethno-cultural groups had concerns that services would lose their ethno-specific orientation: 'If everybody goes through this quote, one-shop-stop [one-stop-shop], then what [does] something like the Federation of Italian Seniors do? And who do you volunteer with?' (C). From the perspective of persons with disabilities, One-Stop Accesss represented a model where professionals still made the decisions; as such, the reform represented the antithesis of the 'consumer-created and consumer-driven' model they would find acceptable (C). Physicians objected that the One-Stop approach to assessment was unnecessary, since they already provided that service, and furthermore, it would cut them out of the loop (P). For-profit (FP) providers believed that the brokerage system used prior to *A New Agenda* had privileged those already holding home care contracts and that the proposed model would do little to change the situation.

P: It was the current way of doing business. There wouldn't be any sets of principles. There wouldn't be a level playing field.

I: So what was the current way of doing business?

P: Just renewing contracts.

I: But how did the contracts get started in the first place?

P: You've got a contract. You keep getting a contract and the percentage that you had last year you get next year. Most communities start their contracts with VON, and the St Elizabeth got in there, and Red Cross, and some of the others. So, as the need grew, they always went to the not-for-profits first. That was the approach thirty years ago. And what happened about eighteen years ago now, with hospitals' discharging clients sooner and sicker, they needed nurses to visit Friday evening and weekends, or night. And the nursing organizations, because they were a monopoly said, 'No, we're not going to do that. Our people don't want to do that. We don't want to set up systems to do that. It's more expensive,' etc. And so Home Care Programs had to find someone to do it, so they called upon the private sector ... It wasn't a competition process of getting [contracts]. We got the leftovers. And we still get the leftovers.

The second main line of attack was that One-Stop Access simply added another layer of bureaucracy without implementing a more comprehensive reform (G).

P: I think that it didn't address the question of 'Are the services that are already there, and that have grown in a very ad hoc way, in fact appropriate services? Is the structure appropriate to the delivery of service? How do we get, not just a coordination of those community services, but some kind of seamless transition from hospital to home and from home to hospital?' ... I think that even then the kinds of grass roots groups that I was involved with were expressing concern that the model would be dominated by the more powerful agencies: the Red Cross, who was providing homemaker services at that point. And some of the hospitals were beginning to tune in to the fact that this might well be a growing field in the future, and beginning to talk the talk without necessarily walking the walk of community-based services.

From a political standpoint, however, many observers recognized that the Liberal-NDP accord favoured a cautious (and incremental) approach, particularly for policies that were not high on the NDP agenda. In addition, forty years of Tory rule meant that the members of the new Liberal government had limited experience. As two respondents captured it, A New Agenda and One-Stop Access represented preliminary attempts at reform while the new government was getting its grounding.

O: The first mandate was a relatively new government, with people who had not been used to governing at all, who tried to articulate general principles ... When they were first elected, '85 to '87, the two-year coalition government with NDP, [they] were establishing values, aims, and goals.

As a result, the first set of reforms was evolutionary rather than revolutionary.

G: I think that it was their way of saying the long-term-care system is evolving; it was not a revolutionary piece.

4.3 Liberal Majority Government, 1987–1990: Service Access Organizations

In the summer of 1987 the Liberal government, which had been gaining in popularity, called an election. On 10 September the Liberals were returned, this time with a majority of 95 seats in the 130-seat legislature. They no longer needed the support of the NDP to form the government. In addition, they were influenced by prominent health policy researchers to attempt to move away from the medical model towards an approach based upon 'population health,' which, if successful, implied the ability to encourage non-medical and less costly means for improving the health of the population of Ontario.

4.3.1 Paradigm Shift through Institutional Change

In the first year of its second mandate, the Liberal government received three major health care reports: that of the Ontario Health Review Panel (chaired by Dr John Evans) (Evans, 1987), the Panel on Health Goals (chaired by Dr R. Spasoff) (Spasoff, 1987), and the Minister's Advisory Group on Health Promotion (chaired by S. Podborski) (Podborski, 1987). All of these groups emphasized in their reports health in its broadest sense and argued that the system should be refocused on community care, health promotion, and disease prevention.

As a result of these reports, the Premier's Council on Health Strategy was formed in December 1987. Chaired by the premier, with the minister of health as vice-chair, the council adopted the World Health Organization's definition of health, which acknowledged broader social, economic, environmental, and lifestyle determinants of health (Premier's Council on Health Strategy, 1991d). The council set up five committees to examine each one of its mandates: Health Goals, Health Care System, Healthy Public Policy, Integration and Coordination, and the Health Innovation Fund. The Premier's Council was an important step towards diluting the power of the strongest members of the health care policy community; physicians and hospitals were counterbalanced by nurses, business representatives, and those with a broader perspective on the determinants of health (e.g., advocates of child development). The council's inclusion of very senior bureaucrats from ministries other than Health also helped members to gain a broader perspective on policy options.

The work of the council and its committees was an important part of the environment during which the early reforms of LTC took place. Although its reports were not published until 1991, the fact that the premier, various ministers, and senior bureaucrats who provided support were involved with the ongoing work of the council and its committees ensured that the thinking of the council and its committees influenced and penetrated government's activities. Indeed, a senior government bureaucrat in that period believed that the council, not the MOH, was the guiding policy body for health and LTC reform.

G: There were a lot of policy ideas evolving and position papers coming out of the Premier's Council that were helping to mould and establish policy ... If you follow the sequence of the papers and the reports that came out of Com Soc [MSCC] on integration/coordination, particularly, you come up with a lot of the policy bases that were being implemented by the ministry. Although the minister had the lead influence in the beginning, as the policy evolved it was ultimately the Premier's Council on Health that had the largest influence in establishing some of the principles on integration/coordination.

The recommendations of the council's committees would be recognizable in the evolving LTC policy. Goal 2 of the Health Goals Committee, with its broad vision of health, emphasized the importance of the social environment and social services to health (Premier's Council on Health Strategy, 1991e). The work of the Healthy Public Policy Committee emphasized the limited role of the medical treatment system for improving the overall health of the population (Premier's Council on Health Strategy, 1991c).

Among the reports tabled was an ambitious plan by the Health Care System Committee, which called for shifting the emphasis and related resources towards the development of community services as an equal partner with the institutional sector in the provision of health services. Recommendations included: the doubling of funding for community services; legislative and policy reforms to allow for the development of community services; enhanced local planning, accountability, and funding envelopes; and new forms of organization and management to be tested by pilot projects (Premier's Council on Health Strategy, 1991a).

Similarly, the Integration and Coordination Committee recommended the devolving or transferring of authority for budgetary allocation, service management, and planning and evaluation to local levels; and responsibility for legislation, funding, and standards setting would remain at the provincial level. Transfer of authority should be phased in after corporate restructuring to integrate MOH with MCSS on a regional basis. Devolution was to make services more responsive to local needs and to give consumers a say in how services were planned and delivered (Premier's Council on Health Strategy, 1991b). Taken together, the reports pointed to a future where less power (and fewer resources) would rest with physicians and hospitals and more with social supports delivered in the home and community.

4.3.2 MCSS Takes Charge

In 1989 John Sweeney, minister of community and social services, was given the lead for LTC reform. In terms of politics within government, this shift was seen by some observers as a pre-emptive move on the part of the line ministries, MOH and MCSS, to abort OSCA's attempt to gain budgetary control of services.

G: One of the big problems was that [OSCA], which was originally designed to be a policy ministry, actually wanted to have line management responsibility for long-term care, that is, ... to have the budget, and that kind of thing ... Health and Com Soc said, you know, 'We understand the policy role, but there's no way that we can give up whole hunks of the two ministries' budget to another ministry and still remain accountable for that budget to Management Board.'

In effect, this move signalled the belief that Van Horne's One-Stop Access model was insufficient to get the job done. As opposed to a pilot project in a limited number of communities, which could be depicted as merely adding another agency to the existing system, Sweeney and Elinor Caplan, the minister of health, were preparing the way for a more comprehensive reform. The decision to place responsibility with MCSS was both strategic and practical. One official indicated that MCSS and MOH had reached a mutual decision, based on the need for an appropriate ministerial culture to inculcate reform and the relative workloads of the ministries, that MCSS should take the lead.

G: Com Soc [MCSS] had the lead, which was Caplan's suggestion because MOH tended to medicalize everything and LTC included both health and social services. We needed something less threatening, particularly since long-term care was going to be community focused. Also, Caplan was embarking on major reforms in other areas and had her plate full.

To some, this decision to de-emphasize the Ministry of Health could be seen as reflecting the prevailing direction of the Premier's Council and other organizations like the World Health Organization (WHO): the view of health being determined also by social and economic factors and the need to diverge from a medical treatment response model to improving health status; the importance of local involvement (as noted earlier, MCSS had a less top-down management style than MOH and already had Area Offices in place for the management of programs); and the need to shift from institutional to community services. A number of interviewees saw the move to MCSS as necessary to bringing about this shift in the prevailing thinking that dominated the policy sector.

G: The Ministry of Health saw care as a very medicalized thing, and everyone understood after they had done their local consultations with the seniors' groups and the regional bodies, that long-term care was, in fact, to be a non-medicalized approach to care of the elderly. Because [if] all we were going to do was medicalize the care of the elderly, then that would be considered a major step back. The view was that medicine was an adjunct to long-term care, it was not the core of long-term care. And that was a decision that was taken fairly high up in both ministries.

P: There was a more generalized belief among people who had concerns about the health sector that the medical model of caring for people had adversely affected many clients of the system. And that something that was more like a social model was more appropriate.

G: And I think that all the time it was with Com Soc [MCSS], they were trying to de-medicalize the system as much as they possibly could, which is in line with sort of the continuing warring cultures between those two ministries.

G: What I'd heard was that they wanted the model to be very much a health and social service model, and that clients did not necessarily want to be treated as patients. And they didn't want a strictly medical model. And so to echo that, at the political level the lead was given to MCSS.

Accordingly, this move was applauded by those who believed that the culture of MCSS reflected the primary importance of social supports in keeping people in the community. This group also stressed that, if one wished to achieve integration of services, MCSS had fiscal responsibility for the majority of community agencies; that is, they had the numbers, in terms of agencies rather than dollars.

P: It may have been when they first decided that the community was, you know, really where health was going, maybe they felt that in terms of being able to integrate, I mean, all of the agency-type stuff, all of the other services in the community were Com Soc [MCSS]. So it may have been trying to figure out how ... can you have this one system, this coordinated thing with all the agencies, all working together in a community if, if it's through three different silos ... And there are a whole lot of services you can't bring into health because they're not about doctors, and treatments.

P: I think the vision [for LTC] was more that it would be in the support service area – community services – that the needs, because it wasn't seen initially, I don't think, as so much a health need as a ... more of a social support primarily, recognizing that there were health elements obviously. But that the focus of what was needed to provide this One-Stop Access would be really this service support system ... and that group had traditionally ... was funded through MCSS.

Other perceived advantages of the MCSS culture were its compatibility with a vision of reform as decentralized, community based and locally driven, echoing the recommendations of the council's Integration and Coordination Committee. According to these recommendations, devolution would make services more responsive to local needs and give consumers a say in how services were planned and delivered. The culture of MCSS was also seen as one that best reflected the dignity and individuality of clients and respected their right to involvement in decision making about their care. The mediation of values through institutional structures and the difference in cultures were stressed over and over by respondents. Interviewees made reference to the difference in clothing styles and work styles, even to the detail that MOH staff wore watches and MCSS staff did not.

G: They [MCSS] were a decentralized ministry, and ... their offices were the ears of the community ... And, at that point, I think the government was looking for a decentralized solution.

G: Com Soc [MCSS] was seen as the ministry most capable of working effectively with the hodgepodge of citizens' organizations and voluntary agencies that were out there doing these services. Whereas Health has no experience, the culture is totally different, and Health is very much a professional and an institution ministry.

P: Com Soc [MCSS] staff brought a lot of influence in terms of dignity of the individual, the idea of consumer choice. Because in Health patients don't have a choice. They're sick people. You have these highly paid well-educated professionals making life and death decisions. Right? That's the head set. Coming from Com Soc [MCSS], you think, 'Well, I wonder what the person will want to do about this' ... The Health culture tends to be, pardon the pun, a bit more prescriptive. The culture comes from wanting to heal, assuming disease in the first place ... Community and Social Services, I think, the culture tends to be more 'What are the consumers saying they need?' ... More of a preventative kind of emphasis, not the same emphasis on expertise, but it's more client centred. So the client is the focus and is very much involved in the planning. So there's certain things we've introduced into the reform that I think reflect that. For example, that the plan of care be done with the client or the client's family; allowing for independent attendant services where people don't have to go through the system and get reassessed.

Another reason offered by interviewees for the shift to MCSS from OSCA was more practical: that it was important at this point to move it to a ministry that administered the programs in order to be able to implement reform, rather than merely listen to concerns and articulate principles.

G: There's no question that the process had become very cumbersome internally, and it was felt that it was appropriate for the lead ministry to be not only a policy maker but an implementer as well.

O: If what they were going to do was implement real changes to the way service was delivered, it made sense to place leadership for those changes with the ministry that was responsible for allocating the dollars for the delivery of those services.

More cynically, the move to MCSS and the emphasis on prevention could be seen as a cost containment strategy. Given the projected demographics, a medical approach to care for the elderly was going to be expensive. Under the existing arrangements, the Home Care Program being run by the Ministry of Health had been set up as a universal 'entitlement' program, which was run by the same program (Ontario Health Insurance Plan (OHIP)) that paid for physician services. This approach was generous of the province: nothing in the federal rules governing transfer payments required comprehensive universal coverage for non-physician services provided outside hospitals. As previously noted, before 1977 provinces seeking to maximize federal funding had had the incentive to move as many services as possible under the rubric of federal cost sharing for hospital and medical insurance programs. However, once cost sharing had been replaced by Established Programs Financing (EPF), with its mixture of tax points and relatively untied cash payments, provincial governments had the reverse incentive to move such programs back to the remaining cost-sharing program, the Canada Assistance Plan. Adding fuel to that fire was the unilateral decision in 1986 by the federal PC government of Brian Mulroney to change the formula: the per capita entitlements were supposed to be indexed to inflation (growing with Gross Domestic Product (GDP)), but Mulroney reduced the escalator to growth in the Gross National Product (GNP) minus 2 per cent (Rachlis and Kushner, 1994); in subsequent years, he removed all inflation protection. Because the federal funding flowed into the province's general revenues, there was no direct link between this reduction in anticipated transfers and spending on health and post-secondary education. Nevertheless, the cuts meant less provincial flexibility overall and affected the province's ability to expand programs. In their second mandate, the Liberals were also becoming aware of the imminence of another recession. In hindsight, it is clear that funding for health care, which had been expanding, would need to be scaled back. Disease prevention and health promotion would be justifications for the shift in the role of the state from fully funded health care towards the more privately funded social model, with its emphasis on the broader determinants of health.

P: There was a significant group of people who felt that the more socially oriented preventative services would be essential to strengthening the system and to find a way to get the system working together. And to prevent just enormous accumulations of need for funding later on. In other words, to control the people getting sicker quicker, you need to find some way to strengthen the more social side of it. It was a way to control the costs, because the health-oriented costs are so much more expensive, the medically funded programs are significantly more expensive than the costs of the home support social service side. There were some folks who thought that if the lead was given to Health, costs would skyrocket. In my heart of hearts I was hoping that the reason was more towards somebody thinking prevention was a good idea, but more realistically, I think there was probably also some significant thought put into the fact that if it was moved to Health, it would become very expensive.

Nonetheless, achieving a better coordinated and integrated system would require the participation of other ministerial players. In June of that year Sweeney made an announcement in the legislature about the formation of an interministerial task force led by his ministry to develop a comprehensive approach to long-term care services. The task force included four ministers – Sweeney (MCSS), Caplan (MOH), Mavis Wilson (minister responsible for senior citizens' affairs), and Remo Mancini (minister responsible for disabled persons). Their mandate was to develop a plan to streamline services by early 1990, with change beginning in the 1990–1 fiscal year. The task force would report to a steering committee of assistant deputy ministers and directors from the four ministries as well as from the Cabinet Office and Management Board of Cabinet. Most interviewees believed that during the Liberal tenure, the bureaucracy was very involved in the reform process and was trusted to lead its development; this bureaucrat-led process was in marked contrast to the process followed by the later two governments, in which policy was much more politically controlled.

4.4 Rationale for and Scope of the Reform

One reason the government remained interested in reform was the burgeoning of the elderly population; in just the previous decade, life expectancy for both sexes in Ontario had increased by three years, to 80.5 years for women and 73.7 years for men. However, the rationale for distinguishing between services to the elderly and services to persons with disabilities was less and less compelling. Based on prevalence rates generated from Statistics Canada's *Canadian Health and Disability Survey* in 1983–4, it was estimated that more than 983,000 adults in Ontario had physical disabilities that resulted in some degree of function loss limiting their ability to carry out routine activities. The likelihood of disability was known to increase dramatically with age. It was estimated that by 2006 the number of disabled persons in Ontario would have increased by about 36 per cent, to 1.5 million (MCSS, 1989).

For these reasons, the planning for LTC reform now included all personal health and social service programs for the elderly *and* for all adult persons with physical disabilities. A senior government interviewee also indicated that the disability community had started to advocate for their inclusion in the reform because they saw that the government was moving more towards population health strategies. They began to recognize that reform 'was going to focus on individual need and was flexible enough to include their preferences with respect to attendant care' (G). Those interviewed from the disability community concurred with this assessment.

As in the One-Stop Access initiative, planning was concentrated upon those who would require chronic services. Although home care would still serve those requiring acute home care to recover from illness, injury, or hospitalization, the emphasis of the planners was on chronic-care services for the elderly and the disabled. Rhetoric focused on prevention, health promotion, and delayed institutionalization of seniors and people with disabilities. (As will be documented in subsequent chapters, this failure to recognize the implications of developments in the acute-care hospital sector led to the 'swamping' of these clients by the late 1990s by those with acute-care needs.)

To bring about integration, the Liberal government undertook yet another institutional change in ministerial structure and set up an unusual dual-reporting relationship. Both the acting assistant deputy minister (ADM), Community Health (MOH), and the ADM, Community Services (MCSS) were ordered to report not only to their own deputy minister, but also to the Deputy of the sister department. It was hoped that this arrangement would encourage better coordination. Indeed, the government was considering eventually placing management responsibility for the new LTC system into a single ministry (without clarifying whether this new home would be the MOH or the MCSS).

Perhaps to avoid an inter-ministry conflict, it stated that this might not necessarily be accompanied by the consolidation of the funding of all LTC services in one ministry. Reform of Ontario's LTC system was now to be guided by seven principles that emphasized efficiency and cost control through cost containment, integration and coordination, emphasis on the least costly service, cost sharing, and strengthening the role of the informal caregiver. The principles were designed to

1. reform the funding system to emphasize individual needs;
2. support caregivers;
3. encourage use of the most appropriate, cost-effective service;
4. emphasize services in people's own homes;
5. establish a single, integrated admissions process for both long-term care beds and formal community services such as Home Care Programs;
6. strengthen the role of the local community; and
7. ensure affordability and appropriate sharing of costs. (See Sweeney, 1989.)

The earlier One-Stop Access approach had centred on a rationalized system for community-based health and social services only, which would eventually move progressively towards the inclusion of other services (e.g., institutional) and other target groups. Now, however, the government felt that a broader approach was necessary, one that would offer a single entry system for health and social services in both the community and the institutional sectors.

The task force reviewed LTC health and support programs as well as the experience in other jurisdictions. Once again, discussions had been held with provincial organizations, consumers, advocacy groups, service providers, and volunteers. Requests by these groups at the time called for communication of more reform details and wider community discussions.

The government had used structural changes to bring about a paradigm shift in the values underlying LTC services at the time. Once a different mindset was established, it would allow for the eventual integration of responsibilities at the provincial level. The shift in thinking also allayed the fears of the disability community, which was now more willing to consider being included in the reform. Ultimately, government hoped that moving from a medical to a health model would also permit greater cost control (and cost shifting away from government).

4.4.1 Strategies for Change *and the Service Access Organizations*

On 30 May 1990 the new minister of community and social services, Charles Beer, announced the release of the next discussion paper about reforming LTC. *Strategies for Change* (MCSS et al., 1990) was intended to outline the strategic directions for reform and to provide a framework for continued community discussions. The announcement was made on behalf of the ministers of health (Caplan), senior citizens' affairs (Morin), and disabled persons (Collins). Beer indicated that over $52 million would be dedicated to the reform initiative in that fiscal year, and by 1996–7 new funding to improve services would increase to $640 million annually.

Strategies was explicitly incremental, in that it was intended to work within the framework of the existing delivery network. The main purpose of the reform as outlined in *Strategies* was 'to build a coherent, integrated service system on the foundation of existing in-home, community support and long-term care facility services ... Fundamental to the reform is the fact that Ontario already has many of the components of an effective long-term care and support system. The reform builds on the current strengths and skills of successful health and social services. The strategies for developing a more coherent system, based on the existing services, are described in this paper' (MCSS et al., 1990, 3).

The document repeated a list of similar reasons for reforming LTC, including the pressures from changing demographics; the lack of integration of planning and service delivery; the growing costs; the variety of policies, funding arrangements, eligibility criteria, and legislation that pertained to the different formal services; inadequate access to services for consumers; changing expectations of consumers to live as independently for as long as possible; the burden on informal caregivers; variable availability of services over the day and across the province; and the changing cultural/ethnic mix of Ontario's population.

Similarly, the principles listed as guiding this new reform effort continued to reflect the thinking of the Premier's Council and the earlier announced principles, with some notable additions:

- individualization (services responsive to individual needs; recognition of the dignity and uniqueness of individuals);
- independence and choice for consumers;
- community living;
- service accessibility;

- support for informal caregivers;
- local planning and management within provincial standards and directions;
- affordability, and sharing the cost of services fairly among levels of government and consumers.

The addition of the reference to individualization, independence, and choice for consumers and to community living reflected the broadening of the scope of reform to encompass the disability community; this community placed a high value on what Stone (1997) termed 'liberty' values. Advocates in the disability community believed that, since the publication of A New Agenda, seniors had shifted towards a similar viewpoint. 'There's a change in the philosophy in the seniors, who are also saying, "We want autonomy." There's actually now more of a convergence again (in the interests of seniors and people with disabilities)' (C).

4.4.2 Service Access Organizations

The new model called for setting up a series of Service Access Organizations (SAOs), one in each of thirty-eight or more areas of the province; they would be built upon the current Home Care Program and Placement Coordination Services. The SAOs were to have the same functions as One-Stop Access.

Existing organizations could become SAOs as long as they were not current direct providers of service. This policy was designed to eliminate the apparent or perceived inherent conflict of interests, which some interests had objected to when direct providers, such as the VON, also managed home care programs. 'I think they wanted a more open process for service delivery. Service providers were lobbying to open up that process. It was seen as sort of a closed shop you know. Home Care had its preferred providers, and there wasn't an opportunity for other groups to get involved' (P). Criteria for the selection of SAOs were yet to be developed and were to be a subject of further consultation (MCSS et al., 1990).

The report also recognized, as one of the essential components of the reformed system, the need to plan and develop community support services more comprehensively. Up to that point, these services had been developed without overall provincial guidance (and often, without much provincial funding). In turn, this had led to a proliferation of single-service agencies, regional variation in service availability, lack of coordination across services, confusing access for consumers, and a multiplicity of funding arrangements, charging policies, and eligibility criteria. Under the new model, resources were to be enhanced to address service gaps and targeted to multi-service sponsors that addressed the needs of both the elderly and the disabled and to underserviced areas of the province. Consumers could continue to directly access those services that complemented both the formal in-home services and the informal services provided by family and friends. However, the SAO would provide information and referral for consumers to these services and could purchase these services on behalf of some consumers. In effect, government agreed to take the slower but less contentious path towards change, seeking to use carrots rather than sticks.

Recognizing that informal caregivers provide up to 80–90 per cent of assistance to people who need personal support or assistance with daily living, the government outlined a number of support services for caregivers. These included respite services, such as adult day programs or the use of LTC facilities for emergency or pre-planned respite care, and information services and support groups.

In terms of costs to the consumer, the government intended to develop a uniform consumer-charging policy for community-based services. The policy would strongly resemble the approach that had governed programs under MCSS, and it exemplified the Liberal view of the appropriate role of government versus the individual in LTC and the related redistribution of costs and benefits to achieve it. The new charging policy was to be guided by beliefs that people are traditionally responsible for paying their own basic living and household maintenance costs, and therefore these costs should not be within the scope of state responsibilities; that people should receive services regardless of their ability to pay for them; and that those who can afford to pay for services should subsidize services for those who need them but cannot afford to pay for them.

4.4.3 Integration of Services through Institutional Change

The desire to integrate and coordinate services, however, had implications for the organization of government, both within the provincial government and at the local community level. The Premier's Council had suggested starting with the province – it recommended that the transfer of authority to local communities should be phased in after corporate restructuring within government, which would integrate the

Ministry of Health with the Ministry of Community and Social Services, and organize the new entity along regional rather than functional lines. The task would be a daunting one. For LTC services, it would be necessary somehow to bring together health and social services that were under the auspices of two ministries with different cultures, legislation, and regulations and different funding, eligibility, and monitoring criteria. Nonetheless, government had already moved part of the way along this path. The acting ADM, Community Health (MOH) and the ADM, Community Services (MCSS) were already in a dual-reporting relationship. Now, government merged the long-term care and support services (MCSS) with the community health services (MOH) into a joint division for LTC, to be made up of staff from both ministries, with a single ADM reporting to both deputy ministers. It was hoped that this new hybrid division could lead to a program that not only reflected the values of both ministries but also created a new amalgamated mindset. Programs from both ministries would be structurally pulled together and would report up through the new ADM.

P: The reality of the day, there was legislation ... under the purview of the Ministry of Health, and legislation under the purview of the Ministry of Community and Social Services. And often, the legislation was contradictory ... or totally unrelated to each other. So there was a decision: 'We've got to sort all this out. We've got to find a way to rationalize how money is distributed, how access is provided, criteria for eligibility or admission.' All of that had to be looked through. So the vehicle that it was seen as, ... to begin to sort all this out was to create this sort of across two-ministry structure.

Government respondents saw the move as a way to get the two ministries to overcome their rivalry and work together. The success of the reform was not possible without it.

G: Health doesn't give much up. And nor does Com Soc [MCSS]. They're both very large ministries that had very distinctive cultures, very large, very competitive with each other. Health ... just didn't give up its budget, because one doesn't give up to another ministry because you never get it back. And I think the same applies to the Ministry of Community and Social Services ... The move to a joint division came from the recognition that they couldn't move forward unless the two ministries worked together. There were bureaucratic barriers. People worried about losing their jobs. This was a signal. The merger was also necessary if you were going to bring the services together in the community. The merged division was to be the bureaucratic structure. It wasn't just an interim step. If we were moving to integrated models such as the CHOs [community health organizations], LTC had to be part of it. And this was going to be easier if the health and social services were together.

G: It was a big move because until then the departments had really been allowed to – you know, at the director level – they were allowed to just fight with each other all the time and erect barriers.

G: The purpose of the joint division was trying to balance off the tradition that had grown up in the Ministry of Community and Social Services and the tradition that had grown up in the Ministry of Health. And at that point, because they had developed, if you wish, on separate tracks, they were distinct.

G: They were recognizing that two ministries were not able to work effectively together, particularly when they were as different as Com Soc and Health. And they needed to pull something out and create at the bureaucratic level what they had earlier created at the ministerial level with Ron Van Horne.

G: It would have been very hard to have made the changes from outside ... It wouldn't have been do-able otherwise. There were so many things that we needed to do that affected both ministries. Our information systems were a mess. And we were dealing with two different sets of legal services, and two different communication branches ... There had to be some way of combining the program areas.

While not contradicting the above stated reasons, others saw the integrated division as a way of allaying the fears of societal interests. Since it had broadened the scope of the reform to include the disability community, one interviewee stated that the government needed to address their concerns regarding the medicalization of their services. Similarly, the government was cognizant of the different cultures within the provider groups that reflected the cultures of their sponsoring ministries. An integrated division was an institutional instrument to manage potential conflict that could derail reform.

G: Among consumer groups you have persons with disabilities. We definitely didn't think that they were to be lumped in with senior citizens.

So when the paper came out, I would imagine that all the Health people thought it was a Com Soc [MCSS] document. And all the Com Soc people thought it was a Health document. And all the Disabilities people thought it was a Seniors' document. And all the Seniors thought that they were importing all kinds of concepts from the disability sector ... And it was decided that it would have been, in order to ease people into the notion of a single division that you weren't going to take it out of one ministry and plunk it down in the other. Simply because, not only inside the ministry, but also in terms of the groups they were dealing with, there might well have been some sensitivity to, for example, if they put everything in the Ministry of Health, immediately the people in the Community and Social Services side would have regarded it as a Health take-over of a part of the social service system .... It was the idea of putting together the two sides in a division that was ... to try and retain the best of both traditions ... and to make everyone comfortable with the fact that, if you're dealing with LTC services, you're dealing with something, which ... has both a health aspect and a social service aspect.

The new division then sought to integrate formerly disparate programs at the local level. In a mixture between the programmatic approach to organization within the MOH and the regionally based approach of MCSS, it established fourteen local Area Offices, where staff would work with local organizations and District Health Councils (DHCs) to plan the implementation of LTC reform in that geographic area. While policy function and program management remained in the division, it was intended that over time even these centralized functions would also be transferred to the local offices. As a senior bureaucrat in that period indicated, this step was essential to the later step of reallocating funds from institutions to the community.

G: One of the basic concepts ... and that I very much feel is the correct concept, is that you need to regionalize your administration, your provincial administration instead of having people in each region responsible for a program reporting to program heads in Toronto in the Hepburn Building [at Queen's Park] ... and their only integration being at the level of the ADM ... So there'd be a long-term coordinator in each region that would be responsible for everything, not just for homemakers, and not just for ... home care, and not just for homes for the aged, and not just for whatever, but the whole gamut. I mean that's the first step. You have to consolidate your budgets as well. That's what it means to do a reform where you're integrating, and where you have the capacity, for example, meaningfully to reduce your budgetary commitment to institutions, and instead bring some of that funding into community. You can't do it, unless those budgets are integrated ... You can't transfer from one to another. It's better to do it at a regional level where it's more local.

The reallocation of funding from institutions to the community was seen as essential to the overall goal of cost control and containment. Operationally, however, without an integration of the two divisions at the provincial level, the creation of a single-budget envelope for LTC community and facility services would not be possible. One key objective was somehow to avoid the enormous capital and operating costs that would be required if those requiring LTC were to be cared for within institutions. 'Anybody that was doing their homework, would do some mathematics, to see how much it cost to build nursing homes. And they'd multiply that by the eighty-five-plus population, and from that, "We've got to find another way to deal with this"' (P).

The integration of budgets thus would serve two purposes: it could facilitate the reallocation of funds from institutions to the (presumably cheaper) community, but it would also allow the LTC budget to be capped. Home Care services would then be reclassified from their current status (as a fully funded entitlement under OHIP) into a new (and capped) budget line from which all LTC community-based services would be funded (G). (This step was eventually taken by the NDP government.) This decision would leave open the possibility that care in excess of what the global budget could fund accordingly would move out of the public realm into the private one of user fees and co-payments. As one interviewee explained:

G: Home Care, which was in the hands of Health, was a universally accessible service. If you established eligibility, the service was yours and it was yours as a right, and there was no cost or cost sharing with respect to that. Com Soc, [MCSS] which funded the home support side, the non-medical side, was a Com Soc'-ish kind of a model where there were user fees, where there was a lot of volunteer participation augmenting their services ... Because behind all of this there was a need to cap the cost, all along people realized that the costs of home care, which was the expensive piece of the formula, were escalating all of the time. In order to cap that, there was a plan, and I don't know when it surfaced in terms of ... being a conscious thing, but there was a need to cap the envelope for Home Care services by moving it into the Com Soc arena. As the lead, they could start to look at that user-fee, shared-cost, more-use-of-volunteers model as opposed to the universal right, like OHIP. And that's basically what our Home Care was. If eligibility was established they had to provide service ... So this was an attempt to shift it from that 'universally paid for, absolutely your right' to a shared responsibility, which was the model that Com Soc tends to espouse, with, you know, a lot of different funders and user fee potentials.

Strategies also dealt with issues regarding workers. There was an ongoing tension between the desire to control costs by paying less for labour (both in terms of using a less professionalized workforce, and in paying less than hospital rates), and the recognition that high-quality staff might be difficult to obtain and retain if wages and working conditions were not competitive. In terms of steering care towards the community, the difficulty in recruiting and retaining community-based professionals to provide in-home services was outlined in the report. The government then tried to have it both ways by suggesting: an evaluation of both the work currently provided by nurses and the ability of other professionals, such as therapists or social workers, RNAs or trained attendants, to perform some of their functions; ways to increase the number of rehabilitation therapists; and improvement of the wages, working conditions, and training of homemakers. Some people with physical disabilities cautioned the government against over-professionalizing homemakers. The anticipated Health Professions Regulation Act would eventually allow greater flexibility in service provision by different types of providers, a way to further reduce costs through the use of lower-skilled professionals. The government also indicated the need to train professionals in community settings, presumably in the hope that they would then be more willing to remain in the community sector.

The government declared its intention to introduce time-limited legislation in the spring of 1991 to implement a number of critical elements of this reform model; it would then introduce subsequent legislation to create a single, comprehensive statute governing the whole LTC system. However, the initial legislation would provide the mandate, funding, and governance for SAOs and their facility placement committees, as well as for the new, consolidated in-home services programs. The legislation was also to include provisions protecting the rights of consumers.

4.4.4 Influence of Societal Interests on the Development of the SAO Model

4.4.4.1 Providers

The feeling among societal interests was that the ear of the Liberal government continued to be attuned more to providers, both for-profit and not-for-profit groups, than to any other societal interests. In particular, the government was said to have listened to those involved in the Home Care Programs and agencies like the VON that administered them. These were the agencies that were credited with developing the idea of the SAOs (5P, G, O).

Although there was an easy relationship between the Liberal government and provider agencies, one interviewee felt that by the end of the 1980s the relationship between the government and providers had begun to change. Towards the close of the decade, the government was beginning to worry about its ability to continue its past spending trend on programs. In hindsight, it would become clear that the Liberals were very aware of the coming recession. Fiscal control would put greater strain upon the cozy relationship between the government and providers.

P: Our relationship with the government until 1989 was quite good. It was so good that we never even thought we'd have to get into government relations and lobbying activities at all. The funding for us was open ended. Members were able to secure anywhere from 70 to 90 cents on the dollar from the province if they felt the need was there ... The province began to change the funding mechanism ... began to introduce 70 per cent funding, and the cap was introduced in 1989. Up until '89 it was almost a partnership relationship. It was only with the sort of move towards fiscal control in '89 and '90, and that whole era in our relationship changed.

4.4.4.2 Labour

There continued to be no coordinated effort by unions to influence reform. The community, unlike the institutions sector, was not a heavily unionized sector. The SAO model was introduced before massive restructuring of the hospital sector and before the recession hit the province in the early 1990s. In addition, because of the incremental nature of this particular set of reforms, there was no imminent dislocation for community workers. One union spokesperson also argued that the silence of organized labour was due more to the lack of recognition afforded them by the Liberals.

P: I don't think the Liberals thought of the union movement as a group you would consult. They were just the workers. They are irrelevant. [They would say], 'Oh, we're talking to the people because we're talking to the user, the community people, and we're talking to the employers. So we're covered.' So it was only under the NDP that we finally broke through in terms of being taken seriously as a group that had to be consulted.

4.4.4.3 Consumers

Many felt that the Liberals, as one interviewee put it, were not as 'wired to the consumer' (P). One reason was that seniors were also not as yet a well-formed lobby group. The disability community was beginning to play an important role, however, particularly as they recognized that the government's intention to reform LTC services for seniors also affected the services they used. Accordingly, there was an effort by the two groups to meet together to discuss common principles for reform and to see if they could form a lobbying coalition.

C: What we tried to do with that was to come up with a set of common principles and say, 'Look, you can recognize that there are going to be differences. You can respect the differences, but is it possible to come up with a common set of goals and principles that we can agree on to get over the hurdle and to really get the government moving on something, and then deal with our differences [when] you have to deal with them?'

However, this was a short-term coalition. As the second Liberal model developed, the disability community did not want to talk about the issues that were of concern more to seniors, namely, institutions, professional assessments and referrals. After the publication of *Strategies*, the disability community accordingly began to lobby government to be removed from the SAO reform.

C: Again, it was pretty much saying to government, 'You've got to take us out.' Even the service providers were on side. So you had the March of Dimes and Easter Seals and the MS Society, Cheshire Foundation, saying, 'We're different.' In a sense, the Liberals never really took them out. But that was the battle, and they did get agreement in principle to get direct funding. So it was sort of an alternative plan proposed. Now, the Liberals never really followed through with it. They [disability groups] did a huge lobby campaign essentially. It was at that point in

1990 that a group which came out of the Attendant Care Action Coalition, and the Centre for Independent Living, and others were meeting on a regular basis and really lobbying hard. So all of the energy from the disability side went into direct funding. That was really what they wanted to talk about ... Once the government sort of agreed that they didn't have to be part of it, they dropped out of the rest of the discussion. There really isn't any active discussion with the government on the other kinds of issues in the SAOs.

Although the disability community got only agreement in principle for direct funding, they felt they did influence government in other ways.

C: I think in part that's the reason that under the Liberals, you never saw the full move of long-term care into Health formally ... I think part of that was the disability [groups], both within the government and outside said, 'We don't want to be part of the Ministry of Health. We're not sick' ... There was a real fear of going into the Ministry of Health, because they'd been in the Ministry of Health and fought to get out, you know, during the Davis years, and didn't want to go back in. And they had their own office at that time, the Office for Disability Issues ... and a minister for disability was around, and I think that also played some part.

The multicultural community remained interested in retaining their own ethno-specific programs. Based on the argument that the population of Ontario, particularly Toronto, was notably multicultural, they lobbied to have diversity of services for different ethnic groups be considered the norm for the sector rather than the exception. They felt that they had more influence with this government, because 'the Liberal governments traditionally, at least for the last several decades in Canada, have been much more attuned to the interests of ethnic communities than the other two parties. This Conservative government [Harris] – not so much the tradition of Conservative governments pre-1985 – but this Conservative government and the NDP are much less attuned to and sympathetic to the issues and concerns of ethnic communities. Frankly, they owe much less to them in terms of their electoral success' (C).

Overall, however, during the Liberal period societal interests were neither very vocal nor very active in trying to influence government. 'My understanding of that era was not much of that [interest-group lobbying] was going on. They weren't organized in a way that would allow for that' (G). Many organizations did not have the necessary resources to lobby – either an executive director (ED) to speak on their behalf or someone within their organization who had the time to review government proposals. However, one government official indicated that, had the groups lobbied, government may not have listened. From this person's perspective, none of the groups truly influenced government, because none was able to rise above its own interests to put together a model that encompassed the whole system. In answer to the question of which groups were influential, the official answered as follows.

G: Well frankly, the answer's, not many, or any that I could think of. Because who sees the whole system? And who conceptualizes it? And how many of them know about what it is to come in and run a huge apparatus encompassing several thousand people and have an idea of what it means to reorganize in a comprehensive way. And the answer is, most of them don't. They're looking at the elephant, and they see a leg, or they see a tail, or they see a trunk, because that's what they deal with. So you ask them what to do. They say, 'Well we need a bigger trunk' – or whatever they happen to be looking at. They don't see the whole animal.

4.4.5 The Mobilization of Interests

Although the SAO proposal began the process of mobilizing groups such as seniors, the disability community, and the support service groups in order to strengthen their positions by joining resources and forming alliances, this process would not gather steam until the NDP mandate. The germs of alliances such as the Senior Citizens' Consumer Alliance (SCCA) can be seen at the end of the Liberal period, however, sparked by concerns that these groups were not having much effect in moving the government forward in their preferred policy directions. Consolidation among the policy community was also enhanced by the recognition of government that it was far easier to deal with coalitions than with a plethora of unorganized groups. The need for alliances was especially pressing among those agencies providing community support services. In contrast to agencies providing professional health services, which had large paid staffs and were better able to lobby government, the support services tended to be small, not for profit, and heavily reliant on volunteers. The organizations providing support services felt undervalued and underpaid. They also were beginning to feel increasing competitive pressure from FP agencies who were being attracted to the sector by the increased demand for services. The volunteer-based groups felt that they were likely to become victims of 'cream skimming,' since the FPs provided the potentially lucrative services, leaving those groups most challenging to serve for the NFP sector. At the end of the Liberal period, the various NFP support services accordingly came together to form the Ontario Community Support Association (OCSA). As respondents noted:

C: And the seniors got together because we were very unhappy. We had responded in writing, attended all of the meeting for *A New Agenda* and for *Strategies for Change*, and we had responded in brief form, and we had meetings with the minister of health and people ... but we were getting nowhere. We were hoping they would implement it, that they would do something. We've been talking to ministries, we've been talking to people, service providers, and we're getting nowhere. So, we decided that the time had come when we were getting nowhere doing it this way. So we had to do something else. And we decided to talk to a consultant and see if they would help us either write a better brief than we were doing, or something. And this is where the idea came in that we would work with other organizations and we would form an alliance.

P: Well, I think we felt that we actually hadn't had a voice at the province. You know, hospitals had a strong voice, physicians had a strong voice, but the community-based services didn't. We were also feeling very threatened by ... a growing threat of the for-profit homemaking sector taking over what traditionally had been a not-for-profit sector. So it was kind of a wake-up call. [While demand was growing and the agencies were not able to keep up with the demand], we were looking at increased competition from the private sector ... And basically, most of us had always thought that because we'd done nice things and had God on our side, that it was fine ... Homemaking and home support and meals on wheels, we saw ourselves as the poor cousins, and we thought, 'This is silly, you know. We do hundreds and hundreds of hours. We're sort of the meat and potatoes, you know, so that everybody can whip in and do fancy stuff. And if patients don't get fed, don't get bathed, don't get their houses cleaned, and so on, you know, it's impossible for a nurse to float in for fifteen minutes and poke somebody in the arm. So why don't we actually do something about it?' It took three years to get those organizations together.

P: There was a time, as there is in a lot of things that happen in life, that you come to a crossroads and it's a good thing to do. But then there's an outside force such as the government, who are about to bring changes, and you realize that you better get together and start to work together and start to really make sure that your voices are in unison first of all.

The group of support service agencies had hired a consultant to help them to write a position paper and to lobby government. The seniors' groups would later hire the same consultant to help them form an alliance and to lobby the next government. As will be discussed in greater detail in chapter 5, the consultant proved highly influential; the two alliances (SCCA and OCSA) would put forward models similar to those of the NDP government.

4.4.6 Assessment of SAO by the LTC Policy Community

The Liberal period was viewed as the period of balanced reform by providers, consumers, and government officials, where balance is defined as meaning that the new model would not greatly disadvantage any societal interest.

P: My sense is that it was a balanced viewpoint. It was just a balanced position of all the stakeholders to come up with something sort of mutually agreeable and seemed to balance out all of the perspectives.

A government official involved in this reform indicated that the reason that there was general support for reform was that it was principle driven and flexible and did not represent a drastic change from the status quo.

G: The important feature of *Strategies for Change* and the SAO model was that the principles were accepted; that is, it was a principle-based reform and there was wide acceptance of the model. The model was flexible. An essential feature was that it was a partnership model without being overly prescriptive. Built into it was a strategy for dealing with conflict of interests between the manager and deliverer of services; that was the idea of community management to monitor conflict of interests ... The government didn't believe that a large monolithic model like the NDP model proposed later would lead to innovation. It was envisaged that the model [SAO] would vary across communities. We decided on the continuation of profit and non-profit agencies in roughly the same balance as existed, because we thought it would be less threatening. We recognized the difference between the two sectors and that there was value in having a balance. In many cases non-profit is more expensive, and for-profit could be more innovative. Therefore, we wanted the best of both worlds.

Service providers on the whole supported the brokerage model, which was seen as non-threatening to their organizations. They also endorsed the concept of independently governed SAOs that were not run by direct service providers. At the time, the policy community tended to be cooperative rather than competitive. Indeed, the elites in this policy community often served on the boards of a number of different agencies. This cross-pollination of boards ensured that board members would not back a reform that threatened another member's agency.

P: It didn't feel like a hell of a lot. It wasn't anything that you couldn't support, because what they were really talking about is creating better access, ... not developing mechanisms to have more services available in the community to support people ... We were feeling frustrated just because there were lots of planning and not a lot happening, but there was no negative sense of what was trying to be accomplished or any major worry about it ... [For-profit agencies] just saw it as opportunity. They felt the demographics, you know, the ageing population, they saw an opportunity to grow their business. And there was nothing that we know that was going to be created in Service Access Organizations or anywhere else that threatened that growth. We didn't feel any threat being an issue.

G: I think a number of [our members] liked the brokerage model because it didn't blow up all of the individual local agencies ... You know Betty doesn't want to be blown up. Charlie on the [Board] won't support blowing her up. So there was a certain amount of support for the brokerage model.

Although the Liberal government's intention in incremental reform was to have a balanced approach, which would keep all happy, there were some criticisms. Senior consumers felt that *Strategies* was not a big enough step forward from *A New Agenda*. The proposal also met the customary resistance to organizationally based changes: money was being spent on restructuring government rather than on direct care where it was needed.

C: We were repeating what we'd done before in the *New Agenda*. Now we're spending hundreds of dollars that could be spent on services. And by now they're turning people out of hospitals early; they're sending them home, to the community; and they're not improving the community care ... All this money being spent setting up another new office [fourteen area offices] to do what? And we had the sense that nothing was going to happen. And you realize how right we were. 'Cause I'm talking about 1985, and now we're into 1990, and we're still talking about one-stop shopping. It's still a good point. It's one we want. But let's get on with it!

P: Because it was still separating health and social services. It was still fragmenting. It was not dealing with the fundamental issue, which was the difficulty of access, that's resulting from the enormous fragmentation. One-Stop Shopping was moving in that direction. The Service Access Organizations moved a little bit further along in the direction. I don't think that many people had at that point in time really believed that it was possible to really integrate the system.

Similarly, the focus on greater coordination and accountability could be seen as a reduction in patient choice and autonomy. The disability community objected.

C: It's still the problem of: it's great if you fit in the mould; if you know what you need, it's a waste of time ... If you have one provider, whether it's the one-stop shopping that actually provides services or they broker for services, you're actually giving people much less choice and much less flexibility in what can be delivered.

Another contentious provision of the SAO model was whether the SAOs should act as case managers. Not surprisingly, views on this issue depended upon existing interests. Thus, Home Care Programs (many of which would become SAOs) agreed that this function should rest with the new organizations, while the direct service providers resisted the potential loss of professional autonomy and control, often arguing that they would still have to perform their own assessments. Hence, moving case management would lead only to waste and duplication. Nonetheless, once reform had gone beyond the narrow informational model in One-Stop Shopping, all models included some form of case manager. How it was defined was critical to its acceptance.

G: The role of the case manager was being defined year by year. And the importance of the success of that role was significant in the eyes of, I think, those who worked in the system. There had been quite a struggle to define what case management's function would be without having to compete with the service providers on occasion ... In the very early days of Home Care Programs ... there was a resistance from the service providers to have this new type of worker, called a case manager, parachuted in on them; where the case manager was viewed as having the authority to decide who, first of all, was eligible for Home Care programs at all. And then the case manager would essentially decide who of the service providers – the nurses, or therapists, or homemakers – which service would be appropriate for this client's needs ... So there was a fair amount of power resting in that position. And it created tension in the relationships among the other professional or paraprofessional team members.

P: The professional social work approach is to have the same individual assessing needs and delivering the services, or the same organization assessing and delivering. Rather than an organization that does the assessment and then tells agency A or service B that is what their decision is and this what they [should] do. The problem with the latter is that then agency A does their own assessment, agency B also does an assessment. And you end up with a minimum of three assessments.

P: The problem with brokerage is the fragmentation of the care delivery, in that the client may have the Red Cross homemaker, the VON nurse, and Paramed for the shift nursing, and someone else for something else. It mitigates to chimneys of care, as opposed to consistent, provider-driven care coordination. Now the Home Care Programs would argue, 'Well, the case manager is in effect managing all this different care.' But the reality is the caseloads with case managers may be 150–200. I mean they're not coordinating care.

Another theme that would become more pronounced in later reform models was the issue about whether competition among agencies (as was inherent in any brokerage process) would lead to the sacrifice of quality in order to obtain cheaper services. One respondent argued that the Liberals were trying in this way to introduce more for-profit agencies, especially into homemaking services. This sentiment would be raised more broadly from a majority in the policy community during the later Harris Conservative period.

P: We had great concerns with the brokerage portion of it. It's the same as the brokerage concerns now, where, although the request for proposals is supposed to be based on quality and on cost, our fear is the drive will be the cost only. There'll be movement to agencies that provide a cheaper service ... It will be of lesser quality.

Yet some FPs felt that the SAO model did not level the playing field for them, and that the SAO would continue to issue contracts more or less in the same informal fashion that the Home Care Programs had been doing (P).

4.4.7 Beginning the Implementation Process for Strategies for Change

Strategies for Change was intended to provide a focus for the next phase of the reform, a move to the local level, where the new regional offices would review directions, resolve concerns and begin the local implementation planning process. A series of consultations was planned, to be coordinated by the local managers of the new division, working with local DHCs, municipalities, and MCSS area offices. A series of information meetings as well as issue-oriented local meetings would take place; in a bottom-up planning process, they were to culminate in a provincial conference. Interested parties were invited to send in written comments on the report. Although the full process was expected to take several years, the first forty or so community meetings were scheduled for September 1990 (Beer, 1990).

Before these plans could be implemented, the Liberals pre-empted any formal response to their model. In the fall of 1990 they called another election, only three years into their second mandate.

Among the items in the Liberal platform was the expansion of community-based care and home care, with a $2 billion, six-year plan to develop these services for seniors and persons with disabilities (Liberal Party of Ontario, 1990). However, the people of Ontario were cynical about why the government had called this election, since there was no obvious rationale. The call was seen as an opportunistic move on the part of the Liberals (and it was rightly suspected that economic forecasts were less optimistic than announced), and the result of the election was unexpected. With a minority of the popular vote, the NDP led by Bob Rae had won a majority government. The SAO plan was in limbo, pending review by the new government.

4.5 Conclusions

Reform during the Liberal period was very much incremental in nature. The LTC system as designed by the Liberal government remained more or less the same as the status quo, adding only a mechanism for introducing coordination of referral and assessment. The main policy output would have been increased public financing for the services provided by this sector, intended to improve equity of access and strengthen seemingly less expensive forms of care. The existing balance of FP and NFP organizations would continue to deliver services, with no dramatic shifts in the existing mix of public/private delivery. The coordinating agency (One Stop Access or the SAO) would be governed by a local board that would not be a provider organization, thus removing the concern of competing providers about potential conflicts of interest in those few jurisdictions where providers also ran Home Care Programs. The new agencies would issue contracts more or less in the same informal way that they had done in the past. Rather than changing the system in one sweep, the Liberals were also planning to introduce reform through pilot projects, allowing local conditions to determine the eventual shape of the model in each community. While more cautious, this approach allowed for greater flexibility.

Rather than revamping delivery, in retrospect, one can view the real agenda in LTC reform as the positioning of government to control an increasing demand for services from an ageing population. The old ways of caring for seniors were perceived to be too expensive and in need of transformation. New ideas were coming forward on the importance of focusing upon the health of populations (rather than simply individuals) and on the determinants of health, rather than on sickness care. Rhetoric emphasized the importance of prevention and the need to shift away from the medical model (Premier's Council on Health Strategy, 1989a,b, 1991c; Rachlis and Kushner, 1994).

The provincial government introduced a number of institutional changes in both the structure and the process of LTC reform development in an attempt to ensure that reform would be guided by this new set of principles. The shifts of lead for reform first to OSCA and then to MCSS (but not to MOH) allowed for the development of a model that was not dominated by medical care. The creation of capped budget envelopes for LTC services could allow both for the reallocation of funding from more costly to less costly services and for cost containment. The future transfer of the budget for the Home Care Program from OHIP to the LTC envelope would transform a universally insured service to one where eligibility criteria could limit government exposure to increased demand (and, in the process, gradually shift the public/private mix towards greater reliance upon privately financed services).

The integration of services was first brought about through the step-by-step amalgamation of the two different cultures of MOH and MCSS. This was first accomplished by having the two assistant deputy ministers responsible for community services in MOH and MCSS report to both deputy ministers. Eventually, the two divisions were joined but separate, with one ADM for the new division reporting to both deputies and both ministries.

While creating the structure that could potentially allow massive change, however, the Liberal government's reform in the SAO model remained incremental. The new system continued to provide professional home care services as a fully insured entitlement under OHIP, while it strengthened the ability of the informal private sector to continue to provide for individuals; and it retained consumer co-payments for services not classified as medically necessary, while providing a safety net for those who were unable to pay.

Although reform was incremental and did not elicit passionate responses from societal groups, it did not mean that there was full support for the Liberal models. Potential opponents of these models did not have the resources (or degree of discomfort) to raise their concerns to an audible level. Nor were there other contingencies that would bring together disparate groups and galvanize mutual interests. However, as groups started to recognize the limitations of stand-alone lobbying, they began to mobilize into coalitions. In the next five years the new NDP government's belief in consumer and worker empowerment and its fiscal strategies to restrain spending would provide the context for the merging of interests.

Without well-organized societal interests during the Liberal period, however, government ideas on reform were allowed to prevail. Institu-

tional changes within government reflected these ideas and were introduced in the service of those ideas to advance reform. Balance and
incrementalism, the hallmarks of the Liberal reforms, would soon give
way to pressures from realigned groups supported by a new government
with a new agenda.

CHAPTER FIVE

Long-Term Care Reform under the New Democratic Party, 1990–1993

5.1 The First Attempt at Long-Term Care Reform under the New Democratic Party

Election of the first New Democratic Party (NDP) government in the history of Ontario was as much a surprise to the party as it was to the rest of the province. Most observers had believed that Peterson's Liberals would easily be re-elected, but the combination of a summertime election and the popular cynicism concerning an early election call proved fatal. Many NDP candidates had run in the belief, and perhaps even the hope, that they would not be elected; other highly experienced candidates from that party had declined to seek re-election. The NDP was accustomed to playing the roles of social conscience and vocal opposition and had never had to reconcile potentially conflicting policies. Most observers agreed that, at least initially, the NDP was not well prepared to assume the role of governor of the province. To add to their difficulties, once in office, the New Democrats discovered that the finances of the province were not as healthy as the Liberals had led everyone to believe. Their first two years were marked by a deepening recession, which further eroded their freedom of action.

The Ontario NDP was a social democratic party, with strong ties to organized labour. Although many of those actively involved in supporting health reform were allied with the NDP, those individuals had not stood for elective office. Indeed, very few members of the new government were experienced with or knowledgeable about health care issues. In consequence, they brought to LTC reform a set of principles that went beyond the emerging consensus reflected in the Liberal models. The NDP favoured community participation, greater sensitivity to visible minorities, support for 'equity' and 'diversity,' a desire to have greater uniformity (often translating into more centralized control of programs), along with support of organized workers and preference for not-for-profit delivery of health and social programs. Never having formed a government, the NDP had not scrutinized whether these values might be contradictory in practice and, if so, how trade-offs might be made. Perhaps believing that they would form a one-term government, the New Democrats moved quickly to reflect their values in the organization of government institutional structures and the relative access of societal interests. Formerly marginalized interests were given voice in this period. In particular, consumers, unions, and community support services were encouraged. As meat was put on the bones of reform, however, certain interests became threatened, and formerly supportive groups joined the ranks of the dissidents. This was a period of considerable dynamism in alliance formation and breakdown, which modified the policy community. Like the Liberals, the NDP would propose two separate models, neither of which would reach the implementation stage.

The first year of the NDP mandate, 1990, marked a period of education for its members, many of whom had been elected for the first time to provincial parliament. Although the Service Access Organization (SAO) model had been placed on hold until the new government could re-examine the policy, the New Democrats quickly released yet another consultation document, *Redirection of Long-Term Care and Support Services in Ontario* (Ontario Ministry of Community and Social Services (MCSS), Ministry of Health (MOH), and Ministry of Citizenship (MC), 1991), in which it was recommended that government set up a Service Coordination Agency (SCA) model. Developed by the same bureaucracy that had produced both *Strategies for Change* and the Liberal SAO model, there was little in the values, proposed structures, and models in the two successive documents that differed. Although *Redirection* carefully did not mention any activities of the Liberal government, many in the policy community recognized the SCA as the Liberal model with a new name. The document, however, was to be the basis of a far-reaching and intensive consultation of all members of the policy community and, in particular, the voices that had not been heard in the past.

Implementation of reform was stalled when the Ontario economy entered recession. The first NDP budget had been expansionary, in hopes that increasing government spending would bring about greater prosperity and help the province to ride through the recession. When this approach failed to do much other than inflate the deficit, the government rapidly changed direction and put the brakes on spending. To the horror of its allies in organized labour, it attempted to cloak restraint within a model of sharing the pain. In particular, rather than lay off civil servants, the Rae government introduced what was called the 'Social Contract.' Under its terms, both the civil service and the broader public sector would be forced to accept restraints on their total reimbursement. Since the NDP was reluctant to reduce wage rates, in many cases this took the form of compulsory time off (which in turn had negative implications for service levels). The Social Contract pleased no one and deeply offended labour by contravening existing negotiated agreements. The Social Contract would erode labour's support for the NDP government, be only marginally effective in its efforts to control spending, and lead to the mobilization of certain interests, all of which had unintended consequences for the process of LTC reform.

5.2 The Early Days of the NDP Government, 1990–1992: Delay, Then More of the Same

Governments have to pick their priorities, and long-term care (LTC) reform initially was not high on the new government's agenda. One of their priorities was the 'diversity agenda'; it set up a new Ministry of Citizenship, which subsumed the previous offices for seniors and persons with disabilities and added to it responsibility for mutlticultural and anti-racism issues. Accordingly, the only immediate change within governmental structures concerned with the proposed reform of LTC services was the involvement of the new MC instead of the former Office for Senior Citizens' Affairs (OSCA). MCSS retained the lead for reform, working with MOH and MC. In turn, MC, under the NDP, was developing a more proactive approach to dealing with racism than had been characteristic of the previous government.

The continuation of MCSS as lead ministry reflected, as before, the continuing distrust of MOH, the fear of medicalizing this sector, and the need for cost control.

P: It was a matter of the government of the day having the philosophy that the social services – I shouldn't put it so much in terms of social services as preventative services – needed to be considered most significant ... The health services were much, much more expensive, and it was a never-ending thing. You could fund them and fund them and fund them, and it would never be enough. And somehow or other, something had to be done to find a way to fund services that might prevent people from getting too fast into that high-end system.

G: Because behind all of this there was a need to cap the cost. All along, people realized that the costs of Home Care, which were the expensive pieces of the formula, were escalating all the time. In order to cap that there was a plan, there was a need, to cap the envelope for Home Care services by moving it into the Com Soc arena. As the lead, they could start to look at that user-fee, shared-cost, more-use-of-volunteers model as opposed to the universal right like OHIP ... So this was an attempt to shift it from the universally paid for, absolutely your right to a shared responsibility, which was the model that Com Soc tends to espouse ... Again, it was an attempt to demedicalize that ... formally as well.

However, no self-respecting new government can adopt the policies of its predecessors without review. Accordingly, the reform, well under way within the fourteen Area Offices (which had already been staffed by the Liberals), stalled. Instead, the minister of MCSS announced the intention of the government to review LTC services and programs before making any further announcements. On 11 June 1991, after a year of internal review, the MCSS minister, Zanana Akande, announced the NDP government's intention to reform LTC (Akande, 1991). The year of review had produced remarkably little change. The minister's speech briefly acknowledged the work of the previous Liberal government, took note of the province's difficult fiscal situation, discovered when the NDP assumed office ('the enormous economic challenge Ontario faces in this time of recession'), and announced the investment of $647 million into LTC services by 1996–7. Astute observers might have noted that the same funds had been announced by Liberal minister, Charles Beer, in 1990. Almost $440 million of this funding would go into community programs, continuing the effort to shift emphasis from institutional care into the community (Akande, 1991, n.p.). The NDP were deeply committed to participatory democracy, however, and felt uncomfortable with a bureaucratically led policy. Accordingly, Akande also promised that the government would produce another consultation paper, this time based on a much broader and more far-reaching consultation than had characterized the previous consultations. She stated that she and her colleagues, ministers Lankin (MOH) and Ziemba (MC), 'believe that the consultation process is an important part of the product' (Akande, 1991, 2, 4). To the NDP, the content of reform itself was not the only product;

procedural justice required that equal attention be paid to how one got there.

5.2.1 Redirection *and the Service Coordination Agency Model*

In October 1991 the government released *Redirection of Long-Term Care and Support Services in Ontario: A Public Consultation Paper* (MCSS, MOH, and MC, 1991). The principles and goals guiding reform continued to be the same as those that had appeared in the previous Liberal documents, with some minor variations in emphasis and additions such as racial equity, enhanced protection of workers, and a preference for shifting the existing mix of for-profit (FP) and not-for-profit (NFP) providers towards an even greater emphasis on non-profit delivery. The goals of reform, as stated in *Redirection*, were

- integration of long-term care, health, and social services,
- improved access to quality services,
- creation of community alternatives to institutions,
- greater consumer participation and control of the services they receive,
- promotion of racial equity and cultural sensitivity,
- realization of funding equity across the province,
- enhanced protection of the rights and security of service workers, and
- continued preference for a not-for-profit service delivery system. (MCSS, MOH, and MC, 1991, 7)

The reform continued to focus LTC services for both the elderly and the disability communities. The government intended to establish approximately forty new SCAs across Ontario. These agencies were to replace and consolidate the services provided by the Home Care Program and the Placement Coordination Services Program. Employees of these two programs would transfer to the new agencies. The SCAs, like the SAOs, were to act as a single point of access for Health and Personal Support Programs (described below), respite and adult day programs, and institutional care. They would assess and monitor the individual's needs, provide information and referral to community support services, and purchase services for consumers from delivery agencies. Each agency would have a local representative board of directors, the membership of which would be subject to consultation but was to reflect the racial, cultural, and linguistic diversity of their communities. Integration of services was to begin within government through the creation of new program structures. The health and personal support services provided through the Home Care Program, Integrated Homemaker Program, Attendant Outreach Program, and the Homemakers and Nurses Services Program (which were administered by different levels of government, provincial ministries, and community agencies) would be integrated into the new Health and Personal Support Program with consistent eligibility criteria and service standards. Access to these essential services would be coordinated through the new SCAs. One major victory for MCSS was the removal of professional gatekeeping. Previously, access to publicly funded support services, attendant care, social work, and nutritional services required that clients also receive professional services (nursing, rehabilitation, or social work). This restriction had been justified on the grounds of demand limitation, but it had also led to potential waste (e.g., case managers prescribing marginally necessary nursing services in order to make clients eligible for free homemaking). Now, access would be de-medicalized and would be unlinked from receipt of professional services. There would be no charges for services delivered under the Health and Personal Support Program (professional, homemaking, and personal support services). Homemaking services that were not classified as 'essential' but were nonetheless wanted by clients could still be accessed directly; clients would be expected to contribute to the cost of the service according to their ability to pay.

The NDP connection and commitment to grass roots organizations were reflected in the decision to expand and increase the funding to community support services. Echoing the previous Liberal policy, priority for this public funding was to be given to underserviced communities, with the aim of improving geographic equity of access.

The government suggested that there should be uniform guidelines to ensure greater consistency in eligibility criteria, consumer fees, service delivery, and administrative standards. In recognition of community support agencies' varying ability to raise funds, the government changed the funding formula from 70 per cent provincial funding and 30 per cent local funding and consumer charges to funding 100 per cent of the agency's approved budget after deducting revenue from these other sources. As a result, some agencies would receive more funds and some less than in previous years, a policy interpreted by agencies with entrenched community support as penalizing them for their success. Services would be accessed directly by consumers or through the information and referral service of the SCA.

Recognizing the gradual change in the site of care, the government indicated its intention to shift funds from hospitals to community-based services. They announced that they would reallocate annually for the next five years $37.6 million from the provincial hospital budget to LTC. Each area of the province was going to be given a funding envelope for community-based services that would be allocated by area offices under provincial guidelines with the assistance of local planning groups. While communities were not expected to have the same priorities for services, the government would establish criteria to determine the basic level of services that must be funded in all areas. In response to the desire of the disability community to retain independence, government also introduced a pilot project to provide direct funding to persons with disabilities who wished to purchase their own attendant care.

As would befit a government with strong ties to organized labour, a key focus of *Redirection* was the attention paid to front-line workers. An ongoing dilemma in the sector was the considerable disparity between the wages paid within hospitals and LTC institutions and those paid in the community. In general, hospital workers were unionized; workers for most community agencies were not unionized (with the notable exception of the Victorian Order of Nurses [VON]). The 'progressive' agenda in health reform called for the reallocation of resources from institutions to the community; however, reformers paid less attention to the fact that this also meant the elimination of well-paid unionized jobs and their replacement by lower-paid, non-unionized jobs within the community. This plan was untenable for the NDP, and the government accordingly indicated its intention to protect the interests of those in the unionized workforce who might be displaced from hospitals. Provisions were included that would give priority to these workers, including training and upgrading programs and human resource planning. In recognition of the fact that most LTC workers were women and, in particular, immigrant women and women from minority groups, the government intended to revise funding so that agencies could provide more secure employment under improved working conditions. It intended to extend pay equity requirements to the private sector and to public sector workplaces that weren't already covered. Wages for homemakers also were to be adjusted.

In turn, it appeared that workers for existing community-based agencies could lose their jobs (and seniority) unless they were union members. In addition, these agencies provided a mix of services, many of which would not have been reimbursed by the proposed community-based LTC program (e.g., services to the frail elderly who did not meet eligibility requirements). The established community workers felt that this proposal devalued their experience; many vehemently claimed that there were major differences between the requirements of community-based care and that provided within hospitals, where many more services (and more supervision) were readily available. In addition, the proposal did not appear to include resources to increase wages of those already working in the community. The attempt to solve one problem, that of displaced institutional workers, in turn would create considerable tension between community and institutional workers, a tension that would become greatly magnified once the New Democrats again revised their model.

5.2.2 Service Coordination Agency: A Liberal Model in NDP Clothing?

As noted, there were fundamental similarities between *Strategies for Change* and *Redirection* and between their proposed models, the SAO and the SCA. Our respondents confirmed this fact: 'It seemed to me at the time that it was just ... some minor changes to give a new government a label' (G). The similarity between the Liberal and NDP models was attributed to the government's grappling with the very new tasks of governing, being ill informed about the issues, and indifference.

G: They never expected to win the election, so they weren't ready to govern. They were suspicious of the bureaucracy; even individual ministers were not trusted by the Premier's Office. It was a government in chaos.

Many felt that this inexperienced government did not have a position on community-based LTC, did not view it as a priority item at the time, or were not prepared to take risks.

G: I think in the first year they didn't want to change a whole heck of a lot until they understood it. And even when they understood it, they still didn't want to change a whole heck of a lot ... They recognized that they ran the risk of losing a whole lot of support if they changed too much too quickly. And I think the brakes were on all kinds of things ... while the new political masters and their senior civil servants, their deputy ministers began to get their heads around things.

G: When it came to long-term care, the folks who were doing the changeover said to Stephen [Lewis, who was managing the transition for the NDP], 'you know, this is a program for seniors, and just leave it alone unless you want to get into trouble.' And so, you know, it was just given a new spin.

Many were of the opinion that, because of its naivety around issues, the government left the development of the LTC consultation paper to the bureaucracy, which had been given a great deal of autonomy by the Liberals. Without a well-formulated policy of their own, the NDP continued to rely on the bureaucracy, which, not surprisingly, came up with a variant of their earlier model, modified with elements to reflect the new political order.

G: I didn't see a heck of a lot of difference between the Liberal approach [and that of the NDP]. And I think it was because it was owned by the bureaucracy in both cases. The minor changes reflected some of the policies and principles of our party in terms of not-for-profit and those sorts of things, inclusiveness, but ... there probably would have been language around the treatment of the workers, you know, those sorts of things ... There was not, I think, strong support in the government for it one way or the other.

P: They [bureaucracy] were asked to rewrite this [*Strategies for Change*]. But they just rewrote it, calling it something different, called the Service Coordination Agency instead of Service Access. They're both the same ... The bureaucracy created the SAO, the SCA model. So it was kind of their birthchild. And furthermore, before that, they [bureaucracy] were the ones that, in years back, supported, created the brokerage model.

G: My interpretation of that first document was really that it was a reiteration of the Liberals' commitment that something needed to be done and a better coordination was essential. And, 'here's our take on what the Liberals have done at a fairly preliminary level. Let's put it out and see what the response is.' And [it] was the best that could be patched together at this point. And so the solution was, 'Okay, let's put it out there, see what the response is, and that will give us the time and the opportunity to make it right.'

Within the provincial bureaucracy, it was still intended that the new LTC programs would be managed by the integrated Community Health and Support Services Division and its fourteen LTC Area Offices, as set up by the former government. The decentralization of the division into the fourteen LTC Area Offices would continue to reflect the ethos of MCSS, whose other programs (outside LTC) were already administered by Area Offices. Once again, structure reinforced ideas, a commitment to community.

5.2.3 Consultation with the Community

True to their principles regarding the inclusion of marginalized voices, the government made it clear that the priority groups for consultation were consumers, their families, and front-line workers; this approach was markedly different from the Liberal consultations, which had given the primary voice to those who delivered services. Emphasizing the importance of process as product, on 12 September 1991 the NDP convened a province-wide focus group to consult on how best to run the consultations. The process was to be open, broad-based and comprehensive; input would be obtained at both the provincial and the local levels. The local consultation processes would determine feelings 'on the ground' and would be assisted by the fourteen area offices of the Community Health and Support Services Division; the area managers would be responsible for relaying community input to the lead ministry and the three concerned ministers. The central LTC Division at Queen's Park was to lead the consultation with provincial associations.

The NDP, strongly believing in public consultations as a part of governing, would also go to the citizens of Ontario to obtain input for a number of other proposed policy initiatives, such as employment equity, social assistance reform, and an advocacy office to ensure that the rights of vulnerable individuals were protected. In its attempt to include citizens in policy making, the government exhausted the capabilities and resources of most community-based groups.

G: It [the consultations] was very ambitious. It certainly let everybody who wanted to be heard be heard. I think it was necessary. I mean, reform of long-term care had by that point been around for about ten years and there was a huge frustration. And as I said at the beginning, nobody had ever, sort of, gone back to square one and said that, if we were starting with a brand-new, clean slate, how would we design this. And the hearings provided an opportunity for that.

To ensure that professional providers would not dominate the advice given to government, the NDP would provide financial resources and access to institutionalize the participation of seniors and support service providers. The seniors would mount an ambitious consultation process that would parallel that of the government. The question on many lips at the time was whether the NDP's support for these groups was designed to correct a previous wrong or to legitimate their own interests by creating a like-minded voice in the community. Both answers reflect the truth.

P: I think when the NDP got in, they had to prove that they were out for the disadvantaged, marginalized groups and had to have signals that reflected that ... So I think that they probably felt they had to provide resources to these groups that previously lacked the infrastructure to have a voice or be at the right tables, or have lobbyists, or know how to participate within the whole political venue. I think some people [political] were probably driven by passion for that and feeling it is about time, these people have been sort of oppressed, and now there's that opportunity. I think they also were very politically naive to how this would really play out. And I don't think they realized that their own would start to eat their young.

What the province did not appear to recognize was that increasing the number of participants would not only change the balance of interests, but also change the likelihood of policy success. Participation raised expectations that voices would be heard. It also did what political scientists refer to as increasing the scope of conflict (Kellow, 1988; Schattschneider, 1964). The new participants had divergent views and preferences, which would become increasingly difficult for government to manage and helped to stall action (Deber and Williams, 1995).

5.2.4 Mobilization of Interests

Pluralism gives greatest power to those interest groups that can mobilize their resources and be persistent in advancing their agenda. Because all resources – including time, money, and attention are limited, those groups with 'concentrated' interests in a particular area are most likely to participate. In the previous consultations, this had meant the providers, whose survival or growth would clearly be affected by government policy. Most potential consumers of services would instead be classified as 'diffuse' interests; the possibility that one might make episodic use of services would usually be insufficient to catalyze active participation.

Those dependent upon LTC services, in contrast, were often too ill or frail to participate, while their caregivers were often overwhelmed by the demands of caring for their family members. Similarly, the small volunteer-based groups providing community support rarely had the resources needed to even know that a consultation was under way.

These previously unheard groups recognized that the election of an NDP government provided them with an almost unique opportunity to mobilize. Indeed, the new government were eager to have a voice to counterbalance that of providers. Two consumer groups accordingly decided to hire Consultant A, a private consultant with extensive knowledge of the provincial government (he had served as an adviser to an earlier PC minister of health and subsequently had been an influential private consultant). Indeed, Consultant A had earlier worked with one of these seniors' organizations to prepare a brief on auto insurance policy. He recommended that the two groups form an alliance with a third organization and create the Senior Citizens' Consumer Alliance for Long-Term Care Reform (SCCA). All three associations were voluntary, NFP organizations, whose goals were to improve the quality of life for older adults by promoting independence and participation. In June 1991 the United Senior Citizens of Ontario (USCO), the Ontario Coalition of Senior Citizens' Organizations (OCSCO) and the Consumers' Association of Canada, Ontario (CAC) combined their respective efforts to develop a coordinated response to the government's proposed strategic plan for the redirection of LTC. The interest of the CAC was specifically to create a 'consumer-oriented health care system' with accompanying rights (SCCA, 1992). USCO, a grass roots organization composed solely of seniors, had received no government funding in the past and had been self-sponsored. OCSCO was made up of seniors' organizations and counted among its members a number of formerly unionized workers who would later inject some conflict into the alliance.

SCCA was intended to be a single-purpose body with a limited mandate to conduct public hearings and to respond to the government on LTC reform. As was typical of what Pross (1975) has termed 'issue-oriented groups,' SCCA had a single, narrowly defined objective rather than broader, long-term objectives. The alliance's focus was limited to those issues that affected senior citizens and their families; it specifically excluded the disability community from its focus (SCCA, 1992). An attempt to bring together seniors' groups and the disability community to form a broad consumer lobby that might 'be able to be a counterpoint to the doctors and hospitals' (C) never got off the ground.

Because seniors felt that the Liberal government had listened more closely to providers, they were determined to be heard this time around and to control the terms of the consultation. Because *Redirection* and the brokerage model were seen as owned by the civil service, these groups argued that a consultation run by the civil service would not be 'authentic.' This sentiment played into the new government's distrust for their public servants; bureaucrats had been too vocal in indicating potential pitfalls of several of the NDP's pet projects. The government was therefore sympathetic to requests from these organizations for funding to run their own consultations. As stated earlier, SCCA sought and received funding from both the Ministry of Citizenship and the LTC Division to consult seniors and to respond to the *Redirection* document. One seniors' organization referred to it as forming a partnership with the government.

C: You [seniors] can probably do that better than we [government] can. You can find, as seniors asking seniors, you'll get better answers. And so we kind of formed a partnership with them [government], and they financed us to do a lot of research.

Other consumer organizations also lobbied for government funding to get people out to the consultations who would back the government agenda (C). Government officials at the time saw that the interests of agencies providing services to seniors were not the same as those of their care recipients and that there were no mechanisms to project the voice of the latter groups. Inherent in the New Democrats' philosophy and their origins, the funding of intervenors created an 'even playing field' with other traditional health providers whose budgets allowed them to analyse policy and lobby to protect their interests.

G: Hospitals, you know, did it [lobby] all the time. I mean the reason they could do that is because they had the OHA [Ontario Hospital Association]. Well, the OHA gets its fees paid out of hospital funds. And hospitals are funded by the public purse. So, you either give it directly to people or indirectly. And I guess one of the things that we thought we were doing was making it a bit of a more even playing field, and we thought it would do everybody good to hear what the consumer wanted.

The SCCA formed a twelve-member panel, which met through the summer and fall of 1991. Shortly after the government released *Redirec-*

tion, the SCCA sent out a public hearings paper to 6,000 decision makers throughout Ontario, outlining what it felt were the right questions about LTC reform. On 17 January 1992 the alliance sponsored a public policy conference attended by 600 people, who were consumers, providers, and experts. It then proceeded to hold sixteen days of public hearings before issuing its 'Consumer Report on Long-Term Care Reform' (SCCA, 1992), which then generated subsequent reports as government responded and the coalition rejoined (SCCA, 1993).

Similarly, three community support associations – the Association of Visiting Homemakers of Ontario, the Ontario Home Support Association, and Meals on Wheels Ontario – had come together; they, too, had hired Consultant A to help them to facilitate a response to the *Strategies* document. Consultant A had originally been hired by the Association of Visiting Homemakers to help them lobby government to increase the wage rate for homemakers. In contrast to the relatively poor connections between health care providers and the new NDP government, a number of the new ministers had had personal experience with community support associations. For example, Elaine Ziemba, the minister of citizenship, had run a meals on wheels program and had been involved in the formation of Ontario Community Support Association (OCSA) in the early days. Ruth Grier, who subsequently became minister of health, had been instrumental in the creation of a multi-service organization in Etobicoke. These groups, accordingly, could expect a rather warm welcome from government. On 1 April 1992 OCSA was formed.

The rationale for coalescing was explained by one interviewee who belonged to these groups.

P: I think we felt that we actually hadn't had a voice at the province. Hospitals had a strong voice, physicians had a strong voice, but the community-based services didn't. We were also feeling very threatened by ... what appeared to be a growing threat of the for-profit homemaking sector taking over what traditionally had been a not-for-profit sector. So it was kind of like a wake-up call. We were getting more and more people requiring services. Home Care service was limited and there were maximum hours. And we were finding we just didn't have enough other services for people. Our home-support programs and our other programs were simply not meeting the need. We had waiting lists ... and many of our customers could not pay their shared costs, and we were absorbing it ... We're sort of the meat and potatoes, you know, so that everybody else can whip in and do fancy stuff. And if patients don't get fed, don't get bathed, don't get their houses cleaned and so on, it's impossible for a nurse to float in for fifteen minutes and poke somebody in the arm. So, why don't we actually do something about it. It took three years to get those three organizations together.

The professional, NFP organizations, such as those providing nursing services, already had either strong provincial organizations or paid staff to lobby government. As a result, they did not see the need to come together with the support services. Unlike professional providers, during the early discussions a number of members from consumer associations had been attracted by OCSA. However, the consumers eventually broke away from the providers.

P: Eventually, what you saw is a breakout between the consumers and the providers, which, by the way, I think is quite proper. It's a much purer kind of thing when consumers are talking about needs for themselves. But when they're all tangled up with providers, you wonder if they're being manipulated. And it's – the word is bad optics ... How does the government know that we haven't manipulated them into just singing from our song book?

5.2.5 The Coalitions Propose a New Model

Consultant A became the hub of many connecting spokes. Within the government, there was interest in developing a model that would be less provider dominated. Seniors, the disability community, and community support agencies agreed. With the help of Consultant A, both the seniors' and the support services' coalitions recognized that they would prefer an alternative to the SAO model that might put more emphasis on non-professional services.

One government official, who had been involved in hiring Consultant A when she had worked in the community, stated that the government was more than pleased when SCCA sought government funding to pay for this consultant.

P: The NDP had figured out that the consumers really didn't know enough to help them answer the questions they needed to have answered. So when the consumers' group got themselves formed and they submitted to the government for a grant to pay for [the consultant], they [government] were only too happy to pay it, because they realized [the consultant] was going to get them educated ... They couldn't say, 'Hire Consultant A.' They could just say, 'Here's the money.' But I think they knew that at that point that this was all going on, they'd [consumers] already been in quite in-depth discussions with him. So, I mean, and I think [the consultant] delivered.

Remembering that some officials in government had previously been involved with community support organizations, some provider groups believed that the seniors were encouraged to hire Consultant A by government because he would promote the model being developed by OCSA.

P: There are many who believed that the management consulting group that was hired by the Seniors' Alliance really was reporting to someone other than the Seniors' Alliance. The Seniors' Alliance was the front, in a sense, for what other groups wanted, but they couldn't hire the ... firm because it would look too close for comfort. So it was the consumer group that was given funding and suggested, 'Well, why don't you hire [name of the consultant]' ... Some believe it was the Ontario Community Support Association's key people ... There was a sense that it (the model) would be viewed like, 'it's their model,' and it needed to come from a more neutral grouping. And strategically, if you place it with consumers ... consumers, especially with an NDP government, are more likely to be viewed as the neutral group versus one of the players, the stakeholders.

Even seniors who saw the creativity and value of this consultant recognized his access to government

C: He was a very political person. He played a very strong role in influencing the development of the planning that the Alliance did. In many ways, he was a very creative person. I would never have conceived of the magnitude of the things that we did. As I say, they [activities] were historical because before we had gone when invited and participated as we were allowed to. So he was very creative in that sense, and he was very good at getting money from government for another project that we oversaw ... There was a lot of very direct communication between the government and the Alliance through the consultant, who was always reporting what somebody in the ministry had said, what they thought we should do, and what we thought they should do. And they would give us money to pursue particular aspects, and so on.

OCSA had argued that the government's own consultation process would not tap into the specific needs of their sector since the sector, was new and underfunded. The association, furthermore, wanted to do more than merely respond to *Redirection*: they wanted to suggest an alternative. With the government's financial assistance, OCSA also held parallel consultations, facilitated by a consultant who had previously worked with Consultant A. The fact that both SCCA and OCSA eventually would produce the same model was therefore not surprising. As one professional provider stated, 'I don't think it's coincidental that the two models were similar' (P). They emerged with a model that integrated assessment and service delivery, the predecessor of the MSA.

When concern was expressed about funding senior consumers but not others, the government, towards the end of the consultation process, also provided funding to the Consumer Coalition of People with Disabilities to carry out consultation with their members (Deber and Williams, 1995; MOH Long-Term Care Division and MCSS, 1992a,b).

Up to this point, unions had little involvement with LTC reform. They kept a watching brief on the government's activities in this sector on certain key issues, in particular, the direct funding project for persons with disabilities and collective bargaining rights. However, nothing at this point spurred them to action. As one respondent from a union stated,

P: One was the idea of how attendant care and services for disabled adults were going to fit in ... And the whole notion of individualized funding, where the individual would broker for their own services. So we were interested in that. And then the other piece that we always monitored was whether it was going to be kind of a massive privatization, or de-unionizing of the units we had. It was probably primarily at that time watching to make sure our members were okay and then watching for what was going to happen to the sector overall ... So, fairly broad at that point.

Other established providers in the field, such as the professional providers, were not dissatisfied with the brokerage model. Most were concerned with the inherent conflict of interest in existing arrangements, where some provider organizations also ran Home Care Programs, a conflict that was addressed by the SCA model. Many approached the consultations as nothing more than an opportunity to promote their organizations: 'I remember looking and thinking, "This [another organization's submission] is saying nothing but selling [the organization]"' (P).

A number of these organizations, however, were beginning to realize that the ground was shifting during the SCCA consultation. They viewed the emphasis on consumer empowerment, justice, and an anti-medical approach as metaphors for reducing provider authority. The SCCA and OCSA consultations were converging on a similar model, which rejected brokerage in favour of uniting the financing and delivery of care. The health professionals quickly realized they would not be able to find common ground with these alliances.

By 31 March 1992 the entire public consultation process was completed. It had been a massive undertaking. Over the five-month period, according to the government, more than 75,000 people and 110 provincial associations had participated in approximately 2,900 meetings held at both the local and the provincial level across Ontario.

Further to its commitment to community consultation and participation, the government had also distributed 87,000 copies of its *Redirection* plan in English, French, audio cassette, and Braille. An information pamphlet had been translated into thirty-three languages. The government hotline had received more than 2,200 requests for information, and 1,800 written submissions had been sent in from societal groups. Widening the scope of conflict, however, brought in new voices, with new demands, which would prove difficult to reconcile.

5.2.6 Institutional Changes within Government: The Shift from MCSS to MOH

One key pillar of the attempt by government bureaucrats to redirect resources from institutions towards the community was establishing MCSS as the lead ministry. In the spring of 1992 this strategy unravelled for reasons unrelated to LTC reform. Zanana Akande, minister of community and social services, attracted the attention of the press (and the Opposition) for her role as a landlord, which was seen as ill befitting a member of a social democratic government. A member of her family also fell ill. She soon resigned as minister and was replaced by Marion Boyd. Frances Lankin, formerly a union leader, and the newly appointed minister of health, was one of the most powerful (and capable) members of the government. She took over the lead for LTC reform; the new LTC Division now reported to her. The move was unexpected. The reasons cited for the government's decision to transfer the lead to MOH ranged from the capabilities of individual ministers, to expediency, to a shift in ideas about the nature of LTC.

G: The premier fairly arbitrarily handed this [LTC reform] to Frances in Health. And said, "for God's sake, take it." And it was a product of frustration and inability to, in fact, move it at a pace that met [NDP] priority at that time. And so it was seen as, 'let's put Frances in charge and get it moving' ... [It was a reflection of] confidence in her and frustration with Com Soc.

This respondent also believed that the policy was now confronted with the results of the parallel changes under way within the institutional sector. As a cost-saving measure, hospitals were under pressure to discharge patients early, reduce length of stay, and increase the proportion of day procedures. Ontario reflected the Canadian trend to reduce both absolute and relative availability of hospital beds. (In 1985, the year the Liberals had formed the provincial government, the Organization for Economic Coordination and Development (OECD) 2001 database indicates that Canada had 174,424 acute in-patient beds, or 6.7 beds per thousand population. By 1990, when the NDP replaced the Liberals, the Canadian totals had dropped to 173,617, or 6.3 beds per thousand population. By 1995, when the NDP in turn was defeated, the numbers had further fallen to 142,213, or 4.8 beds per thousand population). This led to more, and sicker, patients within the community who would need home care services. While LTC reformers spoke about the need to de-emphasize professional services in favour of support for the frail elderly and disabled, reformers in the hospital sector were taking measures that meant that home care was becoming re-medicalized.

G: The realization was growing that whereas this started with just ... community support services to keep people in their homes, there was growing need for services after people were discharged from hospitals, because hospital budgets were being squeezed and that whole thing was happening ... And there was a growing understanding that this was moving more towards health than it was a social service; that if you were really to reform the system, then it had to be seen as a responsibility of Health, as Health was moving more to the community.

C: There was a consensus developing both among the bureaucrats and among the service providers that what we were dealing with in long-term care were issues that were more health related than they were social service related. Whereas for decades many of the long-term care services were more social service based. People's healthcare requirements were less than their social service requirements. But clearly, as the 80s drew to a close, it became clear that the long-term care issues were more health-related issues.

The trend was reinforced by the unintended consequences of the shift in thinking about disability and ageing. Considerable progress had been made in de-stigmatizing these two conditions and focusing on what such individuals could do, rather than on their limitations. In effect, disability and ageing were 'normalized' and were becoming perceived as everyday occurrences. It was a short step, however, to arguing that government subsidized services were intended for conditions out of the ordinary, not for daily living, and hence that meeting the needs and demands related to those conditions should be in the realm of the private market and individuals, rather than a state responsibility. Acceptance and mainstreaming could shade into neglect of the special needs of such individuals, which were often essential to allowing them to meet their potential.

P: I attribute the change to a greater normalization of the ageing process ... There are many, many people today who are physically challenged who live in the community, who live in their own homes, who go on the buses, who have jobs, who go to school, who have families, who live what we consider to be normal lives, but, who, ten or fifteen years ago did not live among the normal community. They lived in institutions. They lived in group homes. They lived in family homes but they were hidden away. But they weren't normalized within our society. And ageing was a similar thing. In my view, throughout the 70s and 80s, we saw greater, and we continue to see a greater, normalization and acceptance of ageing, and acceptance within our broader society of ageing. So a lot of the needs of seniors, the social needs, of seniors and some of their other everyday needs are being met by businesses, by builders, by pharmacies, by the normalized society. They don't have to be met by specialized government funded services. So contractors renovate homes to provide wheelchair access and banks have specialized services for seniors, etc. So a lot of the reasons why people needed specialized services no longer exist. So it's less of a social service ... So there was a consensus that these (needed services) were health services, and there was no longer the pull within Com Soc to hold onto that portfolio.

Some argued that the reallocation of funds from hospitals to the community was too difficult to achieve if MCSS retained the lead: 'And one of the problems had leadership for long-term care rested with Com Soc [MCSS] was that it was a much bigger gulf for that money to flow across. And therefore, it was less likely to happen' (O). Others argued that LTC required a regional presence and therefore fit better under a ministry that was already highly decentralized; that MOH "thought in head office terms" and was nothing more than "a highly centralized claims payment agency and funder of hospitals" (G).

While recognizing the steering effect of this institutional move, some rationalized it as proving the success of the new LTC Division. One respondent argued that this straddled division had developed into a hybrid creature, dominated by neither ministerial culture. Therefore, the shift to MOH was no longer deemed to be detrimental to reform.

G: There was also a sense at the time that we'd gotten past that Health versus Social Services thing and that long-term care had become a more integrated kind of culture; that we weren't going to get flak from outside groups about going under Health. We talked about it. We thought that the disabled community might say, 'What are you doing moving over to Health? What does that mean?' You know, 'a medical model! a medical model!' We had great assurances that we were going to remain as a separate division within Health; that we were not being incorporated in the other silos. And that we were to be seen as a health and social service division. And I think it was just a feeling that probably the time was right, and the bulk of the bucks was being spent on health care, not the social services aspect. That it was a health minister's problem, if you like.

Another institutional mechanism that government hoped would integrate ministerial cultures and ensure that all relevant interests were considered was also producing less than anticipated. The NDP had built in interministerial coordination by requiring that all cabinet submissions related to LTC be signed off by all three ministers involved in the reform (MCSS, MOH, and MC). This requirement was couched in the language of partnerships.

G: We were trying to get ministries to work together rather than have [them] isolated. And this was a little bit of a test, trying to see if we could actually get bureaucrats and the ministers to be more in partnership rather than take complete ownership and run with an issue.

The dual-reporting relationship of the assistant deputy minister

(ADM), LTC Division, to both ministers, however, was cumbersome, muddied accountability, and slowed down reform. Some believed that further institutional change was necessary to simplify the process.

G: It was a very unwieldy process with the fragmentation that was there. And we had this, in my view, quite unworkable arrangement with a shared ADM between Health and Community Services. And what was happening was there wasn't clear accountability ... Every operational issue has multiple ministers. You just can't work the process where you need three ministers to sign off every piece of paper.

5.2.7 A New Model Begins to Emerge

On 25 May 1992 Frances Lankin, minister of health, spoke to OCSA's annual conference and provided them with a progress report on the consultations (Lankin, 1992a). During her remarks the minister indicated that there had been a great deal of consensus on the government's philosophical values and overall direction; in her view, the major differences concerned the way LTC should be organized. She referred to questions about whether the fourteen LTC Area Offices were too bureaucratic and lacked local flexibility and about the financial viability of the NFP community-based sector in a reformed system. She went on to note that people with disabilities were critical of what they saw as the perpetuation of the medical model of service delivery, and consumers generally were concerned about the lack of trained workers and the burden this created for family members (particularly women). The minister acknowledged that she was in fundamental agreement with the five premises for reforming the system as outlined by OCSA in its own submission to government and to the SCCA consultations: that is, NFP delivery; consumer control and participation; integration of LTC health and social services; balance between health and social needs, between community and institutional services, and between prevention and treatment; and integration of assessment, case management, *and* comprehensive service delivery. She acknowledged OCSA's recommendation for a multidisciplinary, multiservice organization.

In this speech, she indicated the goals that she and her colleagues would use to reform the system: equity in service; community control and accountability; accessibility; choice; prevention and rehabilitation; NFP administration; minimum bureaucracy; and a preference for multiservice agencies (MSAs). Was the brokerage model dead?

OCSA had indeed recommended a multi-service agency model, which it called Comprehensive Community Care Organizations (CCCOs). However, the minister had jumped well beyond OCSA's recommendations. Although the association had recommended that this model be piloted in ten areas that were seen as structurally ready for this concept (e.g., those already funded by the Liberals to put a One-Stop Access model in place), the NDP government was ready to implement it across the province. The failure of the government to take a cautious approach would eventually lead OCSA to withdraw its support of the later MSA model. The seeds of dissent within OCSA's membership were sown in this early NDP period. In the words of one of the association's members:

P: We were so new and we were forming at a bad time. Everything was changing. A brand new organization was expected to forward a policy paper without the kind of credibility and relationship with its members to be able to do so ... There was, I think, a little bit of a difference between where the membership was and where the leadership was. The leadership was far more progressive in terms of where they thought things should go than the membership was.

While OCSA had consulted with its membership to get their views, the leadership developed the recommendations. They had neither the time nor the funds to go back to their membership to gain support for the recommendations. During the consultation, most of the discussion revolved around principles. Moving from general principles to implementation, however, unearths details that raise conflict.

P: Everyone agrees with the principles and the policy of being able to work more cooperatively together, and so on. But I don't think people really realize that the way you do that, or one of the ways you do that, is to actually consolidate the agencies into a larger one. And then, it was sort of like, 'Oh my God, what about us, and what about our board, and what about our volunteers, and what about our jobs?'

The association was also hampered by events unrelated to LTC reform. The Canadian Red Cross Society, the largest member in OCSA and a major deliverer of NFP homemaking, was not heavily involved with the LTC reform at this point because it was attempting to deal with the tainted-blood crisis. The failure to ensure that all members were on board was costly for OCSA; indeed, once the government adopted the model suggested by the leadership of OCSA and by the SCCA, OCSA was forced by its membership, including the Red Cross, to withdraw support from the model.

Nonetheless, the leadership felt ready to move ahead quickly. On 22 June 1991 Jane Leitch, chairperson of SCCA, forwarded an advance copy of 'Consumer Report on Long-Term Care Reform' (SCCA, 1992) to Frances Lankin, to Marion Boyd, minister of community and social services, and to Elaine Ziemba, minister of citizenship. In the covering letter she asked the ministers to indicate, at the SCCA's 6 July Public Policy Conference, the areas of agreement with the alliance's recommendation (Leitch, 1991). Arguing that everyone was weary of continuing debate, she further urged the government to provide some indication at the conference of how it intended to reform the sector.

In its report, the SCCA recommended that planning for LTC services must be done in conjunction with the acute care system, stressing that care for the elderly must focus on the continuum of services, ranging from prevention to palliative care, including primary, home, acute, extended, and chronic care services, and on the linkages between those services. It believed that the fragmentation in the sector was caused by the historical schism between health services funded by MOH and social services funded by MCSS. It urged the government to abandon the concept of an SCA, which was viewed as 'another form of the costly, inefficient and overly-bureaucratic "brokerage model" of service delivery' (SCCA, 1992, 8), and indicated that only two out of a hundred major provincial organizations that made presentations at their consultation had favoured the SCA model. Instead, it recommended a major overhaul of the sector by the adoption of 'single service agencies to incrementally transform – through voluntary mergers of agencies – to form what we are calling "Comprehensive Multi-Service Organizations" (CMSOs)' (SCCA, 1992, 9). Although they credited OCSA with the development of the CMSO concept, the SCCA consumer panel eagerly adopted this new model. In their report they argued that the separation of the assessment and delivery functions distanced providers from consumers, failed to integrate services at the delivery level, maintained the distinction between health and community support services, continued duplication of assessments, and created the need for 'elaborate, costly bureaucratic structures' like the brokerage system.

The CMSO model was described as an amalgamation of existing NFP service providers; these providers could either merge their operations or establish formal administrative linkages while continuing to operate under their separate auspices. Considerable thought went into anticipating objections. As a result, some of the features of the CMSO model were the inclusion of provision of a full range of in-home and community support services, services delivered to a defined population and geographic community and responsive to the ethnic mix in the community, a multi-disciplinary approach to assessment, the integration of case management and service delivery, a process of consumer appeal, establishment of provincial standards, and funding through a global budget and/or capitation rather than a brokerage/fee-for-service model. SCCA rejected a 'cookie-cutter' approach, preferring instead local development of models. It also encouraged efforts to ensure that the unique identity of organizations such as VON, the Red Cross, and others be retained within the CMSO, without clarifying how this might be accomplished, other than by vague references to administrative linkages. Other provisions would buy time; for example, the model allowed for the time-limited external purchase by CMSOs of services provided by agencies reluctant to merge. Not wanting to take on the FP agencies, it recommended that these agencies be allowed to maintain but not increase their market share as the system developed. It appealed to the magnanimity of the Home Care Programs and Placement Co-ordination Services, whose functions would be replaced by the CMSO. It urged the equalization of wages between institutional and community workers and recommended the unionization of workers and collective bargaining on a regional basis. Finally, while there was strong consensus that user fees should not be charged on any health or personal care services, the SCCA could not reach agreement on the implementation of user fees for community support services.

This consumer group also wanted to move control outside the provincial government to 'empower communities.' Rather than devolution of planning and resource allocation to local area offices or civil servants, as recommended in *Redirection,* SCCA recommended the establishment of a permanent Standing Committee on Long-Term Care within the District Health Council (DHC) to assume these responsibilities. Given that DHCs had planning responsibilities for the acute care system, the alliance believed that this recommendation would deal with the major structural problems that exist between the acute-care and LTC systems. To overcome the view that DHCs are medically oriented, it insisted that the Standing Committee have an equal balance of health and social service perspectives. Recognizing the importance and steering effect of institutional structures, SCCA recommended the eventual evolution of DHCs into District Health and Social Service Councils.

In keeping with the thinking at the time about the broader determinants of health and the importance of social services to health status, the alliance rejected what it saw as the artificial distinctions between health and social services. The report called for the government to define a guaranteed basket of health and social services that would be available in all regions of the province. The recommended legislated core services ranged broadly from health promotion, education, recreation, home maintenance and support, transportation, foot and oral health care, respite care, meals, day care, counselling services, rehabilitation therapies, assistive devices, and supportive housing, to in-home professional services. Reform should be guided by principles that enhanced the independence and empowerment of consumers. Consumers should have not only the 'right' to alternative services and the right to make choices among them, but also the right to 'take risks' (SCCA, 1992). As the alliance was silent on the role of private financing in a renewed LTC system, the practical effect of its proposal seemed to be broadening the scope (and cost) of publicly financed services in the guise of integration.

On 6 July 1992 Health Minister Frances Lankin addressed the SCCA policy conference to provide feedback from the government based on its own consultations, in particular, to the report of SCCA. She once again addressed her remarks in the context of the 'hard economic times' and stated that reform must be 'cost effective as well as quality enhancing' (Lankin, 1992b). The government agreed with the seven principles for LTC reform identified in SCCA's report, but it would add three more, namely, commitment to public administration and NFP preference, reform must address the needs of persons with physical disabilities in terms of their distinct needs and preferences, and policies must promote racial equality and respect for cultural diversity.

The minister agreed with the seniors' report that 'tinkering' with different parts of the system was not enough for reform, and she acknowledged that their report was the most comprehensive of the submissions government had received, addressing, as it did, systemic issues and the need for greater systemic reform than envisaged in the government's consultation document. The government agreed that a new model for service delivery was needed and noted that it was seriously considering the Comprehensive Multi-Service Organization put forward by OCSA and SCCA. This model would provide a full range of in-home *and* community support services to communities based on a defined population and geography, operate under one local administration with a community-based board of directors, integrate case management *and* service delivery under one roof by providers who would be employees of the new organization, include an appeals process, and be funded on an enriched global budget and/or capitation rather than through a brokerage (fee-for-service) model. While recognizing that care must move away from the costly medical model and that an artificial barrier existed between health and social services, Lankin was pleased that the CMSO was to work under the direction of the LTC committee of a reformed District Health Council. She was also pleased with the suggestion that wages and working conditions of community workers needed to be improved, and that better wages would improve both the quality of care and the quality of work and family life not only for workers but for consumers as well.

On 26 November 1992 Frances Lankin made an announcement to the legislature that began to put into place some of the pieces for this next attempt to reform the sector. The Long-Term Care Statute Law Amendment Act amended several statutes affecting LTC institutional services and the Ministry of Community and Social Services Act, giving authority to the minister to make direct payments to adults with physical disabilities so that they could purchase their own support services. Support services at the time, specifically attendant care programs, did not permit such direct funding arrangements. Government funding was provided to a service agency, which received a fee for administering programs on behalf of disabled adults (MOH and MCSS, 1992). The government hoped that the directed funding for the disability community would address some of their major concerns and thereby soften their voice in the future.

Lankin also stated that a report on the community consultation indicating the policy directions for reform would be released in January, and that early in the spring of 1993 the government would announce the implementation framework for the reform of the system. Meanwhile the DHCs were to restructure their LTC planning subcommittees to include representatives of municipalities, the social service planning and delivery sectors, and consumers. They were to assume the lead role in planning LTC in their communities (Lankin, 1992c).

On 2 December Lankin announced $133.5 of the $647.6 million for the expansion of homemaker services in seventeen underserviced areas of the province. The government also sought to remove professional gatekeepers: homemaking services would be available to consumers regardless of their need for professional health services. Once this expansion was in place, all areas of the province would have homemaking services integrated with home care. The NDP also sought to placate unionized workers who were losing hospital jobs; those areas that would be receiving the new funding would be required to work with the Hospital Training and Adjustment Panel to facilitate the hiring of laid-off hospital workers. She also indicated that community-based services would 'eventually be provided by comprehensive multi-service agencies, which will be created from existing agencies such as home care, placement coordination services and a range of not-for-profit service delivery agencies' (Ontario Minister of Health, 1992). The purpose would be to integrate assessment, case management, *and* service delivery (Lankin, 1992d).

For many stakeholders the Service Coordination Agency model had been seen as a reasonable approach. The most satisfied were the NP providers of professional services (e.g., nursing, rehabilitation); the SCA had the advantage of being a flexible model that maintained their expertise and market share. Consumers were less happy; the SCA model might improve access, but consumers' groups disliked the imposition of an additional layer of bureaucracy between the provider and the client. The flip side of preserving existing provider agencies was that the reform would not deal with the issue of multiple assessments; neither would it result in major consumer empowerment. Even the limited coordination had its opponents; consumers from the ethnic communities, who, for the most part, had accessed services through their own community organizations, were concerned that SCAs would erode this relationship. Support service organizations were concerned because the model continued to make a distinction between services in terms of essential and non-essential services, with much of what they provided falling on the non-essential side of the divide. This concern led some in the support services to promote an integrated model, believing that their organizations would become the hub of such a model agency. The NDP obliged, giving birth to a model strongly resembling CMSO but now going by the name of Multi-Service Agency (MSA).

5.3 The NDP and the Multi-Service Agency Model

5.3.1 The Recession and the Social Contract

External forces were hardly propitious for a major expansion of service entitlements. Most governments were faced with a growing recession, reduced revenues and increasing costs, rising unemployment, and mounting debts and deficits. To make matters worse, the Canadian federal government attempted to deal with its own deficits by unilaterally reducing the rate of increase of federal transfers for hospital insurance, physician insurance, and post-secondary education. Per capita federal transfers through Established Programs Financing (EPF) now grew at less than the rate of inflation. In consequence, the federal share for spending in health and post-secondary education fell dramatically. Ontario's presentation of the figures at the time spoke of a drop from a high of 52 per cent in 1979–80 to 31 per cent, amounting to a cumulative loss of $12.3 billion for Ontario (Ontario Ministry of Treasury and Economics, 1992). Worse, Ontario's economic picture both decreased its own revenues and increased spending pressures (e.g., for welfare and social services). In May 1993 the premier and the minister of finance outlined Ontario's grave fiscal situation. Without intervention, the government was projecting that total revenues would be 1.4 per cent lower than 1992–3 levels. The debt was $68 billion, with a deficit approaching $17 billion.

Faced with the failure of its earlier decision to spend its way out of the recession, which had only inflated the provincial deficit, the NDP government now proposed an economic package that asked all Ontarians to contribute to control of the debt and deficit while maintaining public services and an investment in jobs. It hoped to achieve savings of $6 billion in 1993–4. The package consisted of a balance of increased revenues (through taxes and sales of assets) and an Expenditure Control Plan that aimed to find $4 billion in reduced expenditures in government ministries and programs. As a union-oriented party, the New Democrats were reluctant to reopen negotiated agreements. Their solution, which pleased no one, was to attempt to negotiate what they termed the 'Social Contract,' which would find voluntary savings in the $43 billion in total compensation paid to the approximately 900,000 employees who delivered the network of health, education, and public services in the public and broader public sector (Ontario Ministry of Finance, 1993). Rejecting approaches that would result in massive lay-offs or wage rollbacks, the government believed that, through negotiations among employers, employees, and bargaining agents, it could save $2 billion of that wage bill in 1993–4 through reductions and containment of transfer payments. The Social Contract was to run for three years, starting on 1 April 1993 and ending on 31 March 1996. A major tool was the 'request' that all employees of the Ontario Public Service and of the 'broader public sector' (i.e., those NFP private organizations that received public funds, such as universities and hospitals) take twelve days unpaid leave per year in each of the three years of the Social Contract; that negotiated and scheduled wage increases and benefit improvements be deferred until 1 April 1996, thereby overruling existing contracts; and that early retirements and voluntary exits be encouraged (Government of Ontario, 1993b; Ontario Minister of Finance, 1993). Soon these unpaid days off were named after the premier: 'Rae days.' Some employers (including some universities) designated certain days between Christmas and New Year's as Rae days, thus turning the policy into a de facto pay cut. Other employers sent workers home; still others were forced to pay overtime in order to maintain mandated service levels. The scheme infuriated public sector unions.

These efforts to improve Ontario's financial position had two effects on LTC reform. First, the Expenditure Control Plan slowed the implementation of LTC because of cutbacks in the flow of funds. Second, the Social Contract put a major strain on labour, the government's largest support group, as well as providing the opportunity for other groups to galvanize into coalitions to oppose its LTC reform.

On the latter point, a number of stakeholder groups involved in LTC reform believed that the Social Contract negotiations not only brought together in one room for the first time a number of disparate interests, but also credited these meetings with the subsequent formation of alliances among provider groups in the LTC sector that would slow the implementation of the MSAs.

P: That whole notion of coalitions came after Social Contract or during the period of the Social Contract. They dragged us into a room and said, 'You've got to talk to us under Social Contract.' It was one of the worst things the government ever did for itself in that it showed us how to work together to fight the NDP government. Not just this [LTC reform], you know, things that we didn't like about the NDP or any government. I said, 'Gee, coalitions do work!' ... It was only when we came together under Social Contract that people said, 'Oh, you've got an association. Look who's in that association. And this is how they conduct business.' We all did things individually. And if we did anything, it was unbeknownst to most others. So literally the government brought the groups together in order to discuss Social Contract, and suddenly we developed relationships with these people ... It provided for a huge bonding experience. You can imagine. Those people were stuck in rooms twelve, fourteen hours on end ... And you had rooms for the health sector, rooms for education. So the health people got to know each other, got to develop relationships and understand mutual issues. 'Oh this is in our best interest too. And we'll work out consensus positions.' And they learned to do that.

As will be seen in chapter 6, to make matters worse, attempts by the New Democrats to repair their relationship with labour led to actions within LTC reform that alienated other groups and mobilized further resistance.

5.3.2 The Locus of Policy Development Shifts

In February 1993 Ruth Grier had replaced Frances Lankin as minister of health. Although the NDP had declared that LTC reform was a priority issue, very little work had been done towards development of the new MSA concept. Relationships between the government and its bureaucracy were often strained. With trust lacking, bureaucratic advice was often resented or ignored. Indeed, predicting potential pitfalls was hazardous; the NDP government was apt to believe that such pitfalls, if and when they arose, had been generated by bureaucratic resistance. LTC reform was no exception. The government assumed that inaction was a result of bureaucratic resistance to the proposed model and moved responsibility for developing reform initiatives away from the bureaucracy. MSA development and implementation was now spearheaded by the minister's own political staff.

G: Nothing had been done in the intervening six months [since the announcement in September of the MSA model by Lankin]. The policy staff, some of whom had been with Frances were just terribly frustrated with the bureaucracy because there had been no work to put flesh on the policy announcement that had been decided in September. And so we felt six months had been lost ... So we scrambled madly, and what became known as the first of the partnership documents was driven by [Grier's] office completely, written by her policy staff, and edited by her chief-of-staff, who came from a social services background, with some help from people within the bureaucracy, but no leadership.

One government official saw the battle as resulting in the erosion of the traditional role of the bureaucracy and blamed it on the shifting sands in government of ideology and ministers.

G: I felt the whole process of the bureaucracy became very distorted and undermined, and that the bureaucracy was not any longer in a position to give the best advice to government, but rather the government told them what they wanted and it was the bureaucracy's job to figure out a way to make it happen ... And in fact, I remember quite clearly when there was certain advice and saying, 'No, that's not what we want to hear. You go back and give us other advice' ... The primary purpose ... should be non-partisan, and that's not how it worked. I mean it worked for forty-two years because we had one government and everyone was singing under the same tempo, and there was stability. But once we had these constant changes, it became very difficult for the bureaucrats to shift with whatever the ideology of the day is and the players of the day, and then the different ministers – all different approaches to how you make this happen.

5.3.3 The Partnership Documents

As promised, starting in April 1993, the ministries of Health, Community and Social Services, and Citizenship released the first of the four Partnership documents on LTC reform, which added considerably more detail to the earlier announcement of an MSA model (MOH, MCSS, and MC, 1993a). These documents, which had colourful covers, were commonly referred to as the 'Rainbow' documents.

5.3.3.1 A Policy Framework
The first of the series was subtitled 'A Policy Framework' (MOH, MCSS, and MC, 1993a). It was developed by a planning group that included representatives of DHCs and staff of MOH, MCSS, and MC and signed by three ministers (Ruth Grier of Health, Tony Silipo of Community and Social Services, and Elaine Ziemba of Citizenship). It began with the statement that 'four major factors are shaping policies for long-term care.' Specifically, the arguments were as follows.

1. *Traditional methods of planning and delivering services are not effective.*
   The ministers called for a change of emphasis, shifting from the existing (and expensive) medical model to one 'in which health and social service providers operate on the basis of an integrated approach.' They mentioned the need for greater stress on the social determinants of health and on moving from institutional care to a full continuum of care and support. The document thus indicated support for an integrated rather than a brokerage model and gave

hope to the community-based sector that it would receive more attention and more resources. As stated earlier, in 1989–90 almost 80 per cent of the LTC budget was spent on institutional services and 20 per cent on community-based services.

2. *Consumers want more involvement.* Consumers expressed a desire during the consultations to have a formal voice in allocating services, priorities, and methods of delivery.

3. *Changing demographics.* The elderly and the frail elderly constituted a growing proportion of the population in the province. Meeting their needs in the community would prevent future, more costly institutional intervention.

4. *The current and future economic climate.* The government repeated its concerns about rising costs for health care (an increase of 10 to 12 per cent each year over the past decade, which it attributed to the focus on medical services and high-technology acute hospital care), drops in provincial revenues, and less-than-anticipated federal transfers.

The document summarized the major findings of the provincial consultations. While there was agreement on the principles and goals of a reformed LTC system, different views were expressed on the mechanisms and models of consumer empowerment, planning and accountability, coordination and delivery of services, and funding and human resource strategies. It was indicated that the new system required more comprehensive system-wide solutions than were proposed in the *Redirection* report. 'Tinkering' or incremental reform was no longer enough.

In the framework document earlier comments from consumers' groups were repeated. They indicated that consumers wanted a more meaningful role where empowerment had to extend to more than shaping their own existing services. It also had to include input at a higher level in shaping the design of the LTC system and its programs. Those with physical disabilities raised major concerns about equity in decisions given the relative organization and political strength of seniors' groups vis-à-vis disability groups. They were critical of the perpetuation of the medical model of service delivery and wanted to be able to plan, arrange, and manage their own services.

It was recognized in the document that the two umbrella groups, Ontario Community Support Association and the Senior Citizens' Consumer Alliance, had rejected the brokerage model of the SCA and had suggested instead that services be delivered through comprehensive multi-service organizations, which would be planned by integrated health and social services LTC committees of DHCs. The alliance also rejected the idea of the fourteen LTC Area Offices. By maintaining the distinction between the Health and Personal Services Program and the Community Support Services Program, the SCA model had failed to integrate health and social services at the delivery level. Improved wages and working conditions for workers were also advanced in the consultations.

According to the policy framework document, the new system would provide services to adults with physical disabilities, elderly persons in need of LTC and support services, and people of any age who required health services at home or at school. Not-for-profit multi-service agencies would provide access, offer case management services, and decide on eligibility for community support and long-term health care; decide eligibility and admissions to LTC facilities; reflect the needs and features of communities (including geography, region, language, and culture); and deliver community-based services funded by and accountable to government. For the first time, in-home health and personal support services as well as community support services such as meals programs and transportation were to be provided by one agency, the MSA. Physician referral would no longer be required. There would be no charges for those health and personal care services or homemaking services considered essential to keep people in the community. Nor would there be charges for respite care services, adult day care, and support programs for family caregivers. Charges for community support services would be based on ability to pay. A provincially defined minimum basket of services would be available in each community.

Concessions were made to workers in the new system. MSAs would offer potential for regular employment rather than hourly contracts. The government also proposed improved training for workers and involvement in planning the programs, staffing, and budgets of LTC facilities and MSAs. The planning of MSAs would also ensure that succession rights of workers were addressed. Hiring priority was to be given to displaced hospital workers.

5.3.3.2 A Local Planning Framework
One month later, the new LTC service system, the principles for the local planning process, and the guidelines for representation on LTC planning committees were described in the local planning framework document. Suggestions were also made for community development and roles and responsibilities (MOH, MCSS, and MC, 1993b). The planning group reiterated the government's intention to have newly constituted

LTC committees of DHCs lead the planning process in each community. To forestall criticisms that DHCs were too oriented to the existing medical system, it was insisted in the document that the LTC committees would include representatives of the social service side of LTC and would also be representative of the community (culturally, linguistically, and spiritually). Membership would consist of one-third consumers (people who receive or have received LTC services, their direct caregivers who were family or friends, and persons with disabilities), one-third service providers (evenly distributed between health and social services), and one-third other (representatives of municipal governments, social planning councils, seniors' councils, labour groups, women's groups, multicultural groups, advocacy groups, and members of the general public, also balanced between health and social services). This model was only marginally different from the existing arrangements for DHC, which specified similar groups, albeit in slightly different proportions.

The DHCs and their committees, however, would not run LTC. Instead, they would provide advice to the government (MOH and MCSS) on the allocation and reallocation of LTC resources, while leaving the MOH and MCSS to provide policy direction, set and maintain standards, and establish LTC funding envelopes for each district. The local planning role (and the resources to support it) would be transferred from the fourteen LTC local Area Offices to the DHCs. Although the Area Offices would not be abolished, they would assume a (rather undefined) 'supportive role' to the local planning and implementation process. By 1995 many of their responsibilities were to be incorporated into the central LTC Division, the DHCs, and the MSAs. The plan thus left itself open to the same charges of 'additional layers of bureaucracy' that had been levelled against the earlier models.

5.3.3.3 An Implementation Framework
The third in the Partnership series, *Implementation Framework*, was released in June 1993 (MOH, MCSS, and MC, 1993c). In this document the government intended to provide details on how the province saw implementation proceeding, so that individuals and groups could get involved. The expectation was that MSAs would be up and running across the province by 1995, with a three-year transition period (1993–5) planned. In the description of the responsibilities of the MSAs, it was indicated that MSAs would be expected to provide most services themselves; purchase of services, whether from commercial (FP) or from NFP agencies, would be the exception to the rule. Moreover, if an MSA had to purchase services from a commercial agency, by 1995 it would be allowed to

do so only to a maximum of 10 per cent of its homemaking and professional services budget, or to the existing level (i.e., no expansion in the FP component would be permitted).

The Integrated Homemaker Program (IHP) was to expand across the province from its current level of twenty sites to thirty-eight, and Placement Coordination Services would expand from twenty-three to thirty-six sites. The same bias against FP providers was explicit; NFP health and personal support agencies would provide all services delivered in the new IHP sites, all new service in existing IHP sites, and all new growth in the Acute and the Chronic Home Care Programs and the School Health Support Program. LTC area offices were to establish a steering committee to help communities to make the shift to a new NFP in-home delivery system. Registries were to be established to help match displaced workers from commercial agencies with NFP employers.

Indeed, implementation plans were already under way. An internal steering committee of staff of the LTC division and an external resource group with consumer, service provider, and union representatives had been meeting since the spring of 1992 to advise on the development of a funding system that government expected would be in place by the 1994–5 fiscal year. The government also established a resource group with consumers, workers, unions, educators, and employers to look at developing provincial training and curriculum standards for workers who provided personal care and support.

5.3.3.4 Guidelines for the Establishment of MSAs

The last of the Partnership documents, subtitled *Guidelines for the Establishment of Multi-Service Agencies,* was released in September 1993 (MOH, MCSS, and MC, 1993d). Provincial expectations for MSAs and topics for discussion for MSA development were outlined. The development process for MSAs was to be public, open, and inclusive (within the context of the MSA design features). Each MSA would operate at arm's length from the provincial government and would be governed by a board of directors elected by a voting membership that included consumers, family caregivers, volunteers, and interested individuals.

Because the MSA would unite existing services and provider agencies, it would affect volunteers and staff in agencies whose services were being integrated into the MSA. It was suggested that, to ensure fairness to workers, a human resource strategy for both staff and volunteers would be developed as part of each MSA's plan prior to the establishment of the MSA. Workers transferring from existing service agencies would become employees of the MSA. Unions would have to be involved in the planning to discuss and resolve various labour issues arising from the transfer of staff with different collective agreements, benefit packages, job descriptions, and salary levels into the MSAs. Other issues that would need union involvement included employment and pay equity, the role of volunteers, job security, existing contracts, successor rights, and impact on non-union staff. In the summer of 1994 the government provided two years' funding to the Ontario Federation of Labour to consult with all the health-related unions (not only those affiliated with the OFL) on these changes.

5.3.3.5 Further Details

In August 1993 the director of LTC policy released a draft manual for community-based services provided by multi-service agencies (MOH, 1993). The document was circulated to approximately 100 professional, consumer, and service provider associations to get their views on the direct services that would be provided by MSAs, eligibility criteria, and service maximums. Policies for personal support and professional services were fairly well defined. For community support services, the government sought input about which services should be considered core, consumer fees, and funding policies.

The new LTC Community Services Funding Envelope for any district was to consist of the existing base transfer payment funding for community services and any new funds allocated on the basis of an equity funding formula to equalize regional inequities. This formula, based on population and need factors, was to form the basis for allocating new community services funding to districts. The mandatory basket of core services that MSAs had to provide was further identified. They included meal services, homemaking services, transportation, care provider support, adult day programs, personal support services (homemaking, attendant care, respite care), professional services (nursing, occupational therapy, physiotherapy, social work, speech and language pathology services, nutritionist services), goods and services under specified circumstances, and admission to LTC facilities. By listing community support services first and including them in the mandatory basket of services, the government was indicating a new importance: new power relationships would arise. Discretionary services included social/recreational services, friendly visiting, security checks, and wellness programs. Although this categorization did not mean that these services would not be provided, it did signal that they were seen as a lower priority.

The document was clear in the frequent reiteration that financial resources provided to the MSAs would be limited and that, in consequence, clients could be eligible for services with no guarantee that those services would be delivered. This marked a major change from the principles of the Canada Health Act, under which individuals were entitled to receive all 'medically necessary' services (as long as they were delivered in hospitals or by physicians). In practice, of course, barriers to access for hospital and physician services, particularly waiting lists, might arise. But they had rarely been spelled out as a matter of policy. In addition, although home care services were never included under the Canada Health Act's definition of comprehensiveness, the presence of home care under the OHIP umbrella carried with it the assumption that home-care services were an entitlement. Now, government made it clear: the shift to the community meant a shift out of the terms and conditions of Medicare. In some cases individuals might be able to receive some but not all services or to go on a waiting list; that is, the needs of all persons who required services might not be met, nor might all persons receive the maximum amount of service. The next (Progressive Conservative) government would seize upon this provision to bring in strict eligibility criteria and limits on service maximums, unrelated to issues of medical necessity or patient needs.

Nonetheless, although the Liberals had been planning a similar action, it was the NDP reform that set the precedent that home care services would be offered within fixed budgets and that the costs would move from the OHIP vote (which was volume based) to the LTC vote (which was more easily capped). These budgets would be set regionally (for each MSA), based on estimates of the number of persons with long-term care needs. The authors of the document attempted to have it both ways, arguing that funding for persons with acute-care needs and those with resource-intensive needs would not be capped, but also that resources were limited. As they stated, 'Receiving services is not an entitlement. Local administering agencies must provide service within the available funding. Consequently, priorization criteria have been developed for local agencies to use when confronted with difficult and competing resource allocation decisions' (MOH, 1993, 118). The criteria for service priority, in order, were risk of hospitalization or being placed in a LTC facility within twenty-four or forty-eight hours, services required to enable individuals to engage in competitive employment or attend post-secondary schools, individuals who have moved to another area of the province who have been identified as a priority in the new area, individuals awaiting discharge from hospital, and individuals in the community with multiple personal care and or medical needs who were not at immediate risk of institutionalization. Cost containment through prioritization, waiting lists, and denial of services was clearly going to be the way of the future. Additionally, government would restrict hospital capacity (through hospital restructuring and budget cuts, which in turn dramatically reduced bed availability) and move people more rapidly into the community through reducing length of stay and emphasizing day procedures. These reforms – which, on the one hand, could be interpreted as increasing the efficiency of the hospital system – would mean massive increases in demand for home care services from individuals who formerly would have been treated in hospitals. The implications for the health care system will be addressed in chapter 8.

The MSA planners accepted that there would be means-tested user fees for consumers of particular community support services – specifically, meals, transportation, home maintenance, and some homemaking services. The rationale for consumer fees for community support services was that they relate to basic costs of community living or basic community services that normally would be undertaken by individuals or their families in the course of living in their own homes in the community. Seniors would benefit, however, because the means testing would be based on income rather than on assets. Asset-rich seniors living on fixed incomes would not have to liquidate their estates in order to pay for home care. The principles guiding the development of a fee system were equity (consistent fee across the province, based on consumers' income, not assets, and levied for services related to usual community living costs), affordability/accessibility (reasonable, simple to administer, allowing for maximum service provision), and importance of family and community (fees would not be charged for special support services to family caregivers). No consumer fees were to be applied to friendly visiting, security checks, support services for family caregivers, hospice volunteer visiting services, programming/supervision in Adult Day Programs, and some unspecified goods and services.

As had occurred with previous reform efforts, support for general principles tended to evaporate once governments moved beyond comfortable generalities into operational details. Release of the documents, coupled with the announcement that these comprehensive delivery agencies would actually be set up, mobilized societal groups as the impact on their interests became evident. Informal linkages among provider agencies had already been established during the Social Contract process. Now, concerned about the viability of their organizations, NFP and FP agencies started meeting to plan a joint strategy. Volunteer organizations, worried that there would be no role for them in the new MSAs, joined with organizations that delivered services through paid staff.

Community support service agencies joined with health agencies offering professional services. Multicultural groups feared that government's emphasis on anti-racism left little room for the specific concerns of particular ethnic groups (e.g., the provision of particular types of food or services in particular languages) and became more vocal. Unionized workers were pitted against unorganized workers and community workers against institutional workers; and everyone was pitted against the government plan.

5.3.4 Anticipating Objections

On 11 January 1994 the NDP health minister, Ruth Grier, was a keynote speaker at a two-day conference of DHCs. In her remarks she took the opportunity to address some of the criticisms that had been voiced about MSAs. She indicated that the government was not completely in control of the timing and development of MSAs: 'I have to sound vague because that will be up to you. This really is a partnership. There isn't a cookie cutter at Queen's Park ... that this will be same all across the province. We are doing this to ensure that the system reflects the diversity, the history, the experience and the individual needs of each community.' She went on to say that MSAs would be independent community – not government – organizations. They would not be huge, bureaucratic institutions. The integration of services was to ensure primacy of the consumer and achieve administrative efficiencies. She asked the DHCs to 'ensure that the citizen-consumer perspective – what we usually refer to as the public interest – becomes and remains the driving force of LTC reform.' She referred to the above-mentioned manual as being key to bringing about a rational planning and allocation process that treated all parts of the province fairly. She reinforced both the importance of volunteers, indicating that they would have an enhanced role, and the fair treatment of employees. She believed that, owing to the expansion of the LTC sector, there would be an expansion of jobs and therefore job security (see Grier, 1994a, 2, 4).

In January 1994 the government released a series of 'Questions and Answers' (MOH, 1994) in which its hope that the establishment of MSAs would remove systemic obstacles to cooperation was noted. Under the current system, service agencies competed with each other for government funding. The elimination of this competition was intended to be the incentive for current agencies to amalgamate with MSAs. The government's position, however, was somewhat disingenuous. Granted that agencies could not compete if they did not exist, existing agencies felt that they provided valuable services, and they resented having their concerns dismissed as 'turf protection.' The government's plan could be interpreted as meaning that existing FP and NFP agencies would cease to exist or that they would no longer be offering their existing mix of services. The government argued that, especially in times of fiscal restraint, tax dollars should be directed towards services and wages rather than profit. In addition, these services should be accountable to the communities they served through volunteer boards of directors. It argued that the limit of 10 per cent for external purchase of services for the government represented a balance between its philosophy of an NPF system and the need to minimize the impact on consumers and workers, adding that this NFP policy was not to be seen as reducing consumer choice, because the consumer would continue to have the choice of worker. In reality, however, not only was it unlikely that vulnerable populations would be choosing particular workers, but organizations argued (with some justification) that choice went beyond particular employees to questions of organizational vision and performance. Government and providers were talking past one another, using similar language to convey dramatically different meanings.

The FP providers were even more uneasy because of the stated preference for NFP delivery. Many believed that the eventual goal of the NDP was to eliminate all FP providers from LTC.

The government was soon to table legislation that would provide the legal framework for LTC community services. The legislation would integrate community service programs into MSA agencies designated by the minister and would apply consistent rules, standards, and criteria; it would provide rights and appeal mechanisms for consumers similar to those for facility residents; it would limit the external purchase of services, thereby enabling the shift to an NFP delivery system; and it would restore takeover powers and subrogation rights that were lost in the transfer of programs from MCSS to MOH. More ominously, however, in terms of the government's successful execution of its blueprint for reform, the legislation once again provided a focal point for the expression of concern and attacks by societal interests, attacks that would be successful in stalling implementation of the MSA plan.

5.4 Conclusions

LTC reform in the first three years of the NDP mandate was transformed from a pseudo-Liberal incremental policy to one that more closely reflected this government's ideology – community participation and empowerment, NFP delivery, support for community support services, and integration of service delivery under one agency. The NDP had no commitment to its first model, a minor variation on the previous Liberal model. Because the government was busy still learning the ropes in their first year, the SCA model was developed by the same bureaucracy that had given birth to the Liberal model. *Redirection of Long-Term Care and Support Services in Ontario* (MCSS, MOH, and MC, 1991) was clearly used as a launching pad by the New Democrats to gather support for their own vision.

The period was marked by the mobilization of formerly marginalized groups through the financial assistance of government. Both the Senior Citizens' Consumer Alliance and the Ontario Community Support Association had concerns with the brokerage model. The former wanted health and social services to be integrated into one agency to improve access. The latter wanted to remove the distinctions between professional and support services that always left it as the poor sister. For OCSA an integrated model that removed the distinctions and delivered all services was the solution. Although the SCCA and OCSA had been credited with giving birth to the MSA concept, its origin was debated by most in the policy community. The entwined relationship between seniors, support service provider organizations, and members of the government's political staff gave rise to suspicions that government was pulling the strings. The fact that the Partnership documents were developed by the political staff rather than the bureaucracy gave credence to these views.

The massive public consultation on the *Redirection* document was an exercise in democratic participation. Despite the noble concept, the consultation approach would turn out to work against the NDP by considerably slowing down the process. The Partnership documents, in which the MSA concept and the process for implementing the model were outlined, shifted the boundaries of reform. The new contours of the reform would alert providers who, through the Social Contract process, found new allies with common interests and discovered new strategies to have themselves heard. As will be documented in chapter 6, the conflict between the NDP and labour brought about by the Social Contract would impel government to make concessions under the LTC legislation that would further alienate provider groups, including OCSA, and create conflict between community-based and institutional workers.

CHAPTER SIX

The New Democratic Government and the Multi-Service Agency, 1994–1995

6.1 The New Democrats and the Multi-Service Agency

By 1994, near the end of its mandate, the New Democratic Party (NDP) was finally ready to introduce legislation to implement its new vision for long-term care (LTC). Bill 173, An Act respecting Long-Term Care (Government of Ontario, 1994), generated a further set of interest group submissions to the standing committee process, which in turn resulted in several amendments to the act. The legislation as passed reflected the central-planning elements often associated with social democracy. Within each designated region, the array of agencies currently delivering services would be largely displaced by the new Multi-Service Agencies (MSAs); services would now be delivered by quasi-public sector employees. Unions and their members would be protected and their rights promoted within what formerly had been a largely non-unionized sector. Community support services (although not the providers of those services) would move from the margin into the mandated basket of services, albeit without guarantees that such services would be provided or publicly paid for. Consumers were to be given enhanced autonomy, protection, and control. The sector would be weaned from for-profit provision, while costs would be controlled by moving the home care services budget out of the open-ended universal entitlements of OHIP into a capped home care envelope.

Introduction of the legislation was accompanied by a second round of 'consultations' with submissions from groups in the policy community to the Standing Committee on Social Development. The committee deliberations provided a forum for groups whose mutual interests had been awakened by the Partnership documents and the Social Contract. The NDP were now facing the consequences of having widened the scope of conflict; both the supporters and detractors of the legislation took this opportunity to make further demands on the government. Although some of the demands were for changes within the LTC policy arena, others represented a spillover from other policy communities as interest groups attempted to obtain concessions to deal with undesired consequences of NDP policies in other sectors.

The legislation accordingly evoked far more opposition than the NDP had expected. Possibly lulled by the results of earlier consultations, the government found unexpected alliances emerging. Both for-profit (FP) and not-for-profit (NFP) provider organizations felt that their continued viability was threatened and opposed what they saw as the expropriation of their business activities by the MSAs. Even the providers of community support services could no longer be counted on for support. Although their sector of services was elevated and protected by the legislation, their organizations were not; indeed, the Ontario Community Support Association (OCSA) membership were sufficiently divided in terms of their support for the reform that even that coalition, one of the main sources of support for the MSA approach, would eventually turn against the MSA model. As a result, the New Democrats were confronted by opposition from all provider organizations, for-profit and not-for-profit, as well as professional and support service providers.

Similarly, the legislation exposed the divisions within the 'consumers' constituency. The consultations had primarily brought out healthier seniors; the most frail individuals and their caregivers had not been mobilized. Now, it became clear that the interests of frail seniors differed from those of the well-seniors; providers were able to argue that the sickest individuals were less interested in 'wellness' than in obtaining 'necessary' professional services.

Another source of controversy was the provisions in the act relating to the workforce in this policy sector. The NDP's attempt to appease the labour movement by giving union members preference for positions in the MSA over non-organized workers had both intended and unintended effects. Many community-based organizations were not unionized; accordingly, there was increased unionization activity within the sector in order to protect the jobs of experienced workers who might otherwise have lost their jobs to displaced hospital workers. However, within labour itself there was conflict. Even unionized workers in the community sector believed that they were going to lose positions to unionized workers from the institutional sector with greater seniority who had been displaced through hospital restructuring.

The forced amalgamation of providers under the MSA, the labour concessions, and the 80-20 rule for MSA-provided versus externally procured services were the parts of Bill 173 that evoked the most vociferous opposition. Meanwhile, the potentially most significant element of the legislation in terms of the overall development of the sector – the transfer of the Home Care budget from OHIP into a capped envelope, thereby removing the universal entitlement status for those services – received hardly any notice. Bill 173 removed one of the few remaining impediments to the passive privatization of health care in Ontario, clarifying that as care shifted out of hospitals, it would indeed be removed from the protections of the Canada Health Act.

Although the NDP did manage to pass Bill 173, the MSAs would join the long list of Ontario's non-implemented LTC models. The government's emphasis on community participation delayed the process sufficiently to move implementation into an election cycle. It was evident that the unpopular Rae government was unlikely to be re-elected. Failure to address fiscal issues early in their mandate had forced the government to make unpopular decisions late in its term, which is usually fatal to electoral chances. In particular, the Social Contract process, which was designed so that employers and workers could reach an agreement with government on how to deal with the debt and deficit crisis, had brought together an unlikely coalition, which actively sought to defeat the LTC legislation (unsuccessfully) and to work against the NDP during the election campaign. The bill's opponents also successfully lobbied both opposition parties; it was clear that neither would fully implement the MSAs as planned. Accordingly, the the new PC government, led by Mike Harris, could claim a mandate to modify and effectively undo the legislation. As will be shown in chapter 7, Bill 173 was drafted in such a way that the Harris government could use it to implement a completely different model, which eliminated most of what the NDP believed to be its critical elements. The fact that this was new legislation – outside the entitlements that, although not required by federal legislation, had long been features of Ontario's earlier models – proved to be a mechanism by which the Progressive Conservatives could radically alter the shape of LTC. 'Reform' would prove to have many meanings; in this state-centred policy community, changing the legislative framework in effect meant the removal of one more constraint upon government action.

6.2 Bill 173, An Act respecting Long-Term Care

On 6 June 1994, during Seniors' Month, Minister of Health Ruth Grier introduced Bill 173, An Act respecting Long-Term Care, in the legislature for first reading (Government of Ontario, 1994; Grier, 1994b). Her statement and the accompanying press release highlighted the consumer Bill of Rights and the Appeals Process (Ontario Ministry of Health (MOH), 1994a). On 15 June the bill received second reading (Wessenger, 1994). Paul Wessenger, parliamentary assistant, who moved second reading of the bill, continually emphasized the aspects believed to be important to the government's supporters – consumers, community support service organizations, and unions. For example, in keeping with the NDP's respect for diversity, his speech highlighted requirements that boards of MSAs must reflect 'the diversity of persons to be served by the agency in terms of gender, age, disability, place of residence within the geographic area to be served by the MSA, and cultural, ethnic, linguistic and spiritual factors' (Wessenger, 1994, 1019).

In listing the mandatory services to be provided by MSAs, the NDP also showed an affinity for grass roots organizations. Mr Wessenger began with the 'softer' social services, such as community support services, not mentioning professional services until the end of the list. He indicated that the mandatory service scheme would put all four types of services and providers 'on a level playing field.' 'Community supports provided by volunteer agencies such as Meals On Wheels are equal players with homemaking, attendant care and professional services' (Wessenger, 1994, 1018). However, while the government mandated the basket of services to be offered by MSAs, it made it clear that these services, while potentially on offer, would not necessarily be provided (Ontario Minister of Health, 1994); rather than expanding services, the bill could be read as marking a shift from universal entitlement to restricted access, the criteria governing resource allocation remaining somewhat murky. As noted above, acute home care services previously had fallen under the Health Insurance Act as an insured benefit to Ontario citizens; the home care program provided approximately 90 per cent of the total provincial spending for community-based health and personal care. Now, home care would move outside the entitlements under the health insurance program; it would be governed by its own act and its own approaches to priority setting.

The NDP had made a minor concession to the existing providers: MSAs would be able to buy services from external agencies with up to 20 per cent (rather than the 10 per cent previously stated) of their approved budget, but this restriction would apply independently to each of the four categories of services. Similarly, although these services could be purchased from either the NFP or the FP sectors, the government made clear its intention that any new spending in LTC services would be directed to the NFP sector. Indeed, by this date there were only a few regions in Ontario that exceeded the 10 per cent limit of their current in-home budget on purchasing services from the commercial sector (MOH, 1997). The shift to an NFP delivery system had begun. Indeed, to protect their volumes of business activity some commercial agencies were seeking NFP status (MOH, 1997). Nonetheless, the funds available for external purchase would not be sufficient to preserve existing organizations; were the bill to be implemented, many would lose some or all of their government funding as activities they had been paid to provide moved to the MSAs. As a nod to the disability community, Wessenger reminded them that on the previous evening, the minister had announced a $4.4 million pilot project for direct funding to persons with disabilities, implying that they would not be directly affected by the shift to MSAs.

A Bill of Rights for consumers of LTC services was part of the act; its terms included consumer dignity; respect; autonomy; individuality with respect to cultural, ethnic, spiritual, linguistic, and regional differences; the right to information, including written notice of rights; the right to give or refuse consent to the receipt of services; the right to raise concerns or recommend changes to services; the right to launch appeals regarding service decisions; and the right of individuals to have their records kept confidential. However, the only individuals with rights under the Act were those who were in receipt of services. The government made it clear that the Bill of Rights did 'not represent an entitlement to service; the rights apply only to consumers who are receiving community services funded under the Act' (Ontario Minister of Health, 1994). The bill did, however, provide rights to appeal the determination that a consumer was not eligible for a particular community service, exclusion of a particular service from or amounts of service in a service plan, and the termination of service. This appeal would be heard by the same body that adjudicated denials of coverage under the Ontario Health Insurance Act: the Health Services Appeal and Review Board, an independent body made up of members of the general public, albeit appointed by the province, and mandated to decide only whether or not the ministry's decision was correct and in accordance with the relevant legislation and regulations. Although, as stated earlier, the subsequent PC government would be able to implement their reform without constraint from the NDP legislation, the Bill of Rights and its appeal process would prove to be a thorn in its side.

Under the legislation, the minister had the authority to provide community services directly, to establish and operate facilities to provide services, to make agreements with others or make payments to others to provide services, and to provide financial assistance regarding capital and operating expenditures incurred by others in providing service.

Although the NDP rhetoric stressed local control, the approach remained centralized. The minister of health was given broad powers under the act, which included the approval and designation of agencies as MSAs. Boards of health and municipalities, which in many regions had been providing home care services, did not receive preferential treatment; indeed, they could be designated MSAs only after the suitability of other approved agencies had been considered. The minister's powers included imposing terms and conditions on the designation of an agency as an MSA, as well as approving the premises chosen for the MSA and setting terms and conditions on the approval. One of the factors that the minister was directed to consider when designating an approved agency was the composition of the agency's board of directors, which was expected to reflect the diversity of the community. It also had to include persons experienced in both the health services and the social services fields. No employee of the MSA could be on the board, a clause that would aggravate labour. The minister could also appoint directors and program supervisors. The minister had the authority to revoke approval of an agency and designation of an MSA. The act also included takeover powers of both an approved agency and a designated MSA and the removal and replacement of some or all of the directors of an MSA.

There was a long list of matters that were to be set by regulation, including duties, functions, selection, composition, and powers of directors; additional services that could be added to the mandated basket of services; the development and implementation of a plan for the recruitment and use of volunteers; eligibility criteria; the amounts of different classes of services to be provided; the development of plans of services and waiting lists and the ranking of people on them; the termination of services to a person; consumer charges and how they were to be determined; and the purchase of external services. The extent of matters left to regulatory powers would concern those who wanted their rights and entitlement protected by legislation and would concern others who felt that their individual liberty was encroached upon. It would also prove useful to the PC government of Mike Harris, which was able to use this wide-ranging regulatory power to reverse, in effect, the intentions of the act in the implementation process.

The proponents of the act also used the legislative opportunity to clean up other, rather unrelated issues within the health care system.

One notable inclusion was an amendment to the Ministry of Health Act to normalize the operations of District Health Councils (DHCs), which had been acting under the provisions allowing ministers of health to seek advice. Now, for the first time, DHCs were given legal authority for their ongoing activities: to advise the minister on health needs, to make recommendations on the allocation of resources to meet those needs, to make plans for the development of a balanced and integrated health care system for its geographic area, and to perform any other duties assigned to it. Even this reaffirmation of the status quo was not uncontroversial; the codification of DHC powers concerned those who worried about the medicalization of the LTC system and others who worried about giving too much authority to regional bodies.

The act left other issues to the implementation process. A key omission was its silence on human resources issues such as the rights of employees in existing agencies, the transfer of employees to MSAs, and the status of collective agreements. This omission would be key in subsequent conflicts between labour groups and management.

6.3 Government Interests

Although some of this legislation was incremental, the bill included a number of design decisions that sharply departed from the status quo. These decisions include those related to direct service delivery by the MSA, human resource issues, NFP preference, the 80-20 external purchase rule, the inclusion of community support services into the mandated basket of services to be provided by the MSAs, the decision to remove Home Care from the OHIP vote, and user fees. How were these decisions perceived?

6.3.1 Direct Delivery

On one level, the shift from the brokerage model to the MSA could be viewed as a pragmatic solution to the fragmentation of the existing system, analogous to business efforts to achieve vertical and horizontal integration. Certainly, in its public statements, the government defined 'one stop' as going beyond an integrated information, assessment, and referral nexus to 'a functional integration of information, referral, assessment, case management, *service delivery* and *follow-up.*' By integrating these services under one agency, the government stated that it recognized the interrelationship of a person's health care and social support needs. Government also believed that it could achieve the further integration of health and social services by the participation of persons from both fields on the boards of MSAs and on the LTC Committees of DHCs (Ontario Minister of Health, 1994, 7).

G: All governments were trying to deal with the same thing – fragmented services. How do you coordinate the services? And the two approaches that emerged were obviously the brokerage approach, where you have the single access point and the referrals are made. But it seemed that there was an incredible duplication of administration ... and you still ran the risk of fragmentation and of people's need not being completely met. The Multi-Service Agency approach ... contrary to the criticism that arose afterwards that [they were] big bureaucracies, etc., that approach actually would allow, in catchment areas, an organization to be there with all the different basket[s] of services ... either on a purchase basis or direct delivery ... and that it would be a more seamless delivery of service to relate to the institutional side ... Seniors move in and out of hospitals, and to have the right connection back to the community for the home support ... So integration, we thought would take place a lot better with the Multi-Service Agency approach at the community level.

The government's approach was accompanied by a belief in 'the community'; 'community governance' and integrated service could be obtained only if the existing plethora of service agencies, each with its own board of directors and interests, was removed from the picture. As a bonus, the MSA model was seen as encouraging cooperation, rather than competition, and ensuring that public funding would go towards services for consumers and wages for workers rather than to profits and organizational 'waste.'

G: The (project) was a coalition of a whole lot of agencies, and we had naively at that point dreamed that you went from co-location, getting them all working in the same building, to coordination, which meant sharing services, to integration. And here I was twelve years later ... and that [project] had never moved beyond coordination to integration because for each partner in the coalition to justify their own existence to their own funders, to their own board, they had to have their own intake, they had to have their own files; they had to have confidentiality releases, and these were barriers to integrated service delivery.

From this technocratic perspective, direct delivery could be sold as a model that would further the values of efficiency (integration) and equity (consumer empowerment and access). Politically, however, direct delivery also had to do with more centralized control and allowing labour to organize the community-based sector.

6.3.2 Human Resource Issues: Unionization and Protection of Collective Agreements

The NDP's legacy was that its initiatives tended to be viewed within the context of the party's ideology. Accordingly, some believed that a key reason for shelving the brokerage concept was to assist labour in unionizing the sector. At the time of the reform, most hospital-based workers were unionized. In contrast, fifteen unions represented at least some workers in the heavily non-unionized sector of community-based services. The Canadian Union of Public Employees (CUPE) represented almost half of them, with the Ontario Nurses' Association (ONA) representing a further 25 per cent of workers in home care programs (MOH, 1997). To these observers, the MSA structure was an attempt to institutionalize the government's ideas regarding markets and employer-employee relations and to secure the interest of its major support group. The fact that unionization of workplaces increased during this period provided support for their perceptions.

P: I suspect that a good part of it [MSA] would have had to do with the NDP's agenda. The other piece concerned the displacement of unionized workers. The MSA model better suits the labour movement. The NDP made it very, very clear ... that one of the objectives was to unionize the entire health sector. As you know, while hospitals are heavily unionized – I forget the number; we're talking a figure of 80 or 90 per cent – it's the reverse at the community level. Most of them are not unionized. And the MSA model, more easily, was a better vehicle than the brokerage model. Because the brokerage model has kept everything ... split up and it's straight contractual arrangements ... I think that was a conscious decision of the NDP. Fair enough, I mean, it was part of their philosophy.

P: During the hearings when they put in the clause ... that non-unionized workers would basically be at the bottom of the rung and unionized workers would go job to job into the community ... that's when I could not believe how profound[ly] the ideology had prevailed. I could not believe that that's what this was all about ... Really, it was absolutely clear that unionization was the issue, absolutely clear.

P: The reason why I'm saying this is because [the respondents' organization] underwent incredible amounts of unionization from the time that they announced the MSA to the time when the PCs got elected. Because people thought, 'If I don't get (into) a union, I may not have a job.' So I think with the RPNs [Registered Practical Nurses], the unionization at least doubled, if not more than that. And with ONA there were a significant number of bargaining units, and some other[s]; CUPE got a couple, and OPSEU [Ontario Public Sector Employees Union] got a couple.

The creation of a unionized environment was viewed not only as part of NDP ideology, but also necessary to placate labour, which had been alienated by the Social Contract process and was further threatened by upheaval in the public sector, owing to the recession, and by the restructuring that was taking place in the hospital sector. This view was held by both provider groups and those within government, albeit with slightly different emphasis, the former emphasizing the rebuilding of relationships and the latter emphasizing recognition of negotiated rights and justice.

P: The theory was the unions agreed with this [Social Contract] and went along with this because they had sold them the concept that unionized positions would emerge in the community to offset the downsizing in the hospital system. And that's how they got them to the table to accept some of the concessions for the Social Contract ... and the premier had got the hospital unions to be quiet through the Social Contract activity by guaranteeing that they would create an infrastructure in the community that could accommodate them.

G: I think that in a complicated way it is related to all of that. But the fundamental issue [was] ... recognizing that we were in a major way restructuring, that would cause displacement of workers, and that there had to be some way of fair treatment of workers and ... recognizing that where there are unionized workers and there are rights that have been achieved through collective bargaining – that there has to be a way of some recognition of that.

At the time, unemployment was a critical issue, and many health care workers feared for their jobs. The definition of seniority and successor rights accordingly presented workers with a 'zero sum game' – preferences for some workers might mean that others were out of work. Not surprisingly, this 'no win' situation caused conflict between labour groups. Although the government saw itself as pro-workers, the perception from the outside was that not all workers were equal. The divisions consisted of unionized versus non-unionized workers, community versus institutional workers and skilled versus less skilled workers. There were strong feelings about the hierarchy of claims.

G: The home support side was non-unionized. The Home Care [Program] ... was unionized ... the jobs that were going to open up on the home support side, you were going to be displacing people who had been working in that field in a non-unionized environment who would be [in second place to] ... some orderly or some nursing attendant [from the closed Brockville Psychiatric Hospital], I don't mean to be pejorative, who was unionized ... [They] would have first dibs on that community care job over the people [already] in that work. It was unconscionable.

These complaints were dismissed by some within the government bureaucracy who argued that unionized and non-unionized workers were not equal. From their viewpoint, both sets of workers had made choices that structured their relationship with their employer. One group paid for their legislated rights through organizing, bargaining, and dues; the other did not. To these policy makers, non-unionized workers were not entitled to the same protections as their unionized counterparts until or unless they unionized. Ironically, this championing of the rights of labour followed on the heels of the disregard of negotiated collective agreements shown during the Social Contract process. The recession tested many of the government's principles.

G: They are not unionized and they are, therefore, represented by their employer. And so in terms of conditions of employment, they have by default, designated their employers. So, [government] will talk to their employers, but [government] is going to talk to the unions. And those are the two people [government] is going to deal with. And if the employers don't do very well for their workers, that was a choice that was made by their workers.

G: Well, unionized workers have a collectively bargained set of rights. They have, you know, traded off things to get rights like job security and other sorts of things. And to simply, in my view, to simply ignore that and say that has no special status is to look at union busting ... And so, I think, that while there was a response from people who had workplaces that were non-unionized saying, 'Well, what does this mean about me?' from a trade unionist point of view, the answer would be to organize and, you know, to collectively bargain for those rights. It wasn't a diminishing of those individuals or their rights under statute, but there is a recognition of the statutory right to organize and to collectively bargain, and to ascertain rights that are above and beyond what the statutory minimum are.

One government official begged the question by insisting that there would have been enough jobs for everyone, even with hospital restructuring. In reality, the job loss was grossly exaggerated and exacerbated the division between the institutional and community sectors of care.

G: Both the Hospital Association and the health-bargaining agents had, I think, done quite a disservice to the community by advancing enormously preposterous estimates of the number of displaced workers. If I recall, in '92, both of those groups forecast job loss at 14 to 15 thousand ... Actual job loss across the sector that year – it was a sector of 160,000 people – was about 2,500. And of those, most were handled by early retirement and other measures. There were actually very few people who were displaced and needed employment. The consequence of that was to convince the government that it needed to make significant efforts on labour adjustment – the HTAP [Hospital Training and Adjustment Program], later expanded to the whole sector. And the bargaining agents made a forceful case that there were going to be massive shifts out of institutions into the community. The community sector was absolutely resistant to accepting anybody that worked in an institution, to the point of saying even if their skills were equivalent, you know ... we don't want them. So, I think, the government was pushed from one side by the bargaining agents, but also found the attitude of the community sector – and I would say personally, I found the attitude of the community sector somewhat startling.

Among the unionized/non-unionized and community/institutional divisions, little attention was paid to the legislation's provisions allowing MSAs to substitute lower-skilled (and lower-cost) workers. The Act did not specify what professional or trained non-professional had to be employed to provide a particular service. In conjunction with the redefinitions of controlled acts under the Regulated Health Professions Act, the door was opened for lower-cost personal support workers or attendants to provide some highly personal procedures and treatments that formerly would have been provided by higher-cost nurses. This was presented as a mechanism for freeing nursing staff to be able to provide care for which only they were qualified (Ontario Minister of Health, 1994). The substitution of lower-cost workers may have been fiscally prudent, although evidence collected subsequent to this period suggests that less skilled workers may be less efficient and provide lower-quality care, particularly where direct supervision is less feasible (Baumann et al., 2001; Hall et al., 2001; O'Brien-Pallas and Baumann, 1999; O'Brien-Pallas, Baumann, and Lochhaas-Gerlach, 1998).

Regardless of the clinical implications, however, labour substitution clearly had the potential to exploit already low-paid workers and to erode the wages and benefits of higher-skilled workers. This was yet another provision that would be used by the Harris government when it came to power.

6.3.3 For-Profit versus Not-for-Profit Delivery

At the time the New Democrats introduced their reform, the FP sector received 33 per cent of all government funding for in-home services, largely, but not exclusively, for homemaking services, with a smaller proportion directed to nursing and therapy services. The NDP had a strongly rooted preference for NFP service delivery, believing that public dollars should go towards services and should not end up in the pockets of private investors. The argument was couched in terms such as not allowing the misfortunes of others to be used to actualize profits. The commercial sector was also viewed as exploiting easy markets rather than meeting needs in unprofitable locales.

This debate tended to further polarize the organizations delivering care. Conceptually, much of this discussion was remarkably non-nuanced in its treatment of the term 'for-profit.' It is evident that organizations are heterogeneous: all FPs are not alike; neither are all NFPs. Clarifying the nature of differences within and across the private subsectors and their impact on the quality of care and the efficiency of the system are empirical questions for which there was not much evidence. Even within the FP sector there is a distinction between FP organizations that are investor owned and those that return an income to providers (Deber, 2002; Deber et al., 1998). Virtually all physician services, for example, are provided by FP providers. The rhetoric of 'not profiting from illness' was accordingly unconvincing to many, since all were aware that health providers, by definition, earned their incomes from providing such services. Indeed, in some cases, the line between NFP and FP related to nomenclature (was an excess a 'surplus' or a 'profit'?), the uses that would be made of such surpluses (in-service education? charity care? nicer offices and higher wages?), as well as willingness of the organization to comply with the legal provisions (e.g., board composition and reporting relationships) required to acquire NFP status. Nonetheless, government spokespersons continued to object to the concept of profit, assuming (without much evidence) that NFP agencies were qualitatively different in the nature of the care they provided, the clients they served, and the way in which staff were treated. As suggested in the literature reviewed in chapter 2, there are indeed reasons to believe that, in the absence of monitoring and defined standards, there are greater incentives for FP organizations to provide only the minimum care required, particularly when they are investor owned (Deber 2002; Devereaux et al., 2002). Nonetheless, there was remarkably little evaluation of existing service provision, and a number of FP agencies that believed they were making contributions to the community understandably resented the assumptions that they were sub-standard.

G: The service should be provided so that all of the funding that you're going to be using from government will go directly to the service and NFP [agencies], and what profit means is that one person or two people will end up making a lot of money and will be taking it away from the service that needs to be provided ... There's only so many dollars for any service that you're going to provide ... Nobody should be gaining money; it's the philosophy of [the NDP] party, nobody should be gaining on the ill health of an individual.

G: (There was) absolutely a very clear preference for NFP and a desire not to see the FP sector grow. That's both ideological and, in terms of our commitment and also from my point of view, quite practical – what I saw in terms of the FP sector was a lot of skimming of the easiest sort of patient to take care of and the high-density markets where volume could produce profit and sort of a claim of efficiency. Compared to the NFPs that were servicing the longer distances, the more difficult cases, etc., I think there was both a practical and a very strong ideological reason for that.

The desire to eliminate the FP sector was viewed by several government officials as the factor motivating the elimination of the brokerage model in favour of direct delivery of services. For political optics, however, the MSA was marketed as anti-brokerage rather than anti-FP.

G: When the NDP started to think through this and they looked at the brokerage model, they realized that it was very difficult. The private sector was there. They were [developing] an increasing market share. And they [NDP] didn't know how to keep them out. So one of the ways of keeping them out was to say 'no brokerage.' If you say 'no brokerage,' you have to provide service directly. From my perspective that was the driving force for the MSA model. Okay. Because if you didn't have brokerage, and you weren't buying service, but were engaging or employing everybody, then the private sector's gone. Now originally when they came out with that, it became an anti-brokerage model ... and ... my sense of what the drivers were that influenced the shaping of the MSAs was the attempt to drive the private sector out of health care and that arena.

The commercial sector responded to this direct threat by launching a lawsuit rooted in the premise that creation of the MSAs amounted to expropriation of their business without compensation. According to one government official, a potential defence against the lawsuit was that the government, in establishing the MSAs, did not discriminate against the commercial agencies, because their new model would have a negative impact on all existing agencies providing home care services. The services provided by both the commercial and NFP agencies would be subsumed under the MSA.

G: So they had a lawsuit. That was a good lawsuit. It was going to be very expensive. It was going to be very embarrassing. So that's how they got around it, you see. You employ everybody! 'We're not discriminating. We've got a bottom line – there's only so much you can buy outside of the MSA, whether it's private or not-for-profit.'

6.3.4 External Purchase of Services

The restriction on the external purchase of services became known as the 80-20 rule, specifying that a maximum of 20 per cent of an MSA's budget could be used for the purchase of services external to the agency. In addition to discouraging FP provision, government officials had several pragmatic reasons for allowing external purchase, ranging from practical issues to ensuring integration and continuity of services and political expediency.

G: Well actually, that [20 per cent external purchase] was because we knew that we'd need to do things like vacation coverage, emergency coverage – or where we required a service but only needed it for a few clients and it would have been economically unfeasible to hire a full-time person.

G: It was simply a question of had there been ... no sort of, restriction on it [external purchase] we felt that we would not have achieved a fully integrated service delivery agency.

G: There are substantial quantities of service currently provided or were provided at that time by other than not-for-profit agencies. And I think the ministers were convinced that to move to eliminate that would place an unreasonable burden on clients and patients ... that is, if the net result of the long-term care reform was somebody who was getting service would stop getting service that was clearly going to be the headline.

G: My sense is that the NDP would have been just as happy if there was no outside purchase of service. But they recognized that there was probably a need for some political salve. I don't think the 80-20 was calculated on any particularly sound methodological basis. It was just a kind of salve that allowed some purchase of specialized or unusual services ... but still preserved a large enough chunk for the MSA to control. And as salves go, I don't know that it made anyone horribly happy.

6.3.5 Mandated Basket of Services

The NDP model, as indicated earlier, also broke with the previous models by including community support services, such as meals on wheels and transportation, in the basket of mandated services. This policy innovation could be seen as operationalizing government's stated belief in the importance of broader 'determinants of health' and the accumulation of research findings that keeping people in their homes was dependent on social supports rather than solely on traditional professional services. Indeed, two of the ministers involved in reform, Ruth Grier of Health and Elaine Ziemba of Citizenship, as well as a number of their political staffs, had worked or been involved with community support services before they came to government.

G: When you think about what people need to keep themselves in the home – well, meals on wheels and friendly visiting, somebody just to check that you're okay, and supportive ... And [Britain has] done a lot of amalgamation of health and social services, and it was really success- ful because you don't know where health stops and social service begins. And so [the government was] really trying to make an effort to sort of put them together so that, in fact, if you're the client you don't care which ministry funds you. You just want to make (sure) that you've got it ... So we were trying to do that kind of continuum, and trying to think more about the customer than sort of established cultures.

G: The problem is, you know, with what is perception. And the reality is that those [services] in, get to be the services, and those outside, get to be the add-ons that can be pushed away. And we wanted to ensure that if we're going to have a continuum of services, it was all going to be in one place ... So you didn't end up in a situation where because this was meals on wheels and it was off on the side [outside the basket], it got underfunded and marginalized. Because our concern was that a lot of the literature was telling us that very small interventions were really important to maintain people in their own homes.

Within government, there was a considerable debate as to the likely implications of integrating traditional home care and homemaking ser- vices with support services. On the one hand, integration of budgets would allow reallocation of resources based on changing needs; on the other hand, resources for support services could be absorbed by the mainstream professional services.

G: I mean, on every move of funding you get both arguments being advanced. One that, by combining things you were permitting shifts that were more sensible; that is, people would tend to allocate the resources to their highest and best use. You'd also get the 'defenceless program' argument, that you would get the stronger programs cannibalizing the weaker ones, and that would disadvantage clientele of those programs. That debate raged on certainly the whole time I was there. I don't think I ever saw a single shred of evidence either way on it. So it was a very strong rhetorical debate but with, you know, nothing underneath it.

6.3.6 Entitlement to Home Care

Most of the debate around Bill 173 focused on those issues directly affecting providers – direct delivery, the NFP preference, and the labour issues. There was virtually no mention of the elimination of Home Care as an entitlement by removing it from the OHIP vote. The NDP sought to justify this transfer in the language of equity and efficiency– as an important way of rectifying the geographic inequity in funding allocation across the province (G), or in achieving integration of services and flexibility in resource allocation by placing all public funding for LTC services in one budget envelope. No longer would there be multiple avenues to the same service resulting in multiple assessments, where the mix of totally publicly funded services versus services that entailed a user fee depended less on the need of the client than on the luck of the draw and the knowledge (of either the client or his/her physician) of how to navigate the system.

G: There had to be a continuum of care. And as service providers we discussed this so many different times that it just was not realistic for the person in the home to have to go through all of these different barriers. And also to see some people not getting the service because of lack of information or whatever.

This official went on to say that the move out of OHIP was actually a decision to protect the Home Care budget. Home Care services would be less susceptible to budget cuts under a separate vote than if it remained the 'weaker sister' in the existing OHIP vote.

G: Under OHIP the funding was starting to diminish. There was starting to be a concern that it could be something that could be eliminated eventually. [Because] people do not think that the people living in their own homes require essential services ... there was always the concern that under OHIP, that at some point in time there might be a decision that this isn't essential.

G: As we began to discuss eligibility guidelines, it became clear that having very specific eligibility rules for the part that was funded by OHIP and the ability to construct our own eligibility criteria for the rest would be very difficult. And because we were fully committed and had cabinet and Treasury approval for a great deal of new money going into long-term care, we certainly believed that there was in fact going to be more money available through our model than the proportion that was guaranteed under OHIP ... And in the current climate, where everything is being cut, there isn't a commitment or a firm budget; then I can understand the criticisms that are now emerging ... saying, 'Well, at least we were sure of money under OHIP. We've lost that now.' But it [the decision to remove the budget from OHIP] was (a) to facilitate the implementation of our model, and (b) because certainly in our commitment we were talking more money not less, in doing this. And I think that we were all in the euphoria of believing that there would be more money for long-term care. That as hospital budgets were constrained, there would be even more [money] freed up, and as hospital restructuring and health reform began, some of that money from Health would move into that.

Whereas in the latter viewpoint growth in home care funding resulting from the legislation was envisioned, another government spokesperson was more cynical and saw it as a way of restraining growth, particularly given the projected expansion on the community side because of hospital restructuring, population growth, and the ageing of the population. Under the Health Insurance Act, which governed OHIP, denial of service either because of priority setting through eligibility criteria or a limit on total amount of service gave consumers the right to appeal the decision to the Health Services Appeal Board and to the courts. The new legislation gave no such rights to clients, and hence would enhance the government's flexibility in limiting the projected growth in costs. In this view, what was termed 'community empowerment' through community boards could be seen instead as a way for government to shift both the responsibility and the accountability for making rationing-type decisions away from themselves onto others.

G: An important driver, aside from the brokerage was a sealed envelope. Nobody realized that the home care dollars that were going to [be] put on the table were going to be a closed envelope. And that those [MSA] boards would be really working hard to make decisions ... Hospitals ... all of a sudden, having to look at shorter lengths of stay, and all of a sudden in 1993-94 they are waking up and discovering home care. So the fact that you're planning to send many more people [to home care], we're going to have closed dollars. We've got to plan this together. You [hospitals] can't shorten your length of stay. Because if we've got waiting lists [in home care], or we don't have capacity, they're going to be back in emerg. But we couldn't get their attention ... Everybody tried to hush-hush the fact that it was a closed envelope, you see, with fixed funding. And then you'd make tough decisions, whereas before, on the home care side of it, it was just the more demand, the more you had to supply ... Budgets grew by 11 per cent a year. So that was sort of a hidden step ... you're talking about a closed envelope, which is why they need these independent boards who are going to make these decisions on how they allocate the money. And it's basically a managed system as opposed to an open universal system. But that was very hush-hush. But it became critical to do something to stop the growth and growth and growth.

In retrospect, the earlier expressed belief that there would be more money for LTC services appears naive, particularly given the prevailing fiscal pressures of the time. Providers were having to deal with reduced transfers from the province because of the Expenditure Control Plan. They had to achieve further cuts in their budget because of the Social Contract. Within hospitals and organizations funded on a global basis (including universities), employers forced their workers to take unpaid days off. Although this was sometimes not feasible (particularly when there were service requirements that necessitated workers' being on site), the approach was impossible when organizations were funded on a contract or fee-for-service basis according to which they would be reimbursed only if they performed a service. Existing providers were also facing the costs of pay equity adjustments required of all government transfer agencies. Contrary to the government belief that there was more money for LTC, the signs of restraint were everywhere.

6.3.7 User Fees

The other related debate that did not get resolved while the New Democrats were in government was whether there would be co-payments or user fees for support services. While some favoured the notion of entitlement, others saw this as unrealistic and were more persuaded by notions of affordability.

G: I'm not sure that that had been totally sorted out. The preference, and I wasn't sure I agreed with it, had been for no user fees from any of those community-based services ... I had assumed that we had yet to have the discussion about eligibility and that it would depend to a certain degree on what the level of need was at the point when you became eligible. And if you were totally dependent on the service, then I didn't think a user fee was required. If it was perhaps a bit of an option, then I had seen there might have been room for user fees. But I haven't seen that discussion as being finished.

G: I don't know how much realism there was to it. There [were] certainly ministers who held the view that that [no user fees] is what should happen. But the same ministers also accepted budget numbers that wouldn't permit that to happen.

Ideology, with the injection of fiscal reality, was undoubtedly the driving force behind MSA design features such as NFP centralized delivery by quasi-public sector workers, preference for unionized workers and the creation of an environment more conducive to unionization, the elevation of importance for support services, and consumer empowerment and protection. The New Democrats, based on their notions of community involvement, had consulted broadly and from their point of view had listened to the people. Their design, however, had adversely affected a number of groups who, at least before the legislation was tabled, had no common interest. Even the groups representing 'the people' would turn on the NDP.

6.4 Policy Interests of Societal Groups

Hearings for the Standing Committee on Social Development were held between August and October 1994, with amendments to the Act considered in November. The committee travelled around the province listening to and receiving submissions from many groups. The following analysis is based both on interviews and on analysis of submissions to the standing committee from key members from four categories of interest groups: (1) consumers (including seniors, the disability community, and representatives of multicultural and religious groups serving seniors), (2) providers (NFP and FP, drawn from both professional and support services), (3) labour (both unionized workers and volunteers), and (4) other types of interests. The categorization is not fully 'clean,' especially since many of the associations representing the consumer communities, aside from being advocates for their members, themselves were providers of services largely delivered by volunteers. For example, Alzheimer Ontario provided day programs, respite programs, counselling services, family support groups, education programs, and information services for seniors who are cognitively impaired. It is noteworthy that these groups tended to use competing interpretations of the policy goals of security, equity, liberty, and efficiency to advance their different policy interests.

6.4.1 'Consumers'

Although in the consultations the term 'consumer' was frequently used to refer to those who received home care services, there is some debate about its appropriateness or homogeneity. 'Consumer' has connotations of informed clients choosing the services they demand within a competitive marketplace. It has long been known that these conditions poorly apply to health services (Arrow, 1973; Evans, 1984; Rice, 1998), including most home care services. A number of difficulties arise, including 'asymmetry of information' between care providers and care recipients about what care is 'needed,' or about the quality of competing providers, and the fact that those requiring home care services are often too ill to wish (or be able) to play the role of informed consumer.

The submissions from and interviews with representatives from seniors', disability, multicultural, and spiritual groups highlighted the heterogeneity of the 'consumer' sector. They repeatedly stressed that the ability to assess information and make decisions varied between well and frail seniors and between cognitively and physically disabled people; the last group was most enthusiastic about adopting a consumerist role. Clear distinctions arose between the priorities of seniors and those of the physically disabled. For seniors, the key issues were access to services when needed and the ability to refuse unwanted services (particularly institutionalisation). In contrast, the physically disabled wished to be able to choose their provider. Both groups wanted to participate fully in the decisions involving their care and some assurance that services would be ethno- and spiritually specific. Also discussed were issues of representation on MSA boards and to whom MSAs would be accountable.

6.4.1.1 Briefs from Seniors' Organizations

Briefs submitted by the Seniors Citizens' Consumer Alliance (SCCA), the Ontario Coalition of Senior Citizens' Organizations (OCSCO), the Canadian Pensioners Concerned (CPC), and the Advocacy Centre for the Elderly (ACE) were analysed. While supportive of the legislation overall, these groups reflected their organizational roots or mandate in highlighting which issues were of most concern.

In its brief, SCCA, (1994) strongly endorsed the MSA model as an alternative to the then current system, making only some minor recommendations. As noted in the previous chapter, SCCA had a very close working relationship with the government, to the extent that it had been viewed by many other interests as being the government's mouthpiece. Its earlier report had proposed an MSA-type model, and its submission went as far as to include sections addressing and attempting to refute what its members considered common public myths about the MSAs. They remained convinced that incremental reforms, while politically expedient and capable of making modest improvements in the system in the short term, were not in the best interests of the system or the province in the long term. They believed that individual agencies would not be able to adjust to pressures brought on by federal budget cuts and demographic pressures; comprehensive reform through the integration of agencies was the only way to construct a stronger community-based sector that could resist pressures towards the development of a two-tiered system. They believed that the MSA was the only model that dealt with service fragmentation, the integration of health and social services, assessment and case management, and the inefficiency of 30–40 per cent expenditures on administration and overhead by a plethora of small agencies.

The first 'myth' they addressed in their submission was that MSAs would not be more cost-effective. They had commissioned a paper from a management consulting firm, which arrived at the conclusion that the integrated delivery model was more cost effective than brokerage. (This report would come under attack from provider agencies, which eventually led to its withdrawal by the consulting firm.)

The second 'myth' was that MSAs would be large government bureaucracies accountable only to Queen's Park. They argued that MSAs would be no different from other transfer payment agencies, such as hospitals or community health centres, and that they would be independent NFP organizations governed by representative community boards.

The third 'myth' was that MSAs would limit consumer choice. The SCCA argued that choice of agency never existed within the brokerage model, since it was dictated by Home Care Program contracts. For seniors, choice of individual provider was more important than choice of agency, which the MSA would still protect.

The fourth 'myth' addressed was that MSAs would undermine volunteerism. The SCCA responded that volunteer involvement would increase under MSAs because of better-coordinated recruitment activities, that volunteers identified with the consumer they served rather than the agency, and that experience in other sectors did not support the claim.

The fifth 'myth' was that MSAs would devastate fund-raising activities. The SCCA members argued that MSAs through their community boards and integrated structure would be able to mount comprehensive campaigns and eliminate the current competition for donor dollars.

The sixth 'myth' was that MSAs, as both purchaser and provider, would be in a conflict of interest situation. They dismissed this concern, since the dual responsibility was already prevalent in public hospitals.

While strongly endorsing the passage of the legislation, the SCCA members did express some reservations. They felt that the legislation still fell short of addressing issues of fragmentation. Dividing MSA services into four programs, with separate rules for the purchase of external services and user fees, mitigated against the complete integration of health and social services. They believed that the legislation, by not including supportive housing, wellness and health promotion, primary-care physicians, and regional geriatric programs, did not address the full continuum of care.

The members recognized that funding was key to the success of the reform and that the legislation was silent on this issue. They strongly recommended that the bill clearly state that MSAs would be funded on a global and/or capitated basis. The removal of home care from the OHIP budget was seen as important for the goal of integrating services. They recognized that this act threatened those services, however, and recommended that the legislation be amended to continue to insure under OHIP those home care services that were previously insured under the Health Insurance Act. They also focused their energy on removing any mention of user fees from the legislation. The alliance was against user fees within the reformed long-term care system on the grounds that (1) they produced inequitable access to care, thus deterring those at the lower income scale; (2) they were inefficient in that they were often more expensive to collect than the amount generated; and (3) they continued the distinction between health and social services, therefore negating the increasing belief in the essential preventive effect of social services. Other issues raised included a call for establishing and monitoring explicit provincial standards for quality and an explicit process for monitoring waiting lists.

With respect to consumer empowerment, the SCCA was concerned that the governance structure of MSAs would emerge as federated structures dominated by provider organizations; indeed, the NFP provider organizations would put forward such a model to the Progressive Conservative (PC) government after the defeat of the NDP in June 1995. The SCCA accordingly recommended that consumers and members of the community make up the majority of board members, that employees of provider organizations be prohibited from sitting on the board, and that health and social service expertise be provided by a professional advisory committee to the board. The alliance further wanted more sanctions against agencies that violated the Bill of Rights (SCCA, 1994).

Although OCSCO was a founding member of SCCA, its members made a separate submission to the committee. They claimed to represent sixty-six organizations and 500,000 seniors across Ontario, including the Older Women's Network, the United Steelworkers of America Retirees, OPSEU, and Canadian Pensioners Concerned (CPC). Their submission to the committee reflected concerns about liberty (choice), equity (access), and security (availability of service, quality of care). In their submission, they supported Bill 173 but expressed concern that some services were legislated into the basket of services provided by the MSAs, while others, such as attendant care and supportive housing, were left to regulations. They recommended that the legislation, which they believed was too detailed and therefore rigid, should leave the operational details of reform to the regulations. They strongly rejected user fees on the grounds that they were demoralizing and a disincentive for service. They called upon government to ensure that funding for MSAs be secure, so that there would be no deterioration in service because of waiting lists. Fees, where they existed, should not be means tested. They requested more assurances that the bill ensure that consumers have the 'right of choice' of service, whether it be to remain in the home or to seek placement in an LTC facility. In keeping with their view of consumer empowerment, they recommended that half of the board's representatives be consumers. They defined consumers as individuals who are or will be in a position to receive LTC services. They asked that government establish an independent review board for appeals and that Bill 173 incorporate an enforcement mechanism for monitoring care.

Not surprisingly, given the inclusion of organized labour in their membership, OCSCO saw the introduction and expansion of 'generic workers' and unregulated, non-professional care as an issue threatening the quality of care and the safety of seniors and the disabled. The members demanded stricter regulation of providers, which included proper pay scales, pension plans and other benefits. They asked for recognition and support of family caregivers and payment for their services. Recognizing that patients were being discharged from hospitals 'quicker and sicker' than before, they pressed for an assurance that services would be available in the community before discharge. They rejected the government's claim that it did not have the funds to pay for the original vision of an accessible, equitable and high-quality, long-term care system, and suggested that government reorder its priorities to do so (OCSCO, 1994).

Further highlighting the tenuous nature of the coalitions that had formed, CPC (Ontario Division) a member of OCSCO, also submitted its own brief. CPC advocated on behalf of seniors on health, financial, and social issues. Its members disagreed with OCSCO about how prescriptive the legislation should be; in their brief they argued that too many important decisions, such as fees, eligibility criteria, and hours of service, were being left to regulations. They asked that the proposed regulations be tabled at the time of third reading of the bill or before, so that there might be an opportunity for public input. They also expressed concern about the commonly held, yet untested, assumption that care in the community was less costly than institutional care. They feared that the government had oversold the idea of people wanting to remain in their own homes and asked for the option to choose other forms of care. With cutbacks in facilities, however, they feared that without the necessary funding and expansion of services in the community, consumers would be facing at best inadequate care and at worst no care. They called for a definition of consumer to be incorporated into the bill and for consumers to be fully involved in decisions about their own care as well as in policy and planning decisions. They echoed OCSCO's recommendation that at least half of board memberships should be made up of 'real' consumers and that social services should be represented on a par with health services. They also rejected a medicalized model, arguing that social and recreational programs played an equally important role in maintaining health and noted that, despite the government's professed commitment to a broader definition of health and well-being, no reference was made in the Bill to 'wellness.' Their parting words in the brief reflected frustration with the previous rounds of consultation without implementation: 'Let's get on with it!' (CPC, 1994, 4).

Members of the Advocacy Centre for the Elderly (ACE), a legal clinic for low-income seniors funded by the Ontario Legal Aid Plan, submitted a brief on 15 September 1994. They framed their submission around security/social justice issues, based on the kinds of complaints they typically received regarding community-based services, that is, issues of quality, eligibility, accessibility, and adequacy of service types and volumes. ACE argued that MSA consumers are not typical market consumers in that they are often either cognitively, emotionally, or financially unable to exit if dissatisfied. Voice is their avenue of redress – hence the legislation needed to ensure a tight complaints/appeal procedure, a quality management system that included consumer input, and an alternative dispute resolution mechanism. To address these issues, ACE members recommended that the government make explicit in the legislation changes to the Bill of Rights, eligibility criteria, fee issues, limitations on service, rules regarding termination of services, and waiting lists (ACE, 1994).

6.4.1.2 Briefs from the Disability Community

The briefs analysed for this study from people living with a physical or cognitive impairment came from the Citizens for Independence in Living and Breathing, Ontario March of Dimes, and Alzheimer Ontario. These groups rejected any attempt to medicalize their conditions by referring to them as illnesses or diseases. Instead, they lobbied for giving the affected individuals greater independence and autonomy in decisions regarding their own care, including control over how government funds would be used. They attempted to buttress this case by stressing the 'uniqueness' of their groups and the resulting rationale for keeping their populations (and associated funding) separate under the new legislation. Alzheimer Ontario, which has heavy representation from family members of this cognitively impaired population, called for more support for family caregivers and representation on MSA boards.

The Citizens for Independence in Living and Breathing was a consumer organization representing ventilator users and potential ventilator users with neuromuscular conditions who, because of muscle weakness or paralysis, require breathing assistance. Its members considered themselves to be not ill but living with a disability. As might be expected from earlier accounts, their interests focused on classic liberty issues of independence, choice, and rights protection. While pleased with the Bill of Rights under the MSA legislation, they recommended stronger expressions of rights and entitlement, for example, that access to services be guaranteed for all persons meeting eligibility requirements and that contravention of the Bill of Rights be grounds for the revocation or suspension of an agency's approval. Concerns about independence included the recommendation of a *guarantee*, rather than an *opportunity*, for the consumer or his/her agent of the right to full participation in the development, revision, and evaluation of any plan of service. From their perspective, an opportunity to participate left the provider clearly in control, rather than promoting equal partnership and participation. Fearing the loss of independence and the medicalization of their condition, they recommended that hospitalization for initiation of long-term ventilation be avoided. They also requested representation of a ventilator user on the board of the MSAs, asserting that their needs were unique.

With respect to choice, they 'endorsed with enthusiasm' the phrase in the legislation recognizing the importance of a person's needs and preferences. However, they were concerned that service options for minority groups like ventilator users would be seriously reduced, resulting in their 'ghettoizing.' They further recommended that the direct-funding option be available to all consumers capable of directing their own care and that the option be included in the legislation. Choice and independence were seen as inextricably linked, and the loss of choice was seen as leading to an erosion of control and independence (Citizens for Independence in Living and Breathing, 1994).

The Ontario March of Dimes assisted adults with physical disabilities to live independently in the community through the provision of programs and services that included the Attendant Services Program, Support Service Living Units, and Outreach Attendant Services. While member groups supported Bill 173, they too wanted stronger wording, ensuring the independence, choice, and empowerment of disabled consumers, whom they viewed as unique in their requirements. They unequivocally rejected any medically oriented service philosophy that perpetuated the notion of disability as illness and that promoted dependence. They requested greater consumer involvement in establishing service standards and service plans and on governing boards. They feared that allowing generic workers in the legislation would encourage the use of least costly options at the expense of quality. They recommended that their programs not be included under the MSA but continue to be directly funded by the government because of their uniqueness. They recommended that the direct-funding pilot project legislated under the LTC facilities legislation – a policy that allowed individuals with disabilities to hire their own caregiver – be made a permanent option under Bill 173 (Ontario March of Dimes, 1994).

Alzheimer Ontario, whose members estimated that their group represented the second-largest group of consumers of LTC services, generally supported the legislation. However, they felt that the true providers of most LTC services were not recognized, and they recommended specific reference to support for family caregivers in the purposes of the act. They feared that the translation of the goals of LTC into legislation gave way to a '"health model" of rules and criteria driven by the system rather than by the needs of the consumer or even the local community.' They asked that the focus on consumer need and quality of life be recaptured in the legislation. Unlike other consumer groups whose members are not cognitively impaired and who, therefore, wanted direct rather than mediated representation on governance structures, Alzheimer Ontario protested that the legislation, while spelling out inclusive criteria for board membership (gender, age, disability, geography, cultural, ethnic, linguistic, and spiritual factors) left their members without a voice. They requested that the legislation be amended to require representation by family caregivers of people with Alzheimer's Disease and related dementias on all MSA boards. Finally, they recommended that adult day programs, which are crucial for their members to remain in the community, be added to the mandatory basket of services provided by MSAs (Alzheimer Ontario, 1994).

6.4.1.3 Briefs from the Multicultural and Religious Communities

The Multicultural Alliance for Seniors and Aging was an association of more than forty organizations representing the interests of multicultural communities with respect to the needs of older adults and their families. As might be expected from the demographics of the province, members were drawn primarily from Metropolitan Toronto and Hamilton. The focus in their submission was on choice and consumer empowerment. While supportive of the MSA and the requirement in the legislation of recognition of a person's individuality and respect for cultural, ethnic, spiritual, linguistic, and regional differences, they wanted the empowerment of ethnic seniors through their community and the designation of an MSA as a lead agency for a particular ethnocultural community. They further wanted a formal process for soliciting and appointing ethnic representation on MSA boards. They wanted plans of service to take into account the unique needs of their members and staff to be trained and sensitized to their needs. They also demanded the establishment of multicultural services committees in DHCs, which they viewed as notoriously insensitive to their needs (Multicultural Alliance for Seniors and Aging, 1994).

The Catholic Women's League of Canada (CWL), Ontario Provincial Council is an association of 65,000 members, who volunteer time and raise funds to support local organizations. Although the CWL has been categorized as a group representing consumers with particular spiritual needs, they are also a provider organization and echoed, as will be seen below, many of the same arguments expressed by providers. Their brief estimated that, in the Toronto Archdiocese, members spent over 100,000 hours working with organizations such as the Arthritis Society and Meals on Wheels. Their major objection to the legislation concerned the potential loss of volunteer workers, which they believed would occur as MSAs absorbed existing community agencies into large government-mandated bureaucracies. They argued that volunteers needed to identify with a specific agency and were motivated by the belief that they were essential: if they were not doing the job, it would not get done and someone would suffer. CWL did not feel that MSAs, as government (or quasi-government) agencies, could attract the same loyalty. The loss of volunteers, they argued, would have financial implications for government, which would have to replace them with paid workers. They estimated that it would cost $6 million alone to replace CWL volunteers in Ontario. Added to this cost would be the loss of revenues raised by volunteers through fundraising activities, which they estimated would run over $800,000, from their organization. They worried that government resources would not be sufficient to replace these lost funds and that, in consequence, existing services would be cut (CWL, 1994).

6.4.1.4 Interviews with Consumer Groups

In structured interviews, representatives of consumer organizations reiterated and reinforced some of the above issues. The definition of 'consumer' clearly differentiated groups representing seniors, from those representing persons with disabilities, a difference that had implications both for priority issues and for determining models of service delivery.

C: When the seniors' community talks about consumers, what they're really talking about are family members often, because the person who's using their services is often not in any shape to be on the board. And that was, it's a huge battle ... Our final meetings with the NDP bill had to [do] with the governance, because the seniors were saying, 'Well, if you say it's one-third consumer, you have to have a broad definition.' And of course people with disabilities say, 'I don't want my family making decisions. It's me.'

The FP/NFP question was another issue over which consumer groups divided. Issues of choice versus quality played out in this dimension.

C: The disability community is somewhat different in that it actually, except in the area of health care, doesn't oppose privatization because what they prefer is choice ... So I think they couldn't care less, to be honest, about whether the MSA had the not-for-profit restrictions or not. They weren't prepared to go and fight in the same way the seniors were saying, 'it has to be 80-20' and all of that.

C: Our final position was that not-for-profit is the way to go because for-profit at this time does not have the same rules as not-for-profit, and they can hire people with less training and are cheaper as a result than the not-for-profit.

Another set of issues that divided consumers related to whether services should be standardized or allowed to reflect ethnocultural differences. The issue was potentially contentious, since the longer-established communities (e.g., Jewish, Italian, Chinese) had a more extensive set of available services than did more recently arrived (and less affluent) seniors. These disputes regarding culturally sensitive services were represented either as examples of successful integration of services or as the creation of ethnic ghettos.

C: What unifies the services for seniors in an ethnic community is the ethnic community. So you will have these services developed under one umbrella. So you don't need to worry about the issue of having to merge organizations and do away with existing organization ... They were already Multi-Service Agencies ... But where there was an issue was that we were opposed to a strict geographic definition of MSA boundaries. And we wanted boundaries that could be identified on the basis of communities of interest as well as geograph[y].

C: Under the MSA they would respond to cultural sensitivity to the best of their ability, but not set up ghettos of Italians or Jews or whatever, you know. But try to meet the cultural needs to the best of their ability. There should be in the collection of people, they should be able to cater to the religious, and ethnic, cultural things. Somebody should be able to help them. But we could not see that everybody that was Italian no matter where they were ... they should be serviced within their communities with help from the central area, rather than setting up particular multicultural, ethnic groups [MSAs].

On the whole, however, the overwhelming concern for consumers was to get the reform implemented quickly. Governments had been talking for far too long about reforming the system.

6.4.1.5 Summary of Consumer Interests

It is clear from the submissions and the interviews that all consumers are not alike. Nonetheless, both the main coalition (the SCCA) and the government found it convenient to refer to 'consumers' as though they constituted a homogeneous group. To the extent that such claims are accepted, key interest groups are legitimated in their efforts to claim broad representation and power to speak on behalf of such a large interest group, and government can simplify the process of obtaining consultation and support of policy and program development. A less recognized implication of using the label 'consumer' to refer to those receiving care is that the term carries connotations of market relationships, including a notion that providers should be accountable to the person who pays for the service. These confused lines of accountability had the potential to become problematic, particularly for services that would be paid for through tax dollars; how much say would those receiving care have about the quality of care, identity (and skills) of care providers, and volume of services to be provided to them? Appeals mechanisms were seized upon as the blanket solution; this may or may not have proved adequate in practice.

Offsetting the desire to identify homogeneous spokespersons for consumers was the desire of disability, multicultural, and religious interests to emphasize their differences. Their very existence is predicated on these differences. Each community could (and did) argue the need to respond to differences in language, recreational activities, spiritual practices, culinary tastes, and healing practices. These subtleties played out through the varying recommendations for consumer empowerment and consumer representation on governance structures; most groups sought to ensure that they would be at the table directly, rather than have their interests represented by other consumer constituencies. Similarly, some members of the disability community viewed their own disabilities as unique and not comprehensible by others, requiring direct board representation for each affected group.

Other issues arose around identifying the community of interest. In particular, those with the most severe care needs were least able to participate in the consultation process. Instead, those claiming to represent seniors were drawn largely from seniors' organizations, which are run and populated by the well-elderly. In turn, these groups pushed to expand the consumer constituency to include 'people who will require services in the future;' their interests proved to be oriented towards 'wellness' programs rather than the more medicalized services they did not currently require. Cognitively capable people living with physical disabilities had no desire to have family members as representatives on MSA boards, whereas those representing Alzheimer patients did want stand-ins.

Notions of liberty also varied, but not surprisingly, they reflected the interests that made each type unique as a group. Seniors groups stressed the importance of being able to choose their preferred type of service – that is, home, community, or institutional, or by an individual provider – and they showed less interest in being able to choose a provider agency. Persons with disabilities were concerned about being able not only to choose their own individual provider but also to have direct control over the terms and conditions of their employment. (The potential for a clash with unions and other provider representatives was clear.) The multicultural and religious communities were more interested in choice of provider agencies or an MSA that would cater to their unique needs.

Nonetheless, there were shared concerns, primarily dealing with the adequacy and protection of funding, quality and availability of services, the establishment and monitoring of services, an enforceable complaints procedure, and the establishment of standards of care and eligibility requirements under legislation rather than regulation. Those consumer groups that also either provided services or had a substantial labour component to their membership expressed concern on behalf of the security of workers. However, each group, depending on its own requirements, requested the inclusion of certain services. Well-seniors wanted quality-of-life supports. Cognitively disabled groups wanted adult day care and caregiver supports. With extensive resources, the groups might stay content. If resources were constrained and trade-offs were required, there was clearly a strong prospect for dissension within the 'consumer' group.

6.4.2 Providers

When the MSA was proposed, there were approximately 1,100 community-based service agencies that were directly funded by the government. Most of them would lose their government funding. The government appeared unclear about whether they expected these agencies to disappear altogether (amalgamating many of their functions and staff into the MSA), or whether it expected them to revise their mission and continue with other programs and services outside the mandate of MSAs or delivered to other target groups. It did not seem particularly concerned about whether the agencies would retain enough resources to be able to sustain such activities. As such, it is not surprising that provider groups mobilized quickly and became heavily involved in attempting to shape reform directions.

These organizations were also heterogeneous: some were FP and others NFP. They delivered a mix of services, ranging from professional (e.g., nursing, rehabilitation) to support services provided by paid workers (e.g., homemaking) to services provided largely by volunteers (e.g., meals on wheels). Nonetheless, they maintained a common front, at least initially. The submissions of the Ontario Home Care Programs Association and Saint Elizabeth Visiting Nurses' Association of Ontario (St Eliz.) were selected to represent the interests of NFP providers of professional services; those of the Ontario Community Support Services and the Canadian Red Cross Society (CRCS), Ontario Division, were chosen to represent – FP support services providers; and that of the Ontario Home Health Care Providers Association (OHHCPA) represented FP providers.

6.4.2.1 Provider Alliances
Threatened by various aspects of the legislation, a set of unlikely interests came together to form the Community Providers Coalition. The coalition consisted of both professional and support service providers as well as NFP and FP providers, namely, the Ontario Home Care Programs Association (OHCPA), CRCS, OCSA, OHHCPA, Ontario Home Respiratory Services Association, St Eliz., and the Victorian Order of Nurses (VON). The most contentious aspects of the legislation for the coalition were the amalgamation of agencies into the MSA and the 80-20 restriction; both provisions would affect the viability of provider organizations. Although some coalition members were unionized, they were united in their opposition to the government's intent in offering positions in the newly constructed MSAs to unionized staff in order of priority before they were offered to non-unionized staff. They decried the 'one-size fits all' approach of the government in mandating the MSA model, the basket of services, and the forced transition of thousands of workers into 'yet another enormous bureaucratic structure' (Coalition of Consumer and Provider Groups, 1994a).

During 1994, and particularly during the Standing Committee meetings, the coalition expanded its membership in an attempt to have broader-based representation and appeal. Although it added mostly provider groups to the membership (Association of Ontario Physicians and

Dentists in Public Service, Catholic Health Association (Ontario), Federation of Non-Profit Organizations Working with Seniors, Ontario Association of Medical Laboratories, Ontario Association of Non-Profit Homes and Services for Seniors, Ontario Hospital Association (OHA), Ontario Medical Association (OMA), Ontario Nursing Home Association, and Villa Charities), it also recruited a few consumer groups (CWL; Council on Aging, Ottawa-Carleton; and Ontario Association of Residents' Council). As will be seen, this coalition was highly successful in blocking ultimate implementation of the proposed legislation, although it was less successful in shaping a mutually acceptable alternative. The reasons for this mixed record are evident through an examination of the briefs submitted to government about the proposed legislation and an understanding of the internal conflicts within and across these groups as documented through interviews.

6.4.2.2 Briefs from Providers of Professional Services in Home/ Community (NFP)

OHCPA and St Eliz. had somewhat different expectations about the likely impact of MSAs. OHCPA represented the array of thirty-eight organizations that had previously provided home care services. Together, they comprised over 4,500 staff, including case managers, therapists, homemakers, and nurses. The program was established under the Health Insurance Act as an insured benefit to Ontario citizens and provided approximately 90 per cent of the total provincial spending for community-based health and personal care. While in most locations the Home Care Programs would turn into the MSA with a new board of directors, in Metropolitan Toronto the one Home Care Program would be decentralized into a number of MSAs. Only in Metropolitan Toronto had home care been managed by an independent home care agency; more usually, home care had been managed by a local hospital, public health unit, or NFP provider (such as VON). Most of these branches expected that their paid staff would simply slip into comparable positions within the MSA; that is, instead of working for Home Care they would be working for MSAs. In contrast, St Eliz., like VON, faced the outright elimination of that portion of their organization that provided publicly funded home care.

OHCPA, like most other organizations, expressed support for the abstract principles and goals of the legislation, the integration of health and social services, and the standardization of eligibility criteria and assessment process. However, its members raised a number of concerns about the details. They were worried about the 'de-insuring of Home Care Program Services' by moving services out of the Health Insurance Act, the overly prescriptive nature of the legislation, and the implications of amalgamating most existing agencies for volunteers and workers. They recommended a greater flexibility and local determination around the development of the model and the recognition in the legislation of case management as a mandatory service. Aware of growing pressures on the system from the acutely ill, they asked government to reallocate funding so that care for the acutely ill was not at the expense of the frail elderly currently receiving LTC services. As an employer, they asked for the seamless transfer of their employees to the MSAs and that current community workers be given priority for positions over other socio-health (institutional) sector employees (OHCPA, 1994).

Saint Elizabeth Visiting Nurses' Association of Ontario is an NFP agency with a long tradition of community-based nursing care. While also supporting the goals and principles of reform, St Eliz. members were adamantly opposed to Bill 173. They believed the legislation would lead to the destruction of community-based, non-profit agencies like theirs. MSAs were viewed as regional monopolies that would stifle innovation, would be cost-ineffective bureaucracies, would eliminate consumer choice and volunteerism, and would be insensitive to ethnocultural needs. MSAs were seen as a way for government to control and constrain community services. During this part of the NDP period they would join the informal alliance with other provider groups, including VON and Community Occupational Therapy Associates (COTA), an NFP provider of occupational therapy services.

Many of their arguments were couched in efficiency and liberty terms. 'Consumers want choices. The freedom of choice promotes innovation and excellence.' Underlying these claims were concerns that, once under government auspices, MSAs would be under-funded, since their budgets would be based on government priorities (and resources), regardless of the need in the community. Furthermore, they believed the MSA model would shift onto government costs currently being met through charitable contributions, since they were not convinced that private donors would continue to give to what was perceived as a government agency. Other cost pressures would be felt through the health human resources policies, which encouraged unionized workplaces. Not only was it likely that unions would negotiate enhanced salary and benefits packages – arguably overdue, given that Ontario, unlike several other provinces, had not yet moved to equalize wage levels between the hospital and community sectors – but it was also feasible that they would attempt to ensure that many services currently provided by unpaid volunteers would become the responsibility of paid workers. Furthermore, they suspected that the purported savings in administrative costs through reduction of the number of 'duplicative' agencies would not be realized in Metropolitan Toronto, both because many of these agencies provided services other than home support and would therefore seek to remain in business, and because the MSA model as planned for Toronto would increase administrative overhead by dividing that city's single Home Care Program among approximately twenty MSAs.

St Eliz. members also rejected the argument that NFP agencies were no longer needed to provide home care services. They firmly believed that NFP organizations were essential to fill gaps that neither the government nor the FP sector would fill. 'Under Bill 173, the government is tearing down service structures that are proven to be efficient, effective and sensitive to the changing needs of the community, in the hope that the government itself can do a better job. Many non-profit agencies in this province arose out of the fact that the community recognized the need to fill the service gaps that governments had allowed to develop in the first place' (St Eliz., 1994a, 3). They, like many other such agencies, were unwilling to allow carefully formed infrastructures to be demolished in the hope that such gaps would never again arise; instead, they feared that, come the next shift in government priorities, gaps would again develop and not be filled.

In a sample letter for interested persons to send to their MPPs, which was attached to their fact sheet, St Eliz. members revealed what they viewed as the government's intentions. 'The government has gone beyond addressing the issues of ease of access and the coordination of existing services. Instead, the government has chosen to destroy existing community-based agencies and to scrap the excellent services that are already in place because they hope that the government and the big public sector unions can do the job more efficiently and effectively through a large bureaucratic monopoly' (St Eliz., 1994b).

Although government policy was clearly a direct threat to these organizations, the arguments were couched in terms of what would be in the best interests of consumers. Failures of liberty (loss of consumer choice of provider agency), security (not meeting needs of consumers and communities), and equity (destroying organizations that improve consumer access to services in non-profitable areas) were used to buttress claims of the inefficiency of the MSA model. Although these arguments did not stop passage of the legislation, they were instrumental in preventing its implementation.

6.4.2.3 Providers of Support Services in Home/Community (NFP)

The submissions from the OCSA and from one of its constituent members, the Canadian Red Cross Society, Ontario Division, typified the issues raised by the NFP support service sector. These submissions also illustrated the difficulties an alliance made up of organizations with different resources and organizational complexities has in coming to and maintaining consensus.

OCSA made two presentations to the Standing Committee: one on 17 August and one on 3 October 1994. OCSA members claimed to comprise a grass roots organization with 300 member agencies across the province, over 10,000 staff and over 45,000 volunteers. In their 17 August presentation (OCSA, 1994), they echoed most other organizations in supporting the principles, values, and purposes enunciated in the legislation; they endorsed NFP service delivery, community-based planning, equity of access, a delivery mechanism driven by consumer needs and responsive to cultural diversity, the Bill of Rights, alternative models to the MSA that are the result of local planning and meet the requirements under the act, the functions of the MSA, and the integration of health and social services. Again, like many others, they had difficulty with the details. OCSA members expressed six key areas of concern.

First, they were concerned about the preference for unionized workers. A policy document released by the ministry in September 1993 indicated the government's intention to give preferential treatment to unionized workers in the MSAs. Moreover, Bill 173 was silent with respect to the protection of NFP community-based employees in the implementation of LTC reform. They recognized that the development of MSAs in the context of Social Contract reductions and constrained finances would have an adverse impact on employment in the health care sector. Fearing the transfer of staff from downsizing institutions that were largely unionized, they argued that the skills of community and institutional workers were not comparable, and therefore the government could not simply transfer one to the other. Community support sector employees who had been exploited through low wages and long hours of work, precisely because they were not organized, were now going to be disadvantaged once again. Arguing for the security of consumers through continuity of service workers, OCSA recommended that community support service workers from NFP agencies be guaranteed comparable positions in the MSA without loss of seniority and be given priority over other socio-health sector employees (i.e., institutional workers). This clearly put them in opposition to organized labour, which had negotiated terms and conditions of employment and for which seniority was a bargained-for right that did not exist outside negotiated contracts.

Second, OCSA was concerned that the legislation was both too prescriptive and at the same time not detailed enough, leaving too much to regulation. While the province was moving to implement MSAs, major regulations regarding eligibility criteria, program standards, and MSA guidelines and regulations were not in place. OCSA members demanded active involvement in producing and approving the regulations and that caution be exercised in setting retroactive dates for application of the regulations.

Third, they were concerned with the lack of effort and planning spent on the recruitment, support, and maintenance of volunteers, who were the backbone of their organizations. They joined the chorus arguing that, without active volunteers, both the number of services and the private revenue needed to support them would be jeopardized. They called for formal recognition, support, and planning for volunteers.

Fourth, OCSA members were concerned that the government was too rigid in its model of the MSA. They argued that the form of the agency should emerge from the community planning process and, accordingly, might vary from one locale to another. They stated that MSAs must not be allowed to develop into large bureaucracies that they believed could not be responsive to local community needs.

Fifth, they argued that the act's separation and distinction among the services included in the mandated basket of services (i.e., community support services, homemaking, personal support services, and professional services) reinforced the existing hierarchy, which was based on medical need and the split between health and social services and between cure and prevention. They suggested that this distinction mitigated against the development of a 'generic worker' who could perform a variety of non-professional functions, such as personal support and homemaking. For example, if a client needed both a bath (personal support service) and shopping and housecleaning (homemaking), would the proposed MSA model require two workers, or could one worker be used, with separate billing items? It was indeed OCSA's employees who would benefit from the new training program for generic workers. Furthermore, they argued that the four categories in the legislation did not allow for enough flexibility in the community planning process to meet different local needs or to innovate. They recommended combining all the service categories into one category. Although not explicit about this point, they did not favour the separation of workers into what they saw as a hierarchy of skills, which would result in an unfavourable comparison for their workers.

Sixth, they pointed out that while many services, such as their own, were defined in the act, many others, in particular professional services, were not. They recommended the development of these definitions and OCSA's involvement in their development. They ended by applauding the government for their leadership and looked 'forward to working in continued partnership' in bringing about the new system.

Because of a number of intervening developments within their own organization, OCSA members requested another opportunity to address the committee. While supporting the government in August and express-ing willingness to work with it in partnership, on 3 October OCSA mem-bers informed the committee and other organizations that they were now less enthusiastic about the MSA model. They admitted that in 1992 they had recommended a remarkably similar model, the Comprehensive Community Care Organization (CCCO). They argued, however, that they had also recommended at the time that a fund be established to fos-ter the development of no less than ten demonstration models of CCCOs through a phased-in approach over a period of years. They argued that the legislation's insistence on one model for all of Ontario involved too much of a systemic change in too short a time and violated its own prin-ciples of community planning.

OCSA members now indicated that they supported the recommenda-tion of a number of other organizations that Section 13 of the Act, restricting the purchase of external services to 20 per cent be removed. They argued that restriction on external purchase of services needed to be relaxed on the condition that community boards provide or obtain their services from the NFP sector unless this sector was unable to pro-vide them. They reiterated their concerns and recommendations regarding workers and volunteers in their sector.

In an effort to justify their about-face, OCSA members pointed out that since the NDP government had begun its reform, the focus had shifted from an emphasis on simplified, equitable access, a reduction in fragmentation, an expansion of services, and consumer-centred care to a focus on cost cutting as a primary argument for organizational change. This change in focus, they argued, was due to the pressures of cost shift-ing from a downsized institutional sector to the community and the added costs associated with pay equity. As a result the pledge of $647 million by the government was now meeting pressures not originally envisaged. OCSA took this opportunity to discredit the report released by SCCA and prepared by the management consulting firm on the savings that would result from the reduction in administrative costs in the MSA model over the existing community-based system. The report had implied that community-based programs were administratively top heavy and inefficient. OCSA accused the consulting firm of using unexplained assumptions and burying in the appendices the data showing that the administrative costs of community support programs were already on average below the administrative costs projected for MSAs. OCSA's fear was that the government would argue that the administrative savings from MSAs would be sufficient to compensate for the increased service pressures. OCSA contended that the shift to the community demanded a shift of funds as well as clients (Stapleton, 1994a).

The friction within its own membership was evident in memoranda sent by OCSA's executive director to the board. Indeed, the chair of the OCSA Policy Committee resigned over the new position, indicating that she 'could not advocate for the Board's position regarding the MSA and *Bill 173*, when she cannot personally support this position' (Stapleton, 1994a). She had been both the person who persuaded SCCA to hire Consultant A and one of the architects of the MSA model, and she had maintained very close ties to the minister's office. As one respondent said, 'When her own board came out against the model, she was fit to be tied. She had been a prominent creator of the MSA. And to this day, I think, is still pushing for it, or trying to create it in local communities where she lives' (P).

In a 19 October memo the executive director referred to the 'varying levels of support for and against Bill 173 and the 80/20 section in particular' within the association and the board: 'This has been a difficult time for OCSA ... to have had to balance the various, sometimes competing, perspectives.' He recommended that members of OCSA be given the choice to proceed individually when approached by the Ad Hoc Group (described below) in a media campaign. He reminded the association that its creation was the result of a successful amalgamation 'which resulted from three groups negotiating and coming together ... Let's not forget this part of our history during these troubling times!' (Stapleton, 1994b, 1, 2).

One OCSA member organization described the split within the parent organization in the following way.

P: [Red Cross] could not continue to be a very large member of OCSA at the same time that the two organizations appeared to be taking a divergent role in terms of the creation of the MSA. I am probably oversimplifying, but it seemed to me that people who had been involved in the process from the beginning did not realize that the concepts coming out of the NDP policy position were incompatible with organization survival.

A respondent from an organization outside OCSA saw the decision to pull out as quite self-serving.

P: They didn't realize it [MSA] was going to put them out of business too. They initially thought that they would be served by it because they would somehow arrive at being in charge of the system. Because they all wanted to become MSAs themselves. When they discovered that no one was going to be having their own board of governors. It was all, 'We were all going to be workers under one system. Holy smokes!' The board of OCSA said, 'Wait a minute! What are we doing here? We're committing suicide by endorsing that.' So they backed out, too.

Not surprisingly, support for and concern about Bill 173 dealt with those issues in the legislation that had a direct impact on these organizations. They favoured the inclusion of support services in the basket of services that increased their importance, but not the continued distinction of service categories that would foster a hierarchy of care, thereby detracting from their programs. They supported the notion of a generic worker, which would increase opportunities for their employees. However, they opposed the preference for unionized workers, which would disadvantage their largely non-unionized workforce. Understanding that the 80-20 rule would affect their membership to varying degrees, they called for greater flexibility.

The internal discord within OCSA emanated from the disparate beginnings, institutional structures, and interests of their members. The Red Cross was a large agency of long standing, with a complex governance structure, comparably more resources, and a large pool of paid staff; it was heavily vested in home support services. During the reform, it was involved in a dispute over its blood bank, which threatened a substantial portion of its business. It had much more to lose than the other members of OCSA. The latter were small grass roots organizations with small paid staffs and budgets, whose services were provided by a bank of volunteers, for example, individual meals on wheels programs. Although they formed their own provincial association, which joined OCSA, they did not match the Red Cross in resources or longevity. The power differential within OCSA's own membership would account for the group's withdrawal of support for Bill 173.

OCSA's shift from qualified support to not supporting the legislation without change was a blow to the government, particularly since they were fond of describing the MSA as a development of the association's proposal. Given its commitment to consumers and grass roots movements, OCSA's seeming defection was bad optics. It also underscored the government's political tone deafness to the implications of its proposal and the rising opposition among providers. The undercurrent of OCSA's change of heart had to do with its own internal politics, of managing consensus among 300 agencies, many of which found that they could not live with the details of what had been proposed. One example of this opposition could be seen in the brief of OCSA's largest member, the Canadian Red Cross Society, Ontario Division.

The Canadian Red Cross Society, Ontario Division is an NFP charitable corporation incorporated under federal law. As a member of the International Red Cross, which allows only one society in each country, the Red Cross's divisions, regions, and branches are prohibited from being separately incorporated or from having their own boards. The proposed legislation, however, required each MSA to be incorporated under the Corporations Act, Ontario or the Co-operative Corporations Act, Ontario and to have its own board of governors; these requirements were incompatible with the society's fundamental principles and corporate structure. The Red Cross interpreted the discrepancy as meaning that the Society would not be able to become an MSA or even provide services as part of an MSA.

The Ontario Division, at the time, operated 78 branches with 10,000 volunteers and 6,000 staff (three-fifths of staff employed by all OCSA member agencies), who provided community-based services to more than 130,000 Ontarians. Also at the time, the Red Cross had responsibility for managing Canada's blood supply. In addition, the society provided community support services, which included homemaking (about half of the service provided in the province), meals on wheels and wheels to meals, transportation services, home maintenance programs, and friendly visiting. Their Ontario zone accounted for between one-third and three-fifths of their national budget, excluding the amount used to manage the blood supply.

While echoing most stakeholders in claiming support for the principles underlying the reform and the purposes in the act, the Red Cross, not surprisingly, did not support the creation of MSAs. The rationale was similar to that of other provider groups whose organizational viability was threatened by the reform: the legislation went too far and ignored many strengths of the existing system. At the same time, the legislation did not go far enough: it took a bureaucratic approach to reform (addressing 'systemic problems through the creation of a corporate structure') without reforming the entire health care system. As a result, the organization was worried that the powerful institutional sector would shift its costs to the less powerful LTC sector (e.g., by reducing length of stay and shifting the costs of caring for these 'post-acute' patients to the home care budget). It echoed the complaints that the Act was too prescriptive and inflexible, believing that it would quickly become dated. The Red Cross recommended that service categories in the MSA be defined by regulation rather than legislation to allow for adaptation to emerging practice patterns. The society also felt that drawing a distinction between homemaking and personal support services devalued the former services, thus reinforcing the stereotype that homemakers were little more than cleaners. This belied the reality that services in the home were highly individualized and the boundaries between 'homemaking' and 'personal support' extraordinarily blurry. Certainly, providers of such services found the nature of the job to be evolving, incorporating more complex activities such as transfers and mobilization, training clients in activities of daily living, and even assistance with self-medication and with care of the dying.

The Red Cross further stated that the problem with the existing system was not brokerage, but rather coordination and access. The limits on external purchase of service by MSAs did not allow a sufficient volume of services to be provided by agencies outside the MSA to keep more than a handful viable. Somewhat paradoxically, it noted that in some communities the Red Cross was the only provider. If the society was not able to continue, it warned that clients would face waiting lists and a decline in service quality and would be severely limited or have no choice about provider. The Red Cross recommended that the limits on the amount of external purchase of service be removed and that each community be allowed to choose its own delivery model and mix of provider agencies (CRCS, 1994).

6.4.2.4 Providers of Professional and Support Services in Home/ Community (FP)

The Ontario Home Health Care Providers' Association represented FP (commercial) home care agencies in Ontario. Through 115 offices across Ontario, its member agencies employed over 20,000 staff, including nurses, home support workers, occupational and speech therapists, physiotherapists, and administrative staff. Members claimed that 40 to 45 per cent of publicly funded homemaking services in Ontario were provided by OHHCPA members.

In their submission to the Standing Committee on 16 August 1994, they opposed Bill 173. Their arguments were also phrased in terms of efficiency for the system, and liberty (choice) for consumers. They argued that it would destroy rather than reform the system. It would be more costly and less responsive to consumer needs because it would put in place a monopoly that would be both administrator and provider. They drew to the committee's attention the fact that the legislation originally put a limit on the external purchase of services of 10 per cent from FP agencies. When the government later increased the limit to 20 per cent, to placate the FP agencies, they extended the new limit not only to commercial agencies but also to NFP agencies. OHHCPA argued that the limit on external purchase would cripple an agency's ability to retain the critical mass necessary to survive, driving almost all of their member agencies out of business. The legislation threatened commercial, NFP, and volunteer agencies, workers, and ultimately consumers, who would no longer be able to choose their providers. The lack of competition, they argued, would discourage innovation and choice, remove consumer safeguards and rights (consumers would not complain about service because the people who provided the care also determined eligibility and amount of care), erode quality, and increase costs. Not surprisingly, as proponents of the market, they saw the legislation as micro-management of the system from the centre at Queen's Park. They stated that government should not attempt to manage the details of service delivery; in their view, the legitimate role of the provincial government was developing overall policies, defining core services, determining the level of funding, and letting the local communities determine priorities for home care (OHHCPA, 1994).

6.4.2.5   Providers of Services Insured under the Canada Health Act in Institutions/Physicians' Offices

Systems are interconnected, and changes to LTC clearly would affect other services providers. Accordingly, submissions were also made by providers whose services fell under the provisions of the Canada Health Act. Hospitals feared that giving a legislative basis to District Health Councils might be a step towards the regional authorities already in evidence in other parts of the country; these regional bodies had basically replaced independent hospital boards. Hospitals were worried that the government intended to weaken the autonomy of Ontario hospitals. Family physicians also were alert to attacks on their role; they viewed the case management function of the MSAs as envisioned in the legislation as undermining one of their most important roles in the care of their patients.

The Ontario Hospital Association and the Council of Chronic Hospitals of Ontario, made a joint submission to the committee on 12 September 1994 (OHA and CCHO, 1994). Again, they felt it necessary to indicate that they fully supported the principles of reform, but they could not accept the details. Therefore, they could not support Bill 173. Their appeals were also to the values of liberty and efficiency, echoing other submissions in arguing that the legislation was too prescriptive and introduced a 'top-heavy structure of centralized control' representing an unnecessary and unwarranted intrusion on the autonomy of individual organizations, volunteers, and providers. Furthermore, they believed that the proposed MSA model would 'usurp the management and governance responsibilities of community-based organizations, including hospitals.' They drew a distinction between One-Stop Access to services (which they supported) and 'One-Stop Shopping' (which they did not support).

They began by rejecting the premise, inherent in the legislation, that institutional and community-based care were mutually exclusive systems; instead, they argued that they were 'common pathways' to meet needs. They argued that hospitals were already an integral part of community-based care, pointing to existing activities in providing outreach palliative care programs, home care services, respite services, and meal programs. They also joined the opposition to any restriction on the amount of external purchase of services, which they felt would threaten the capacity of hospitals to continue these programs. As an alternative to the MSA model, they suggested an 'interim strategy' of encouraging a federation of long-term care agencies agreeing to work together to provide services for a given area.

While supporting the planning function of DHCs, the OHA/CCHO were concerned about the blurring of the distinction between the functions of planning and management in Section 62 of the act ('the allocation of resources to meet health needs in the council's geographic area; and ... plans for the development of a balanced and integrated health care system'), which would undermine the autonomy of individual institutions. Furthermore, Section 62 allowed the DHCs to perform any other duties as assigned. For the OHA/CCHO, this section was a red flag when viewed in conjunction with the June 1994 final report of the ministry's Regional Planning Steering Committee for Southwestern Ontario, which recommended a regional health council for the area. These provisions could enable DHCs to take on the functions of regional authorities, which had undermined the autonomy of individual institutions in all other Canadian provinces.

The Ontario College of Family Physicians, which represented approximately 5,000 family physicians, submitted its brief on 17 August 1994. From the members' perspective, the bill represented a government attempt to de-emphasize the medical aspects of LTC and write the family physician out of the loop of care. They noted that the legislation as written did not allow for medical input into decisions regarding services for a patient, did not allow physicians to directly access services on behalf of their patients, and did not even provide for a communications link between the physician and the MSA. They were not convinced that the policy direction of shifting care to the community would always be in the best interests of their patients, particularly in rural areas where community services were not available or in cases where there was no family support structure to supplement the care that would be provided by MSAs.

6.4.2.6 Insights from Interviews with Provider Groups

While apprehension about organizational viability was implicit in the briefs, interviews with representatives of provider groups reinforced the inference that this was a paramount concern. Although some organizations placed 'the mission of the organization' (usually to provide a particular service to clients) above their own survival, most were reluctant to allow their activities to become subsumed within the proposed MSAs.

P: The issues were loss of identity, organizational identity ... We would no longer exist.

P: I think some of the stronger not-for-profits who actually had a corporate identity in addition to a public service identity, wanted to hold on to their corporate identity. And it was mainly the smaller community support agencies that had been struggling to death to get funding ... that [would] not have to worry so much about the day-to-day financing and didn't really mind transferring who they were and what they were into an MSA.

P: It was difficult for [organizations], just as an example, to consider dissolving and becoming part of an MSA. It was equally difficult for community 'xyz' that had its own board of directors, that had worked so hard to develop its own world, to even conceive that it could fold and become part of something else.

For some there were also considerable liabilities, associated with severance and pensions, to transferring their services and staff to the new agency.

P: There would be huge costs to the not-for-profit sector around severance and terminations. It was very clear ... We bore the responsibility and I recall having a legal opinion done at the time in terms of what would be the burden, the financial burden, to our organization around the costs of devolving. And it was huge.

Arising from the issue of viability, the 80-20 rule limiting the amount of services that could be purchased externally to MSAs became a major focus of contention. Because this rule threatened all existing providers, it tended to unite the NFP and the FP groups. Many of the existing organizations felt that they might be able to survive if the MSA could contract out enough services, and they therefore sought to remove any possible restrictions. In practice, of course, there would be no guarantee that MSAs would remain willing to work as closely with (in effect) competitors, but the organizations appeared to believe that sufficiently flexible rules would allow them to continue with business as usual.

P: If a lesser percentage than 80 per cent came under the MSA, then it meant that not as many organizations would have to be folded under it.

Opponents were able to cast their disagreement as a mistrust of government and large, public-delivery organizations for home and community services, which, like an infection, would spread to other health sectors.

P: Where you've got [a] Multi-Service Agency, you've got government employees providing health care.

P: MSA is an attempt to really 'governmentize,' if there's such a word, and do away with all of the governing structures ... This whole MSA concept ... was the slippery slope that, you know, first starts in the communities; then you'll start in the hospitals. Then you'll start to erode all of the separate governance of agencies.

P: I just saw the government sitting on top of this thing like a hen on an egg.

P: Because it was so circumscribed by government regulation, it was a defacto extension of the government in the mind of the providers.

P: We're not a wing of the government. That [is a] fundamental, world view difference.

P: What I kept saying to the government was, 'Tell us what the funding model is going to be, or let us help you develop it. And then get out of the way! Let the managers manage!' There isn't a person in the Ministry of Health today that I can think of who would know how to run any of these programs, community-based or institution ... The belief was that these bureaucrats ... had an agenda whereby they would, in effect, tell them [MSAs and their boards] what they could and couldn't do, and so box them in. These boards would be nothing more than window dressing.

Some were opposed to what they saw as an obvious attempt on the government's part to unionize the community sector, an attempt that, whether intended or not, met with some measure of success.

P: This is a government takeover of the health sector. This is a union-driven takeover.

P: At that point in time we weren't unionized. And it was really fascinating, but our workers unionized during that period because again they saw themselves as having an advantage ... They felt that if they weren't going to have a union that some other group would come in and provide the work ... that they wouldn't even be guaranteed the succession into the MSA.

The model created additional difficulties, because whatever group was successful in winning the MSA contract for a district would be placed in an immediate conflict of interest situation, in determining which, if any, services would be contracted out to other agencies.

P: The only concern we had, and that's a continuing theme through-out, was that conflict of interest will become an insurmountable prob-lem; that there will be an agency that will be delivering 80 per cent of services, buying 20 per cent, and at the same time deciding on each indi-vidual case what service this person should get.

The logistical issues of implementing such a massive, largely untested change (described by one respondent as a 'juggernaut') also created considerable unease, even among those sympathetic to the model. For some, the New Democrats' determination, during this difficult period of fiscal constraint, was driven by the need for at least one success story to come out of their agenda. However, their belief in this solution was mis-placed and was hampered by their inability at implementation.

P: I thought it was kind of like taking one major leap, wiping out every-thing and thinking that the next day you were going to set up something new. I thought that was absolutely insane. And of course, you would need some human resource strategy and so on if you were going to be that devastating. I had always thought that the way you would approach it would be in steps ... before you actually sort of just decided to create one employer that would take over everything.

P: We had said, initially, 'We're not sure about this, but we think it's a good idea. Try it, you know, in, say, ten demonstration projects, and then you can adopt it elsewhere.' Senior's Alliance said, 'Forget pilots, they never work' ... And the government opted [for] that approach ... They were getting battered so much on so many different issues that they wanted to have something that would be a good news story ... Only as it turned out, it wasn't such a great news story.

P: I just think that this big leap to the MSA was absolutely absurd. I just think that the NDP was very, very weak on implementation and didn't know how to go to the bureaucracy to help them to work that out. I do think they had a lot of good, you know, policy ideas, and even initiatives. But when it came to implementation, it was sort of like they never were able to think through the detail and how to get from A to B and carry everybody with you.

P: It was a juggernaut ... And they'd come out with these manuals this thick and draft lines for how your MSA will function. They had just

come out, womp! And people ... 'Where the hell did this come from?'
And you start reading it, and it is a nightmare. And one abomination
after another ... It was just like everybody had ripped out their favourite
twenty pages of nightmares.

In particular, many providers realized the inherent conflict between
the cost control imperative of the period and government's desire to
improve wages and working conditions and expand the scope of services
in this sector. The bringing together of workers from organizations with
different compensation packages would raise the thorny issue of
whether to ratchet up or down to equalize wages while honouring negotiated labour agreements. In a sector where the majority of the budget
went to labour costs, these were not small issues. The unlikelihood of a
massive bureaucracy's being able to attract volunteers in a sector heavily
subsidized by unpaid labour would be further deleterious to the bottom
line. Other providers feared that the ultimate result would be the purchase of fewer, higher-cost services, with adverse implications for those
who no longer qualified for assistance.

P: Bringing together of a number of different agencies had significant
HR implications for the workers, because the diversity of the services
provided was so extensive that you had hourly workers with very, very
comprehensive benefit plans side by side with workers like homemakers
that were hourly workers paid somewhat above minimum wages. [Our
organization] was very concerned, first of all, that the system could not
sustain an equalization that would move up the cost of all the service providers. At the same time they did not want the more lowly paid and less
professional workers to be disadvantaged in the process, because
throughout the creation of the MSAs it was always argued that 'Oh well,
no one would lose any jobs. It would be more efficient.' And in a system
that's primarily staff driven and all the funding goes for staff, at least 85
per cent, you can't achieve a lot of efficiency without having implications
[for] the staffing.

P: We felt that while the governments are trying to control costs, at the
same time they're putting in place provisions which will drive the costs up
significantly. We saw some of that happening by that time ... in the facility
sector, [there] was the constant ratcheting of labour agreements. And we
felt that the same process will happen as soon as MSAs are created. All the

costs will go up to ... whatever the highest cost element is. All the wages will go up to that level ... In creating a new agency and bringing staff from four or five different workplaces, no one's going to take a pay cut.

P: I think our key concern was that this new structure would not have the same standards, approach, responsiveness to the current delivery profile we had ... our current home care system with its complications would be simplified to the point of lack of services and actually less responsive to the home care needs.

P: What about our volunteers? They're not going to join this massive MSA. They just won't do it.

P: And for some of these agencies, like VON or some of these neighbourhood services, you know, these groups have been going for 80 or 100 years. They have this whole identity, this whole community persona, this whole tradition. And people who have been loyal supporters for generations and stuff, and they're like, 'If you get rid of us, these volunteers aren't going to go over there.' You know, like they're going to be so mad that you destroyed their organization that they loved that they're not going to want to waltz over and become your volunteers there. And the people who give money to a community-based, local neighbourhood organization aren't going to feel the same way about giving to this kind of quasi-governmental creature that you've created ... You know, it's hard enough to get enough resources focused in here. What you're going to do is you're going to drive away some of them ... They got really concerned when we started talking about – when they found out how many volunteers were actually involved. And they didn't have any clue how many volunteers were involved in delivering services: 'You mean, like to deliver all these things, you need all these people? And it's all contingent on the good will of these organizations?'

Providers, like consumer groups, were not homogeneous in their reactions to the legislation. Providers of professional services had different interests from those providing support services; FP organizations differed from the NFPs. Nonetheless, they quickly became united in their opposition to the legislation. Security of the consumer, choice for the consumer, and efficiency of the system were heralded in support of their arguments, but the bottom line was the security of the organization.

6.4.3 Labour

The government had provided funding in the summer of 1994 to the
Ontario Federation of Labour (OFL) to consult with health-related
unions on LTC reform. The OFL itself, and most of the health-related
unions, submitted briefs to the Standing Committee. In this section we
document the issues raised in submissions from the OFL, ONA, and
OPSEU.

The Ontario Federation of Labour, in its submission to the committee
on 3 October (OFL, 1994), claimed to represent the position of over
650,000 members from many sectors of the workforce, representing not
only front-line workers in the health care system, but also individuals
who on occasion needed to consume health care services. The members
made it clear that they joined with the Ontario Coalition of Senior Citizens of Ontario (a member organization of SCCA that had union roots)
and SCCA to urge the NDP to move the legislation in this term of their
mandate. They attempted to position themselves as acting in the public
interest and the opposition as being self-interested provider organizations: 'The opposition to the Bill is really about power. What is being
played out is turf wars among over 1,000 agencies who want to keep their
control over their piece of the long-term care delivery system' (OFL,
1994, 2).

Because they also represented workers in health care institutions, in
the brief OFL members advocated 'consumer choice' as to whether those
in need of care should be treated in the home, the community, or in long-
term care facilities. They recommended that Bill 173 be amended to
ensure that Home Care Program services currently insured under OHIP
continue to be insured without user fees, whether provided in home,
other community settings, or LTC facilities. From their perspective,
underfunding of the system would result in low-paid workers, over-burdened family members, and exploited volunteers. They expressed grave
concern that the government had increased the potential purchase of
external services from 10 to 20 per cent and had not stated a preference
for NFP agencies. They recommended that the government revert to the
10 per cent limit without exception and mandate a NFP preference. The
OFL strongly opposed the use of volunteers to do work that 'should' be
done by full-time trained staff and asked that Bill 173 be amended to prohibit the use of volunteers to do work previously done by any employees
in the health sector (not only the LTC sector) and that the MOH develop
a protocol on the role of volunteers in consultation with organized

labour. Under this interpretation, one could conceivably argue that, if unionized workers delivered meals within hospitals, community-based meals on wheels programs would be forced to hire unionized workers; the role of volunteers would revert to fundraising.

With the downsizing of the acute care sector, where most of their members worked, the OFL asked that a mandatory redeployment protocol be enshrined in Bill 173. The protocol would include a guaranteed transfer of workers in the community to MSA jobs without loss of salary or benefits, the development of a central registry of laid-off workers with the requirement that employers hire from this registry, and a mandate for the Health Sector Training and Adjustment Program (HSTAP) to administer the registry. The members asked that the Standing Committee urge government to develop a redeployment system ensuring jobs for workers displaced by health care restructuring. Because HSTAP was administered under a board with equal labour and management representation, this was a way for labour to have direct input into job transfer policies. Institutional workers on the whole had better salary and benefit packages than their counterparts in the community. Institutional (and unionized) workers who were transferred into community jobs were liable to receive poorer compensation packages. As a result, the OFL recommended that the Act enshrine the goal of equalizing the wages and benefits in the two sectors.

The members rejected the Act's prohibition of MSA employees as directors of the agency and asked that the offending section be deleted. In the continuing battle to have labour representation on District Health Councils, they asked that Bill 173 be amended by allowing labour to nominate four appointees (two labour consumers and two labour providers) to DHCs. Although DHCs were volunteer organizations, they also recommended 'that Bill 173 be amended to ensure that board members of MSAs and DHCs be remunerated for any lost wages and expenses they incur in order to attend meetings' (OFL, 1994, 17).

The Ontario Nurses' Association claimed to represent 50,000 registered nurses, working largely in institutions. The members' brief contained the mandatory full endorsement of the goals of the legislation in their submission (ONA, 1994) before their areas of concern were discussed: human resources, governance, and accountability. With respect to human resource issues, they pointed out that community health agencies tended to use lower-paid staff than institutions because these staff were less qualified and tended not to be organized into unions. ONA feared that the option of using the alternative, lower-cost workers cited in the Compendium of the Act, in conjunction with the provision under the Regulated Health Professions Act for regulated health professionals to delegate controlled acts, would tempt agencies to control costs by using lower-paid staff. Since most of the approximately 1,700 home care case managers were registered nurses, ONA members urged government to make use of these skilled professionals rather than employ cheaper labour. They claimed that increasing job security and compensation could be justified as improving quality of care through reducing the high turnover rates in some agencies. To further protect themselves, they recommended that volunteers should not do work that might be performed by paid workers. They also asked for successor rights (continuing rights of unionized employees to be represented by their union and to be governed by a collective agreement). Because of the complexities of amalgamating many agencies with different labour affiliations under one organization, they also asked that union representation be included on MSA boards.

The Ontario Public Service Employees Union claimed to represent 110,000 (predominantly female) workers; besides health care workers, their members included teachers and other government workers. OPSEU also claimed to speak for its members in their non-work related roles as consumers, informal care providers, community activists, volunteers, and taxpayers. The 16 August 1994 submission covered ground similar to that of the later OFL and ONA submissions, including the interests of workers in the hospital sector. Accordingly, they expressed concern over the discrepancies between the rhetoric and the 'reality' of Bill 173, arguing that the shift to the community had more to do with cutting costs by creating a cheaper system based on downsizing a 'well-trained, fairly compensated workforce' than with genuine reform. To OPSEU members, the 'affordable community means low-paid, unorganized workers, over-burdened family members and exploited volunteers.' The 'inappropriate use of volunteers' would undermine the 'efforts, and successes, of pay equity and employment equity legislation' and 'erode the quality, accessibility and continuity of services.' They saw government 'offloading the responsibility for negotiating employment adjustment strategies onto communities' and called for a labour adjustment strategy enshrined in the legislation and for labour representation on boards (OPSEU, 1994, 3, 6, 7, 12).

6.4.3.1 Insights from Interviews with Labour Groups
Excerpts from interviews with representatives of various labour groups

reinforce the issues raised in their submissions. Although they were strongly opposed to a greater role for FP providers, they favoured setting up MSAs, which they saw as the best guarantee of unionizing the community sector. They also sought to ensure adequate funding for the new MSAs. Thus, the interests of labour were closely aligned with their philosophical commitment to universal and comprehensive health care. Labour accordingly pushed hard for full funding for a comprehensive array of services, without user fees and with some legislative protection to ensure that subsequent governments could not delist services. For them, necessary care should be funded regardless of place.

P: [We wanted] the MSAs to provide services without user fees ... and the guarantee that the Home Care Programs services wouldn't get delisted under OHIP. We wanted all the traditional community support services to be fully funded under OHIP ... We're keeping them [patients] out there [in the home] longer. If you fund those things properly, why should they be eligible for it [in] a hospital or a facility and not in the home when it's cheaper to keep them in home?

They stressed the setting up of a set of rules to protect unionized workers, including restricting the ability to contract out work, and ensuring that union members (often from the hospital sector) would have the first call on jobs.

P: Our position across the health sector has always been that with increased demand and the so-called fiscal crisis and rising cost, we did not want to see any dollars going out of the system. And there are an increasing number of examples, you know, where that's happening now with the private sector coming in to deliver health care ... our position was not that everybody who's providing service has to now be a direct employee of the MSA ... We just wanted the service to be purchased from not-for-profit providers.

P: [We wanted] zero contracting out. If the Multi-Service Agencies were going to do it, they should do it. Right? [The legislation] allowed people to contract out for different reasons, and it was really like an open gate because you could ... have contracted out for almost anything the way the wording was. And we wanted exceptions [to] be stipulated and maximum limits [to be set] in terms of how much they could contract out. We wanted to make sure that it didn't include things like short-term absence of employees due to illness, vacation. [Contracting out] was supposed to be used for [something] special, a new service or something else but not for regular, ongoing business ... Vacation[s] [sh]ould be seen as regular ongoing business ... Their [MSAs'] human resource plans should include that ... [We wanted] a framework for, that workers who are displaced in health system restructuring are placed in comparable jobs, at comparable wages, in other parts of the health care system ... So as they downsize the hospitals that those workers should – and this was a major bone of contention for the community – that they should have rights to go at comparable pay and benefits in other parts of the health system ... See, labour never had their head in the sand and said we don't want change. We said we want change within these principles. And we want change in such a way that workers who aren't trained and have the skill are moved within the new system and are part of the new system in a comprehensive planned way ... And it would have gone a huge way in dealing with even the issues around the Social Contract if this had, if they had dealt with this thing first.

Unionization, wage parity, and issues of seniority and successor rights were paramount for labour. They made it clear that the rights of non-unionized workers were not their concern.

P: We really wanted ... to secure employment and working conditions for employees and have as part of its approval process [for designating an MSA] a human resource plan. How are they going to make this transition ... Wage parity is a non-starter. But we had to put it in as a principle. And it's still an ongoing fight. And I don't think, until we get the community health workers unionized, we [will] get it equalized. It's atrocious what community workers earn. And mostly because their agencies have been underfunded ... You're taking the skills and in this case even demanding more of the community workers than ever before because they're taking care of sicker and more complex people in the community, and yet you're paying them a third of the salary.

P: So we had drafted into the legislation that it would be considered a sale of business, which we could have probably have argued at the Labour Board anyway. But right in the legislation it said it would be deemed to be a sale of business, and so therefore everybody would have successor rights. And we wanted the seniority to be recognized in terms of these job offers. So it got very complicated. What we were saying was the unionized member would be given job offers and if there was any paring down of jobs, then it would be done in terms of seniority.

I: How would seniority have been determined with non-unionized members? Non-unionized members don't have seniority. They have length of service, which can be recognized for certain things. But the only way you actually have seniority is through a collective agreement that defines how your seniority is counted ... And then your contract goes on to define in what cases your seniority applies and the foremost obviously is lay-off and recall ... The other thing we wanted in the legislation was that [if] unionized members were a minority that [there] wouldn't automatically be a de-certification vote. So it wasn't a massive unionization strategy. What we were concerned about was that it could be a de-unionization of the sector.

Even the suggestion that unionized workers might be given preference over those currently working in the sector led to some changes within existing provider agencies whose workers moved to protect themselves.

P: At that point in time we weren't unionized. And it was really fascinating, but our workers unionized during that period because again they saw themselves as having an advantage ... They felt that if they weren't going to have a union that some other group would come in and provide the work ... that they wouldn't even be guaranteed the succession into the MSA.

Those interviewed from the labour movement expressed their opposition to allowing volunteers to deliver services that might otherwise be provided by union members. Quality of care for patients was often cited as the rationale for using skilled workers. Moreover, the use of volunteers should be guided by principles in order to avoid substitution of unpaid or cheaper labour for paid work.

P: We see it in the long-term care facilities right now with funding cuts. One day a worker gets laid off, the next day they've got a volunteer coming in to feed people. We're saying, 'No, that's a worker's job' ... And our position on volunteers was we wanted them to supplement things that workers couldn't do, like writing letters, doing the social stuff, you know, doing the extra things for people. But not doing the daily work that's required to provide the ongoing [care]. So more the support work, as opposed to the core services. And we were saying that the minister of health should have a protocol of role of volunteers with organized labour.

P: They [volunteer associations] were very concerned around using volunteers inappropriately for doing things that they weren't covered [for by] WCB [Workers' Compensation Board]. They weren't trained properly for expecting them to do more and more. And it's no longer being a volunteer. If you're going to feed somebody, you have to be there every day at 12:00. It's like a commitment for work. You can't miss it.

P: I also sat on a consultation group on the role for volunteers and long-term care. In the training group, what I was really concerned about was that with a little bit of training what they were doing was just widening the scope [of the use of volunteer service] to the point where it was going to be dangerous, using less skilled workers.

In an effort to avoid seeming self-serving, unions attempted to describe their views in terms of avoiding exploitation of volunteers or ensuring that clients received a high quality of care. Security of workers was cloaked in arguments of security for clients and volunteers. The labour position was an effort to expand the use of paid workers into service areas that had traditionally relied upon volunteer labour. Even though they favoured NFP delivery, their stand on union rights, the imposition of legally defined seniority, restricted use of volunteers, and the elimination of generic worker concepts was contrary to the interests of many NFP providers, and it was a key element in awakening opposition from community-based groups, including both FP and NFP providers and volunteers.

6.4.4 Volunteers

On 4 October the Ontario Association for Volunteer Administration, the Ontario Association of Directors of Volunteers in Healthcare Services, and Volunteer Ontario put in a joint submission to the Standing Committee. The primary mandate of these organizations was the promotion of volunteerism and the promotion of the professional management of volunteer programs. Whereas the unions sought to shrink the use of volunteers, these groups sought to expand it. They wanted the legislation to directly address the need for adequate resources in the core operating budgets for agencies and programs to recruit, train, recognize, and support volunteers, 'all of which should be managed by competent, professional, paid staff.' They asked that their members, as 'professionals in the management of volunteers and volunteer programs', be included at the planning table. The associations asked that volunteers be treated with some dignity, rather than as 'warm bodies' that could be moved around on a board to suit the needs of the system (Ontario Association for Volunteer Administration et al., 1994, 3, 6). They wanted volunteers to be given the same kinds of protections as primary caregivers enjoyed. They argued that volunteers should not be seen either as a cheaper alternative to paid labour or as the tail end of a welfare state. Instead, the decision of 'who does what,' from their perspective, should be discussed with labour, management, and volunteers, rather than being left to regulations or to the decision making of individual communities. Their fear was that decisions would be driven by the availability of dollars rather than by rational planning. Volunteers viewed as cheap labour would be an insult to them and a legitimate concern to labour. However, they were most unwilling to have volunteers relegated to the role of fundraising; they saw strong merit in citizens helping citizens. Making contact with individuals (e.g., delivering meals on wheels) was recognized as far more rewarding to volunteers than merely writing a cheque.

6.4.5 Other Interests

The Association of Municipalities of Ontario (AMO) is an NFP organization representing most of Ontario's local governments. At the time, Ontario had 817 municipal governments; approximately 700, representing over 95 per cent of the province's population, belonged to AMO. The members focused their submission on the impact of reform on the role and status of local governments in the new system, in particular, demanding a municipal role on the planning and service coordination functions. Traditionally, local governments were called upon to provide a share of social services to the most vulnerable populations. This role extended to both financing and delivery; local governments were responsible for paying a share of expenditures under the programs funded through the Canada Assistance Plan, and they also directly ran many social services (e.g., public housing, municipal homes for the aged). AMO members strongly believed that municipalities should ultimately make the decision on those health and social services for which they held some responsibility. They viewed DHCs as unelected advisers to the provincial government about resource allocation and the planning of services and strongly argued that it was inappropriate to give responsibility for setting priorities for LTC services at the municipal level to 'unaccountable special purpose bodies' (AMO, 1994, 2). Bill 173, from their perspective, bypassed municipal councils as the representatives of local communities. AMO members believed that the over-prescriptive nature of the legislation was necessary to monitor unelected and unaccountable agencies. They called on government to conduct a formal review of the DHC mandate and structure. AMO recommended that, in the spirit of empowering decision-making at the community level, municipalities should ultimately make the decision on the local authority for health and social services.

AMO members also believed that the province ignored their long history in the funding, management, and delivery of services and programs in LTC. Rather than being a last resort option for designation as an MSA, they recommended that municipalities be given the right of first refusal to serve as MSAs. Furthermore, ever watchful of cost shifting, they pointed out that, while the provincial government mandated the basket of services that must be provided by MSAs, it did not commit to fund these services. In summing up and appealing to values of liberty and efficiency, AMO argued that the legislation would 'not achieve the following objectives: greater community empowerment, decentralized decision-making, integrated local programs and services, accountability, reduced government bureaucracy, or an efficient allocation of limited government resources' (AMO, 1994, 9).

6.4.6 Activities of the Provider Coalition

Subsequent to the hearings, members of the coalition of providers stepped up their opposition to the legislation. Their campaign included writing to the premier, seeking his personal intervention in the reform, with the argument that the reform would result in fewer but more costly services for consumers, decreased volunteerism, and less empowerment of local communities (Ontario Association of Residents' Councils, 1994). They issued press releases and held news conferences (Coalition of Consumer and Provider Groups, 1994a,b). The coalition hired a consultant, who advised on media relations and on the procedure and behaviour required for being present in the legislature during debates (Rhodes and G.P. Murray Research, 1994a,b).

They got a legal opinion on the amendments to Bill 173 dealing with staff transfers, which the government tabled in November following a meeting with the Ontario Federation of Labour. They issued a media release stating that the amendments would force MSAs to offer available jobs to unionized workers before they were offered to non-unionized workers. Despite the government's assurances that the non-unionized workers would not have reduced job security and that the community care sector was expanding, the coalition stated that there would be fewer jobs:

> The announced purpose of MSAs is to reduce duplication and increase the efficiency of service delivery. This is typically done by reducing jobs. Thus, in the MSA former employees of service providers will compete for fewer jobs than formerly existed. These MSA jobs will be given first to unionized workers and then to non-unionized workers. The result is that non-unionized workers will have reduced job security ... This means that a non-unionized long term care worker with twenty years of experience could be pushed out of the system by a unionized worker who has been on the job for four months.

Leaving the media to draw their own conclusions, the coalition stated that the government 'amendments have nothing to do with improving the delivery and access of long term care to the people of Ontario' (Coalition of Consumer and Provider Groups, 1994c, 1).

An interviewee from one of the organizations that joined the coalition indicated that it was very easy to form the alliance once the union issues surfaced, whch provided a common interest.

P: Yes, it was easy. It became really easy when the union ideology came out of the whole thinking. And that's where ideology really started to prevail, and that is when all the forces came together. That is when the commercial agencies provided resources for all of the community agencies, that's when the OMA came into the thing, and that's when we created the LTC Reform Group. ... They got enough people angry all across the board, from physicians to commercial agencies to not-for-profits. Just everybody they alienated. So we all banded together, got two or three really good government relations people, and that when it was going through hearings and all of that. There was tremendous, just tremendous momentum.

Indeed, the union's success in having its pro-labour amendment introduced late in the day prompted the executive director of OCSA to recommend reversing OCSA's previous position of not 'going high-profile in opposition to the Bill.' He justified his recommendation as follows: 'I feel that we need to make an exception in this instance and speak out, because the government has clearly backed away from its previous amendment, which protected unionized and non-unionized employees equally. Our Association represents 12,000 employees, of which, 94 per cent are non-unionized, and I feel that *all* employees should be treated equally under the law during the transition to MSAs ... Therefore, I have agreed to be listed as a contact on the attached news release, which is being circulated today to the press'(Stapleton, 1994a, 2).

After the passage of the legislation, the activities of the Coalition continued under the name The Group for Long Term Care Reform, and its membership was expanded to include Alzheimer Society of Ontario, Association of Ontario Care Therapists, Association of Local Official Health Agencies, Catholic Charities, Lambton Alliance, Ontario Home Care Case Managers' Association, and the Ontario Home Care Medical Advisors. CRCS, OCSA, OHHCPA OHA, OMA, St Eliz., and VON committed either financial or in-kind support (Group for Long Term Care Reform, 1995a). The Group mandated four roles for itself: to act as an advocate on behalf of change in LTC, a clearing house for information, a resource for the media and the public, and a liaison with other stakeholders. One of its goals was to raise LTC reform as an election issue by providing information to the media, being a resource for politicians, and working in concert with the Ontario Health Providers' Alliance in its election strategy. It planned to increase consumer participation in its organization and to 'minimize the apparent government strategy of "divide and conquer" by explaining our position and our activities to consumer organizations, and listening to their views and concerns' (Group for Long Term Care Reform, 1995b, 2).

6.5 A Babel of Values

A review of expressed societal interests clearly highlights the clash in meanings attributed to values or goals. Ideas were appropriated and repackaged to serve different policy interests. In this section we analyse the ways in which the four policy goals – security, efficiency, equity, and liberty – were pressed into service by different groups in support of their own policy interests.

What is the meaning of 'security'? This concept was used in a multiplicity of ways. Many groups defined security in terms of quality or service availability but differed on how best to achieve this goal: through guaranteed government funding without user fees (consumers, labour); through competition of providers (providers); through good salary and benefits packages (labour); through the use of trained staff rather than volunteers (labour); or through elected and accountable versus appointed officials (municipalities). Security was also expressed as the need to mandate eligibility criteria, amount of service, user fees, and so on through legislation rather than regulation (consumers), or to prescribe labour adjustment and human resource plans in legislation (labour, NFP providers).

Similarly, groups variously argued that 'efficiency' could best be achieved through amalgamation of agencies into a one-stop-shopping delivery model (consumers); one-stop access and referral and competition among agencies (providers); job security and compensation packages, which would reduce turnover (labour); or volunteer participation to reduce costs by providing services and increase revenues.

'Equity' was sought through a publicly funded mandated basket of services throughout the province without user fees (consumers, labour); the encouragement and support of NFP agencies that respond to community needs (NFP agencies); the provision of comparable salary and benefits packages between community and institutional workplaces, the recognition and respect for negotiated contracts (labour); or the levelling of the playing field for both the FP and the NFP organizations (FP agencies).

'Liberty' expressed as choice had a number of meanings: choice of type of service – community, home, or facility (seniors, labour); choice of individual worker (seniors, disabled); or choice of provider agency (ethnocultural and spiritual communities, providers, and volunteers). Liberty was often expressed as rights protection; however, groups varied in terms of whose rights needed protection (consumers, providers/workers, or volunteers) as well as in the details about how (if at all) these rights were to be enforced.

Even terms like 'community empowerment' were variously used to argue for representation of particular constituencies on governing boards of the MSAs or DHCs (well-elderly, frail elderly, family caregivers for disabled consumers with cognitive impairments, ventilator users, persons with physical disabilities, volunteers, consumers, and workers appointed by labour) or returning the responsibility for planning and allocating resources to local elected officials (municipalities).

Groups displayed a number of strategies to promote their credibility. Most inflated their voice by claiming to speak for a large number of peo-

ple or groups or for a diverse set of groups. They formed (and disman-
tled) alliances to support their interests. They strengthened their claims
by putting forward recommendations that they claimed were not based
on self-interest but reflected a laudable desire to protect vulnerable
groups in the sector.

To advance their interests, they mobilized the array of public relations / lobbying techniques. They hired management, policy, and media
consultants. They held news conferences and issued press releases. They
provided templates for letters that their members might use to lobby government. They approached opposition members. They forced LTC
reform onto the agenda for the upcoming election.

Reflecting the state-directed nature of the LTC policy community,
which interests were heard depended less upon the inherent power of
particular stakeholders and more upon the compatibility with the ideology and policy interests of the government of the day. As government,
the NDP found itself trapped in a polarized environment: it did not go
far enough to satisfy its supporters, but went too far for the dissenters.
In an effort to ensure passage before the election – and the almost inevitable defeat of the government – the NDP agreed to modify the legislation.

6.6 Amendments to Bill 173

On 17 November 1994 the government forced closure on the debate.
Third reading occurred in December. The Long-Term Care Act, 1994
was proclaimed on 31 March 1995. The proclaimed Act (Government of
Ontario, 1994) incorporated a number of amendments to the legislation
as originally introduced in June. Other than general housekeeping
changes, the amendments reflected an attempt to shore up the government's political base by making concessions to consumers and to labour.

The section in which the purposes of the Act were outlined was
expanded to include statements about the provision of support and
relief to informal caregivers; the integration of health and social services
to facilitate the provision of a continuum of care; the recognition of
needs and preferences of consumers based on ethnic, spiritual, linguistic, familial, and cultural factors in the management and delivery of services; the promotion of not only the efficient but also the effective
management of human, financial, and other resources; the involvement
of volunteers in all aspects of the MSA except their management; the
promotion of cooperation and coordination among providers of com-

munity services and of health and social services; and the coordination of community services provided by MSAs with other health and social service agencies, such as hospitals and LTC facilities.

The Bill of Rights was amended by adding protection from financial abuse by service providers to the earlier provisions requiring MSAs to develop and implement a mechanism to prevent, recognize, and protect clients against mental and physical abuse. The right of consumers to participate in the assessment of their requirements, the development of their plan of service, and the review and revision of their requirements was also specifically codified in the bill. In addition approved agencies were to establish a process for reviewing complaints. The grounds for complaint were expanded beyond the earlier grounds of quality of service or violation of rights to incorporate ineligibility for services, amount of service, and termination of service.

With respect to the designation of approved agencies as MSAs, the minister was given the added authority to designate MSAs for specific geographic areas or for persons in a specified geographic area who could be identified by their membership in a particular ethnic, cultural, religious, or linguistic group, or by any other prescribed characteristics. This would allow MSAs to be designated to cater to particular groups, such as the Chinese or Jewish communities.

The board representation was broadened; now, not only did it need to reflect the community it served and ensure representation from persons experienced in the health and in the social services field, but it had to ensure that at least one-third of the board represented persons who were receiving or had received community service from the agency. Past and current consumers, not merely potential consumers, were empowered to advise on the direction of the agency. The section prohibiting an employee of an approved agency from being a director was deleted.

The act now included specific sections dealing with labour issues. It defined 'previous employer' and 'successor employer.' The transfer of the provision of a community service or a part of community service from a previous employer to a successor employer was deemed to be a sale of a business under the Employment Standards Act, the Labour Relations Act, and the Pay Equity Act. Employees were to be given notice of sixty days before the transfer. A number of sections dealt with job security issues such that a successor employer made reasonable job offers first to employees with the previous employer in descending order of each person's length of service. However, not all employees of the previous employer were equal. The successor employer was to make job offers first to employees of the previous employer who were in bargaining units in order of seniority before making offers to employees of the previous employer not represented by the bargaining agent. The successor employer did not have to offer positions to people who were not qualified to perform the services required or who could not become qualified with a reasonable amount of training. The position offered was to consist of the same work or comparable work and was not to represent a break in employment.

The criteria for the exception to the rule of 20 per cent restriction for external purchase of service were now to include the absence of employees due only to unforeseen, unplanned events; absence due to vacation did not so qualify. To further appease labour, it was specifically stated that absence due to a strike or lockout would not constitute a criterion for external purchase. A specific section was added to require MSAs to develop plans for the recruitment, training, supervising, retaining, and recognition of volunteers.

6.7 Perceived Influence of Societal Interest Groups

Driven by their ideology of grass roots / community empowerment and democratic participation in governing, the New Democrats tried to listen to all interest groups. While all groups may have been given voice, however, not all were necessarily influential. Those interviewed agreed that consumers were given priority. The interests of labour, although always important to the NDP, became more salient as an election neared. Support service providers lost the ear of the government when they withdrew their endorsement from the legislation.

Clearly, the influence was not unidirectional. Particular groups may have influenced government, but government also sought out groups that shared their policy goals to win support for the legislation. For example, not all consumer groups were given the same access to cabinet ministers as the Senior Citizens' Consumer Alliance, whose claims to represent all seniors were open to challenge. Was the SCCA's preferential access to government motivated by an NDP ideological belief in empowering consumers or seniors? Or were the New Democrats orchestrating their voice? Motives are not easy to ascertain, and our respondents differed about the rationale for these links between government and its favourite consumer groups.

P: There was something else brewing there. And there were sides being drawn. And if you were on the side of the Seniors' Alliance and [Consultant A] and the Eunice McGowan group, [you had] access to Frances Lankin and then, after, Ruth Grier. But those lines got drawn very early in the reign of that MSA model ... I don't know why but that triumvirate kind of got formed, and those were the power brokers for the stay of the NDP government ... During the MSA stuff, when you talked to consumers, or consumers being represented, it was Jane Leitch [chair of SCCA], through the Seniors' Alliance group. And there are those who believe that it really was, they were a puppet for [Consultant A's] group, who was funded to promote a policy that the government wanted.

G: Although the seniors' groups didn't seem to me to be as well defined or as well organized then, they got much better organized under the NDP. Can I tell you why? 'Cause [government] funded them. Government actually funded them, to attack them. 'Cause that's what you're supposed to do in a democracy ... They're unfortunately not funded now [under the Conservative government] which is why they're so silent. They simply don't have the money to have the voice.

Government officials took the occasional independence of the seniors' groups as evidence that government was not controlling them; as the reform proceeded, they believed that seniors constituted a barrier to helping government to get the job done.

G: I wish they had been [a government mouthpiece]. They certainly weren't; they enjoyed a close relationship with the minister and her office, but as I say, they certainly didn't agree. They took a lot of persuading around some of the details, to trust us and to let us go. We had huge, hours and hours and hours of consultations around various aspects of it with them, where they were very leery that we could be trusted to do it right. And their consultant became a barrier in a way, as opposed to an aid in moving forward, because of his particular mode of operating and commitment to a particular model ... They lost the ability to be flexible and to just allow us to get on with it as time went on.

G: The were listening to Jane Leitch and the coalition of senior citizens. They were listening to people within their own party, which is not atypical ... I think they listened less to provider groups. They certainly did not hear what the VON or Red Cross, Home Care were saying. They did not hear what the nursing home people were saying.

G: NDP had always been the party of special interests and unions. NDP weren't balanced in who they listened to. The special interests they listened to were all the disaffected, the most radical advocates, the disabled, the mental health groups, the consumer advocacy groups. It was a mentality of us against the establishment. This is our government and they are going to do what we want.

While the SCCA was viewed as most influential, it was not, however, seen as the voice of all seniors or all consumers. It represented a very particular and narrow subgroup of consumers. One respondent from a senior's organization, two from provider organizations, and one within government made the following observations.

C: That to me was not a real consumers' group, at all. It was run by [Consultant A] and a bunch of people who were, I thought, manipulating the whole thing. I'll be honest. We tried to make submission before that [SCCA consultations]; I was ordered by [Consultant A] only to present certain things. I couldn't present what we wanted. I never bought it that that was a real consumer group.

P: One of the challenges we faced throughout, was that the government had the Seniors' Alliance on their side, and we were never able to clearly define the fact that those were not our consumers. If you're able to drive to a meeting in downtown Toronto and hold press conferences and write articles, you aren't the people we're serving. The people we're serving ... can't get out, or they wouldn't be using our services. And I think there was a real concern among a number of groups that the MSA was being driven to provide service for the people represented by the Seniors' Alliance.

P: The consumers and the community groups ... with the ethos of community, grass roots, that whole ideology – and they were being listened [to] by the government. They had priority over the Health [agenda]. And it got to be a battle. Well, it shouldn't have been a battle. But it was 'we' against 'they.' The health providers were seen as the 'they.' And we [consumers] were the good guys and we were going to get all these home supports and we were going to look after our own, and we were going to do friendly visiting, and shopping ... Do you realize ... that 75 per cent of the health Home Care dollar goes to these high-need [clients] ... I mean a failure on the part of consumers to be aware of the

[data] ... Well when they were sick elderly, they weren't at this planning table ... they were well elderly planning services based upon what they perceived their needs to be ... That describes for me, sort of, where things were going. They had a voice, they were listened to.

G: How much broad-base support [was there for the MSA], it was never really tested. But I'd for one be kind of surprised if you could have found one in a thousand seniors that ... had the vaguest idea of what an MSA was, or what a Service Coordination Agency was. So it was ... a debate confined to a rather narrow group who on one side purported to speak for the government, and on the other side purported to speak for all seniors in the province.

Some respondents felt that the real power brokers were the groups in OCSA, rather than the seniors, and that OCSA was using the seniors as a front for its ideas.

P: It was the seniors' group, but within the seniors' group there were members who belonged to the Ontario Community Support Association and they had the ear of the government. They had the ear of the Ministry of Health and the minister of health ... [There were] a couple of key people who influenced her [minister of health] to think about moving to another kind of model, away from the Service Coordination Agency model ... Eunice is the person who was on the board of the OCSA, friend of Frances Lankin. Some believed [she was] the chief architect of the MSA-type model that was then moved forward. And [she] helped also to get [Consultant A] the contract with the Alliance and had close ties with all of that. And right until the end of the NDP era, [she] carried a lot of weight with the Ministry of Health.

While a number of respondents felt that the NFP support sector, namely OCSA, was most influential in the beginning, they believed that balance changed as the reform progressed, resulting in the government's aligning itself more closely with the seniors.

P: I believe it was OCSA who really detested brokerage. The Home Care Programs are, I think, reviled is probably not too strong a word, by many of the community support associations ... The relationship with Home Care Programs across the province, there was very much a perception, it's a servant-master [relationship] ... It was very, very controlling, very arbitrary, and very difficult to accept. And the OCSA membership was very, very frank and very outspoken in its desire not to continue with that ... Originally, they [government] had been listening very closely to OCSA. OCSA had a very strong contact with Ruth Grier in the person of Lynn Grist. But as OCSA shifted its approach, I will tell you, it permanently eroded some of their relationship with the senior bureaucrats and some of the political staff and the politicians. And that I think drove the NDP to cement their relationship with the Seniors' Alliance more tightly.

Even within consumer groups, respondents saw an ideological hierarchy. We have already noted the priority given to the group representing the well-seniors, as opposed to the needs of the very frail elderly. Similarly, as the party de-emphasized multiculturalism in favour of anti-racism, the balance within the cultural communities shifted accordingly.

C: Multicultural community as a whole kind of just collapsed – maybe towards the last part of the NDP's term. Much because there was a bit of a faction growing between the anti-racism and the multicultural contingents. You had a split in the ranks and, as they say, a house divided against itself ... When anti-racism hit, anything with any concept of Multiculturalism was past, and you had to start from scratch with anti-racism.

The other powerful group was labour. The NDP was viewed by many groups as trying to create an environment in the community conducive to unionization and also as trying to placate unions for actions taken on other fronts (hospital restructuring and the Social Contract).

P: I know that labour ... had an open door. They could access the minister of health, particularly, and possibly also other very significant cabinet ministers at will.

P: And I think through Frances Lankin and all those connections ... unions were very powerful. And very powerful with the premier himself, Bob Rae at the time, and the cabinet. I think the union movement was very influential.

P: I think that was again a reflection of the ideological bent of the NDP. I think probably the pressure came from the unions, and the NDP were largely, you know, backed by that group and they had a lot of influence ... And I think in the end, the inability to move beyond some of those labour barriers was what scuppered the MSAs ... In the end, the HR problems became too huge to overcome. And it was even inter-union, you know. The fact that you had successor rights so that unions came into an MSA and you could have multiple unions for the same provider. You know, you could have different unions representing the same worker category ... the MSA would have to inherit that. And different wage scales for the same work. And it was horrific.

Although the NDP sought to please both consumers and labour, at a fundamental level the two groups had diverging interests. These interests could be hidden if enough money were available; in times of economic restraint, however, there would be a conflict between the ability to maximize wages and working conditions and the ability to maximize services. This became most evident to the disability consumer groups, who were pushing to have clients control the recruitment and management of their own care workers. Clearly, direct funding could go farther if clients did not have to employ unionized workers.

C: The real conflict with the NDP came between their balance of labour and consumers ... Labour took a huge role and that probably had more of an impact on what happened than anything else in terms of the development of the MSAs and where the NDP eventually went with long term care. And it created some of the problems from the perspective of people with disabilities in terms of the lobbying and where we had the battle and where we didn't have the battle ... It [MSA] focused on labour issues and it was union driven, and making sure that people had jobs, but not a whole lot of accountability back to the people who are getting services. And it affects a lot, the direct funding model. It was a really clear funding split; by this point we had two tracks going. There was the independent living group that was working on the direct funding. It had gotten pretty far. The government said, you know, 'We agree in principle.' And at the last minute labour stepped in and said, 'No you don't.' Because from labour's perspective direct funding is a huge threat ... [with direct funding], I hire the person. I'm a single employer and they blocked it for a year ... What labour said is, 'We want the agencies. I mean, we want to still have employment standards and contracts.' People can understand that they're concerned that wages would get pushed down, but there also is a really serious problem between labour and consumers, to be honest ... It's not that people don't like the attendants, and it's not they don't like labour, but you've got it set up right now where the person who's getting service and who should be directing ... has literally no power.

In their rush to get the legislation out before their mandate ran out, the New Democrats had not worked out the labour issues, hoping to clarify them in regulation, and they did not appear to recognize the potential conflict. Respondents suggested that the NDP viewed the sector as expanding and able to accommodate all workers, both unionized and non-unionized, from both the existing community sector and those displaced from institutions.

G: Some of those issues (human resource issues) really just began to surface during the hearings because we really were sort of on two tracks. We had the legislation going through ... had to get it through before other things could happen. And in our development of policies and issues we were moving ahead of the legislation in some ways ... It was a case of, we haven't got to that issue before we drafted the legislation and so, yes, it would have regulations and I suspect labour was saying we want some greater [assurances] ... and, you know we're back to our regulations versus legislation debate at that point. We were talking about a growing system, and we were talking about the creation of MSAs in areas of the province where there were very few services. On a provincial level, you were certainly looking at far more jobs for nurses, in home support services. But if you're laid off from a job in Kingston and it's Timmins that is setting up for the first time a nursing service, you know, it doesn't quite fit. So there would have been huge problems in adjustment, but I think overall the number of jobs would not have been less.

G: I still believe that in the future there's going to be probably more need than there will be workers. So probably the issue of who's going to get the jobs will be really redundant.

As mentioned in chapter 5, the government had provided the OFL with two years of funding in the summer of 1994 to consult with labour groups. Our respondents perceived that labour first woke up to their interests during the Standing Committee hearings on Bill 173.

G: And the discussions around Bill 173 were, I think, [during] the committee hearings ... probably the first time when labour woke up to the impact this might have on some unionized members. And I think that that was part – what was happening was not only long-term care but also the whole squeeze on hospital budgets, and nurses were being laid off in hospitals and weren't buying the bland statement that 'okay, there will be jobs in the community,' because they know how different those jobs were going to be. The Social Contract had happened or was happening, and so labour was certainly watching with great interest anything the government did.

The fragility of the coalition supporting the bill became evident. Seniors and labour were the most supportive of the MSA model. As they pushed their own concerns, however, they both delayed the passage and implementation of Bill 173 and lost former supporters. Among the most obvious signs of backlash was the disaffection of a formerly supportive interest (OCSA). More crucially, the delay in passage gave dissenters an opportunity to gather momentum and launch a powerful counter-attack.

6.8 Conclusions

When the New Democrats took office, they put in a structure for developing LTC reform that reflected and would further their ideology of more centralized control of programs, favouring NFP delivery and support services over medical services. This structure vastly increased the scope of conflict and the complexity of managing the bill. For example, their desire to strengthen social supports in LTC resulted in their temporarily giving MCSS the lead responsibility, before reverting to MOH following the consultation process. Their desire to ensure that the voices of marginal consumers were heard led to the involvement of the Ministry of Citizenship, which now covered disability, seniors, as well as multicultural issues.

Although the NDP government's first model was a minor variant of the Liberal SAO model with an NDP spin on it – preference for NFP providers, support of workers, and rights of consumers – it was clear that the government was not committed to this model. Rather, it used the *Redirection* document as a discussion tool, a foil for its later reform. Because members of the government and their political staff had roots in the NFP support services LTC sector, when the New Democrats formed the government, they brought with them the ideas that had been percolating in this sector towards the end of the Liberal period, namely, a comprehensive multi-service organization.

Under this government, formerly marginalized or ineffective groups found or were given a voice. In keeping with their ideological principles, the New Democrats strengthened consumer groups through the funding of the Senior Citizens' Consumer Alliance, and NFP grass roots organizations, namely, the Ontario Community Support Association. Through the rhetoric of giving Ontarians a say in the reform by means of an ambitious and all-inclusive consultation process, they gave preference and financial aid to those who would support their vision. Both SCCA and OCSA had used consultants who had ties to the same firm, and both organizations had received similar advice on recommended models. Given the common roots in the support services sector of key ministers, the government was open to the model suggested by both SCCA and OCSA. However, many felt that, for political optics, it was important that the MSA model be perceived to be the birth child of the seniors. Initially, the approach was successful: SCCA made a series of recommendations that matched the government's policy preferences. Eventually, however, the fragile consensus would fracture under the pressure of attempting to reconcile opposing interests.

The New Democrats were fatally damaged by the economic recession of the early 1990s. Trying to spend their way out of the recession in their first two budgets, they further damaged the economy, restricted their degree of freedom, and left the hard decisions too late in their mandate. With a little more than a year and a half left in their term, they changed their budget strategy, asking for major concessions from workers without enough time to make amends. Their attempts to alleviate the economic pain ultimately cost them many who had previously been their staunchest supporters. Although the Social Contract was an attempt to protect labour by saving jobs, the strategy went against one of their strongest principles: the sanctity of negotiated collective agreements. The Social Contract, along with hospital restructuring, left the NDP beholden to the labour movement. As a result, they made concessions in the MSA legislation that further alienated dissenters and estranged OCSA, one of their staunch supporter groups. The Social Contract and its process created new political cleavages. It provided an unintended opportunity for groups to learn about each other's concerns about LTC and to forge a common strategy against the NDP in this policy sector.

The MSA model raised much opposition based on fears, which

included lack of choice, especially for the disability, ethnic, and religious communities; viability of provider organizations; decline of volunteerism; loss of jobs; and loss of negotiated rights and benefits. In the heat of this dissent all groups buttressed the nobility of their interests with arguments of improving security, equity, liberty, or efficiency. The debate over the merits of the MSA model made visible the contention that the interpretations of these goals are highly contested and constitute political claims to garner support and redraw boundaries in the policy community.

Although the act was proclaimed in early 1995, it was not implemented, because an election was called in the early summer of that year, which resulted in the defeat of the NDP government. The New Democrats' belief in consultative governing and their attempt to listen to their supporters brought together disparate groups that had one common purpose, that is, to defeat the NDP reform. The dissension managed to delay the passing of the legislation and ultimately its implementation. MSAs were an election issue, with the established NFP and FP agencies vehemently opposing a model that would diminish or eliminate their roles. The Progressive Conservatives promised that, should they be elected, they would abolish MSAs. They were true to their word. With so few of the structures of the MSA in place, it was not difficult to achieve. Broad consultations had slowed down implementation. One interviewee made the following assessment.

P: There was a lot of pressure on the NDP from all sides. And one of the things ... in the NDP's era of wanting to please everybody, they pleased no one. They consulted so much, and they tried to bend over backwards to meet the VON, the Red Cross, who were major fighters of this. And in the end they didn't get their support. I mean, now the VON, the Red Cross are probably saying, 'We should have supported the NDP!' Because what's coming down is a lot worse for them than this.

The ideology of the New Democrats influenced the institutional structures that were put in place to fashion reform, favoured particular political interests and processes, and ultimately shaped their LTC model. In the end, following their ideological commitment to an all-inclusive policy development process opened them up to defeat. The incoming Progressive Conservative government of Mike Harris, elected in part on a platform of 'no MSAs,' learned that key lesson from the NDP effort – its consultation would be far more narrow and focused.

CHAPTER SEVEN

The Progressive Conservatives Implement Long-Term Care, 1995–1996

7.1 The Progressive Conservatives

In June 1995 the Progressive Conservatives (PCs), led by Mike Harris, were elected on a platform that advocated less government and more reliance on the private market and market mechanisms. The key promises were incorporated into a document entitled *The Common Sense Revolution* (PC, 1994), which became the blueprint for the new government. Learning from the NDP government, whose consultation processes had delayed action on a range of policy initiatives until late in the election cycle, the Conservatives decided to act quickly and decisively. The province experienced a dramatic change in the nature of governmental decision making. Consultation and participation were no longer valued for their own sake; the government believed it had been given a mandate to implement its Common Sense Revolution and moved with often breathtaking speed. Although the NDP had managed to pass long-term care (LTC) reform, the Harris Conservatives had promised during the election campaign that they would not implement Multi-Service Agencies (MSAs), and they now emphasized their intention to keep that promise. Accordingly, the direction of LTC reform yet again changed dramatically, and the interest groups yet again mobilized for action.

Although the political and policy interests of societal groups did not change markedly in this period, their influence with government did. Previously influential groups, such as seniors and labour, lost ground. Provider groups correctly assumed that a pro-business government would be more sympathetic to their interests. The underlying differences in values and interests between the for-profit (FP) and not-for-profit (NFP) agencies resurfaced. These differences split the Group for LTC Reform, as NFPs and FPs re-positioned themselves with the new government. The reform proposed and implemented by the Conservatives, the Community Care Access Centre (CCAC) model, brought in managed competition among providers and shifted the allocation dimension from a heavily command-and-control model to the market end of the continuum. In the end, the notion of competition for contracts would shatter the already fragmented and ineffectual policy community.

The Conservative model would have ramifications beyond the goal of increasing efficiency for community-based LTC services. The competitive contracting process altered the balance of NFP and FP provision of care in the LTC sector, with care shifting over time to the FP commercial agencies. In an age of international trade agreements and global markets, this has led to the real possibility that LTC services in Canada could eventually be provided by American multinationals.

7.2 The Progressive Conservatives on Campaign

Before the election campaign, the Progressive Conservatives released *The Common Sense Revolution* (PC, 1994). In this document they clearly outlined an ideological shift in the way government would operate should they be elected. Less government, the superiority of markets, and emphasis on individual effort were to be the order of the day. The Conservatives announced their intention to cut the provincial income tax rate by 30 per cent; reduce non-priority government spending by 20 per cent; cut barriers to job creation, investment, and economic growth through actions such as the elimination of 'red tape' and the repeal of Bill 40, the NDP's labour legislation; and cut the size of government by reducing the number of MPPs from 130 to 99 and eliminating 13,000 civil servants. They planned to introduce 'workfare,' a program that would require 'all able bodied recipients – with the exception of single parents with young children – either to work, or to be retrained in return for their benefits,' on the grounds that 'the best social assistance program ever created is a real job' (PC, 1994, 9). The party stated that many of government's activities could be done 'cheaper, faster and better if the private sector is involved,' and that those functions remaining with government should be managed like any other business that provides goods or services. Efficiency would dominate; the language of the document referred to the 'public' not as 'citizens,' 'recipients,' or 'patients,' but as 'customers.' *The Common Sense Revolution* would have a significant impact on the way that the government and its employees did

business on a day-to-day basis, because it would demand that government do business *like* a business – in other words, in an efficient and
productive manner focusing on results and putting the customer first
(PC, 1994).

Jim Wilson, who had served as the PC health critic, indicated in an election campaign speech his party's position on health and LTC. Reflecting
the new provincial order and ideological tenor should they be elected, he
clearly laid the blame for Ontario's lagging economic condition on too
much government, ineffective bureaucrats, conflict in all sectors produced by the NDP's governing style, and inefficient management and
excessive spending by government.

The Conservatives argued that 'a vibrant economy means a better,
more sustainable health care system.' The *Common Sense Revolution* promised a 30 per cent tax cut, which was to lead to 'more jobs, more taxpayers
and more growth' (Wilson, 1995, 6).

The new government clarified that there was a clear divergence of
ideas about the appropriate relationship between state and society.
Where some saw 'participatory democracy,' others saw the triumph of
'special-interest' lobbying. The Conservatives adopted the latter view,
suggesting that the provincial government was besieged by special-interest lobbies and vowing that this practice would end under their government. Wilson went as far as to characterize the province under the NDP
as a 'war zone' and said that a new Harris government would end the
hostilities plaguing the health care system. He referred to community-
based workers 'warring' with institutional sector workers, 'seniors who
support *Bill 173* skirmishing with providers who are justifiably concerned with it,' MOH bureaucrats 'turning on their bosses,' and an
overall attitude throughout government that favoured support service
workers over health professionals. All this 'bickering and back-biting'
had prevented effective health care reform. Solutions were to be found
through cooperation, not confrontation, and through a leaner, but not
meaner, bureaucracy. In stark contrast to the NDP's belief in almost
endless consultation, Wilson depicted a province in a state of anarchy,
which could benefit from more provincial control over the policy
agenda. (See Wilson, 1995, 8–9.)

Wilson promised that the new government would discontinue the
'ratcheting down of the institutional sector until adequate supports are
in place.' He implied that the New Democrats were interested merely in
cost cutting and were incompetent at it, arguing that Bill 173, although
legislating better access and coordination, did so 'at the expense of vol-

unteers and long-standing community-based organizations who will soon be driven from the system.' FP agencies were not mentioned in the description of those who stood to lose from implementation of the MSAs. The PCs noted that their strategy was to spend 'smarter' and included 'empowering people to assume more responsibility for their individual health needs and for the overall management of the health care system.' For critics of their approach, this pledge translated into shifting public costs to the individual and laying blame for the costs of the system on patient demands. The PCs also promised to stop 'payment on cheques which the government has dangled to bribe communities to set up MSAs.' The latter strategy was to save $5 million in start-up funds. They also argued that scrapping the MSA model would retain $37 million annually in volunteer services, which presumably would otherwise have disappeared from the system. (See Wilson, 1995, 11, 4, 10, 13.)

7.3 The Progressive Conservatives and the Community Care Access Centres

The Progressive Conservatives won a majority of seats in Ontario's thirty-sixth Parliament. On 26 June 1995 Mike Harris was sworn in as Ontario's twenty-second premier. Jim Wilson, the former health critic for the PCs, was made minister of health and given responsibility for long-term care.

On 12 July 1995 Premier Harris announced that, in keeping with his election promise, his government was immediately halting implementation of the MSAs, thereby 'undoing the damage imposed on long-term care services by the previous government' (Harris, 1995). In the same press release, Health Minister Jim Wilson revoked the 80-20 rule and the labour adjustment provisions.

Although Harris indicated that over the next sixty days Wilson would be meeting with key people in the policy community to get their advice on how best to coordinate the LTC system, the PCs had decided that he would not meet directly with the stakeholders. Instead, in an attempt to distance the minister from any attempts at lobbying, they hired the ARA Consulting Group, a private firm, to conduct the consultation sessions. According to 'Qs and As' prepared by the Ministry of Health (MOH), they were designed to be 'tightly focussed. Anyone who is not invited to attend these meetings is welcome to make their views known by writing to the ministry' (MOH, 1995a, 2).

Within government, responsibilities were also simplified. The Ministry of Citizenship had been amalgamated with Tourism and Recreation.

Neither the new group nor the Ministry of Community and Social Services (MCSS) was involved in this round of LTC reform. Instead, responsibility was centralized in the Ministry of Health. This move had the practical effect of redefining the policy community, thereby weakening the ability of those interest groups that were client populations of the other two ministries.

As noted above, the government quickly decided not to implement those sections dealing with MSAs, the 80-20 rule, and labour adjustment. However, it was generally satisfied with the other provisions of the act, which had given the minister of health considerable authority over home and community care (MOH, 1995a). The PCs realized that Bill 173 did not prevent them from pursuing their own agenda. Furthermore, repealing this legislation would delay implementation of their preferred model and would reopen debate, potentially moving it beyond their control.

The keen observer could find strong indications in this press release as to what sort of model would be acceptable to the new government. Discussions were to take place within the context of the following principles, which had both similarities to and differences from those of the previous governments. The principles of improved access, consistent eligibility requirements, and consistent and equitable funding for services remained. Added was an emphasis on 'highest quality of services at the best price,' on cutting duplication and red tape to put more money into front-line services, and on provider accountability for how money is spent on services (Harris, 1995). These principles were indications of an ideological shift in focus towards private business (highest quality / best price and provider accountability) and against public government (elimination of red tape).

7.3.1 The PC Consultation

In its request for proposal (RFP) for the consultation, the government indicated that it wanted to move quickly, with the expectation of announcing a new reform model by the fall of 1995. To achieve this end, it planned to avoid the mistakes of the NDP government, which had engaged in extensive consultations, by holding a limited consultation with approximately fifty provincial associations in eight discussion sessions. Like the NDP, the Progressive Conservatives wished to legitimate their own reforms through the seemingly autonomous support of societal interests. However, the PCs decided to hold seven sessions with representatives from various sectors primarily serving the elderly (providers, users, and workers were listed, in that order) and an eighth session for providers and users in the disability community (workers were not included in that session). As discussed above, under the NDP government the labour movement was not in favour of the direct-funding approach for people with disabilities. Their exclusion from this particular session may have been intended to avoid conflict over that issue, which might have further delayed the process.

The RFP also indicated that the consultants were to meet with ministry staff prior to the discussion sessions. In this meeting the consultants were to be briefed on the proposed content of the sessions as well as the preferred format and process for the discussions. To avoid raising expectations it did not wish to meet, government intended to control not only the process, but also the areas in which it sought input (MOH, 1995b).

The consultation process moved rapidly. Each session was scheduled for five hours (including a lunch break); all sessions were completed over a two-week period in August 1995. They were attended by MPP Helen Johns, Jim Wilson's parliamentary assistant. The reasons offered for the government's decision to have Johns rather than Wilson in attendance varied.

G: When the new ministers came on, they had agreed to approximately half the staff of the previous government. They didn't have the office staff ... And then we're [MOH] dealing with so many issues. So they had one parliamentary assistant and asked her to do that [consultation]. It was just a matter of workload.

P: The first sign that all was not well was the fact that Jim did not take the lead on the long-term care [consultation]. Helen Johns took the lead ... I think that the lobbying by the FP sector had continued all along. And that Helen Johns, when she came on – first of all she's a business person, so there was an openness to the idea of private sector involvement ... Additionally, her campaign manager, I remember, was a Home Care administrator. I have to check that out, but I think so, if I recall. Now the Home Care people were very much in favour of maintaining a brokerage model, because, of course, that maintains Home Care and it maintains the case manager role ... Remember I said about the role of the nurse versus the role of the case manager? So they had it in with Helen, and Helen was the lead. So between Harris's own and this government's overall idea that maybe there's nothing wrong with having private sector involvement, and it might in effect be good to improve the system. Helen's link into Home Care. What that all leads you to is favouring a brokerage model competing on best quality, best price.

Among the stakeholders, the consultation was viewed as a formality. It was clear that the government already knew its objectives.

P: I'm not sure how much change came out of the consultation in terms of policy. I think the majority of the input from the consultation was in process.

While the choice of Johns may have been either practical or ideological, or both simultaneously, it also created an institutional barrier to the ultimate policy decision maker for this reform, namely, Jim Wilson. In this way the Conservative government was able to protect Wilson from special-interest lobbies that could slow down reform.

The discussions at the consultation meetings were organized to discuss the following four questions:

What are the major access and coordination problems with the current long-term care system?

From a consumer's perspective what characteristics should the new system have vis-à-vis access and coordination?

How should the new system be organized to ensure access and coordination?

To what extent should government prescribe a model or models? (ARA Consulting Group, 1995, 2)

On the first three questions the previous two governments had already collected copious information. The last question was the opening for all provider groups who felt that the NDP model was far too government controlled and intrusive. In sessions dominated by providers, the consumer and union voices, which favoured the all-inclusive MSA model, were relatively muted.

The compressed time frame, the participation by invitation, the abbreviated invitation list, and the selected and well-managed agenda resulted in a report that, not surprisingly, supported the model the Conservatives intended to develop. Institutions, in terms of government structures and processes, were used to constrain societal interests and to further government ideology and interests.

7.3.2 The Consultation Report

In its report to the government, ARA Consulting indicated that there was agreement on the problems with the current LTC system, namely, poor access and coordination, inconsistency and inequity of services, inflexibility, fragmentation, duplication, multiple assessments, inadequate accountability, provider domination, inadequate complaints and appeal mechanism, lack of continuity of care, lack of recognition of special needs populations, and inadequate staff training (ARA Consulting Group, 1995). Not surprisingly, given the Conservative government's commitment to eliminate the MSA model, the consultants indicated that participants cited service organizations, staff who provide services, and volunteers as the strengths of the current system.

According to the report, the features of an ideal system for participants included minimal layers of bureaucracy; recognition that people with disabilities needed services, not care; provision of service choice; and encouragement of family solutions. Adults with disabilities particularly wanted a system that provided both individualized direct funding and an agency that brokered needed services, maintained choice (meaning that all providers should not be located within an integrated agency), and operated a separate system for seniors. ARA noted that participants wanted a parallel system for adults with disabilities, children with disabilities, and aboriginal people.

It was indicated in the report that, with a few exceptions, most participants were reluctant to recommend a model that would be suitable for all areas of the province. Instead, most participants wanted government to allow communities the flexibility to develop local models suitable to their own needs. The exception was 'a few seniors' organizations and most labour groups, who favoured having one model prescribed for the province' (ARA Consulting Group, 1995, 14). In most cases the latter groups supported an integrated model.

In terms of organizing the system, ARA argued that there was general agreement that the screening function should be combined with the information function. With the exception of special situations, assessments should be independent of provider organizations. While there was no consensus on funding approaches, three were suggested, the last one having the most support: brokerage (an independent MOH-funded organization would purchase services from agencies); ministry-approved budgets (MOH would fund agencies directly); and a local non-ministry authority funded by the ministry, which would in turn fund agencies.

Models presented by participants had a common basic structure, which included a local board, an independent assessment and resource management entity accountable to the board, and a range of independent service providers. Three models emerged from the discussion, according to the consultants: the Federation/Partnership Model, the Augmented Home Care / Managed Competition Model, and the Municipal / Public Health Model. A fourth model, the Amalgamated MSA was dropped. Although this model was indeed suggested by seniors and labour during the consultations, it was clearly not acceptable to the government. Accordingly, the only reference to this model in the report was a note in passing, buried in a different section, that a few participants supported an integrated model.

The Federation/Partnership Model would be a new, local, incorporated, NFP organization with a local community board made up of providers, consumers, and other representatives. The organization would purchase services and administer contracts, maintain a management information system and coordinate assessments. Service providers could authorize services for consumers with straightforward needs and for consumers who would approach them directly. The federation would work cooperatively with the network of providers, and its board would determine which providers would be recognized.

Under the Municipal / Public Health Model local health units would manage resources and care and either provide direct service or contract with others for service. This model was similar to the brokerage system operating in some areas of the province where the Home Care Program was operated by Public Health Units.

The Augmented Home Care / Managed Competition Model (which would eventually become the Conservative government's preferred model) consisted of a single local authority that would merge Home Care, Placement Coordination Services, and Community Information Centres. Although it had the same functions as the Federation Model, it would also house case management and assessment. Services would be purchased from approved providers. Without offering details as to how services would be purchased from providers, the consultants indicated that consumers would be involved in the choice of their providers, thereby fostering competition, and quality standards would be used to encourage competition among providers to achieve high quality care. Curiously, the only aspects of managed competition that were mentioned were those traditionally raised as concerns, namely, consumer choice and the maintenance of quality if price were used as the major criterion on which contracts were awarded.

With regard to implementation, the consultants indicated that the participants had advanced a list of criteria for the development of local models but were reluctant to specify these criteria or how they should be implemented. The participants' list repeated the same criteria that had recurred in each reform effort: clear access points, accessibility, accountability, consumer/community involvement, consumer control and choice, a defined set of mandated services, evaluation, case management for those who required it, simple assessment process minimizing duplication, provision for the unique needs of special populations, continued participation of volunteers, complaints and appeals procedure, human resource planning, standard training, information systems, sharing of resources where possible, cross-boundary access, linkages across providers, and flexibility to create new services. It was now up to government to create a new community-based model. The highly orchestrated report from the consultations gave the Conservatives carte blanche.

7.3.3 Assessment of the Consultations

To many in the policy community, the consultation was generally viewed not as an honest attempt to entertain recommendations from societal groups, but as merely a strategy of 'smoke and mirrors' (P) or 'meaningless' actions (G). One respondent believed that both the Liberals and the NDP were committed to public consultations as process as well as product.

G: But you see, you're dealing with a different mind set with the Tories. To them the consultative process is far less important than getting the job done. The consultative process has far less meaning to them.

Another respondent indicated that the reason for the focus groups was 'to tell us what they were doing was the right thing and that we would agree with it' (C). The constraints put on the consultation were evident in not only the participation by invitation, but also the number of representatives each organization was allowed and the tight control on the agenda for discussion.

C: We were told when we walked in the room there were two representatives only could go from each organization. And they had two different days. so all the organizations were consulted. Johns ... was there, and she started off in the morning by saying that now, 'we want to talk about reforms. There's some things we don't want to talk about. There's no point in bringing up anything about the MSA, because we're not talking about that today' ... There must have been twenty-five of us, and there was a consultant hired to do this and they went through their questions and answers and all this sort of stuff. And we all had about four minutes for one person of the two to make our point. And since we couldn't talk about the MSA, what could we talk about?

C: The problem with them, of course, was, they said, 'Here's what you're going to talk about. And here are the issues.' And we said, 'These aren't really the issues.' And it was such a narrow consultation. For all intents and purposes, it was not a consultation ... Basically there were consultants who said, 'Here's what we're allowed to talk about.' Helen Johns listened. I will give her credit for sitting through every single session all day, asking questions. But it was pretty clear they knew what they were going to do, and what they wanted to do. And it wasn't going to matter very much what we talked about doing.

P: We didn't bother [putting in a submission] because every sense of the issue that we had was that this wasn't a serious consultation. They'd had their mind made up. And they told us it was going to be determined by best quality, best price.

P: It was very staged. The consultation was, 'Here are the four questions ... This consultation is going to be basically, tell us what your answers are to these questions, and thank you very much.'

C: It was a selected consultation of selected individuals representing selected organizations and selected interests. So when you stack a room ...

Some groups, who disagreed with the government's direction, accused the government of distorting their position. For example, one respondent felt that the government purposefully misrepresented the consumer position by indicating that consumers had not supported the MSA model and wanted a different model. This was offered as further evidence that the consultation consisted of mirrors, that is, the government was interested only in views that reflected their own.

C: Contrary to the records from the government, we were very disappointed with the cancelling of the MSA. But the focus groups tend to be where you come and you say your piece and then you get your report saying, 'Seniors all agreed,' which is whatever way the government wishes it to be.

The fact that Helen Johns ran the consultation was seen as evidence of the slant the Conservatives were going to take and that the consultation was merely for political optics.

P: She [Johns] was from the business community ... And it was very obvious that she had very much a commercial marketplace-driven philosophy to everything and that she felt that the health care system needed to be more businesslike. So we kind of knew that the game was over even before we began, especially with her.

There was a feeling, however, that the Conservatives did correctly read the mood of interest groups by consulting quickly.

C: Now what they were right about, however, is that people were sick and tired of consultation ... so they were right to fast-track it.

The tight reins put on the consultation and its product narrowed the participation of groups in the policy community to a selected number, constrained the discussion to permissible topics in a reduced time frame, and distanced them from the policy makers. The Conservatives were intent on bringing the market to LTC and did not want to be distracted. With the exception of a few supporters, the attempt to give legitimacy to their policy model through the consultation failed in the eyes of most of the policy community.

7.3.4 The CCAC Model

On 25 January 1996 Health Minister Jim Wilson announced the LTC reforms, which were billed as simplifying access, preserving existing organizations, and reducing administration. Rather than creating over 100 multi-service agencies, the government was going to amalgamate the existing Home Care Programs with the existing Placement Coordination Services to create forty-three Community Care Access Centres. The CCACs would purchase services from existing providers based on best quality, best price (MOH, 1996d). With the exception of Metropolitan Toronto, service areas generally would be defined by the current Home

Care boundaries. In Toronto, the existing Home Care agency would be broken up, and up to six CCACs would be established.

In making his announcement Wilson remarked that the NDP had developed a model that 'was not supported by consumers or providers.' He argued that MSAs would have eliminated choice, favoured organized labour at the expense of volunteers, and hurt quality of care by driving provider organizations out of business. Through Bill 173 the NDP would have established approximately 130 MSAs throughout the province compared with the 43 CCACs, which he suggested would increase costs and add far too much bureaucracy (Wilson, 1996, 2). The announcement clearly emphasized the Conservatives' preferred interpretation of values: liberty through consumer choice, increased efficiency through less government and duplication, and improved quality from greater competition.

CCACs would constitute simplified service access points and be responsible for service information and referral to all LTC services, including the volunteer-based community services. They would coordinate service planning and monitoring, determine eligibility, and undertake case management and placement coordination services for LTC facilities. CCACs would determine eligibility and purchase professional, homemaking, and personal support services on behalf of consumers. Funding for these services would be allocated by the provincial government through envelope funding to the CCACs and would involve no charges to the consumer. They would not deliver services directly except during a three-year transition period; the purchaser of services and providers of service were to be split. Consumers could access community support services directly. These services would be directly funded by government and would involve a user fee. People with disabilities would be allowed to deal directly with their attendant services and would remain independent of the CCACs. However, they could, opt to apply for personal services through the CCAC. 'Clients' could directly access volunteer programs such as meals on wheels.

CCACs would be governed by independent, incorporated NFP boards of directors accountable to the MOH through service agreements. Board membership would be both a mix of the broader community LTC consumers and their caregivers and a balance of health and social services perspectives. The board would not include service providers under contract with CCAC (MOH, 1996c). In a draft job description for board members it was stated that they were expected to be committed to act in the best interests of all persons served by the CCAC, not to be spokespersons for any particular geographic area or special-interest group (MOH,

1996b). The first board would be selected by the minister, and subsequent boards would be elected by the membership of the CCAC.

According to the government, all providers would have equal opportunity to provide their services on a competitive basis. A transition period would allow providers (in particular, the NFP agencies) to 'adjust to the competitive system.' That is, the market shares of all existing providers would be protected in decreasing amounts for an initial three-year transition period. All existing service providers would have 90 per cent of their 1995–6 home care volume protected in year one, 80 per cent in year two, and 70 per cent in year three. Thereafter, not-for-profits and for profits were to compete on an even playing field. Provider agencies would retain their own identities, governance structures, and volunteer bases. CCACs would administer the RFP process within provincial guidelines, and funding would be based on both cost and quality. Objective methods of measuring quality would be developed in collaboration with providers, consumers, and the ministry, but they would include consumer satisfaction, worker continuity, staff training, and hours of service provision (MOH, 1996a). The Ministry would monitor service contracts on an ongoing basis and provide feedback to providers on their performance. Bill 173 still would provide the legislative framework for managing and delivering LTC community services, but sections pertaining to MSAs, the 80-20 rule and the labour adjustment strategies would not be used; indeed, they would eventually be repealed (MOH, 1996c).

Coupled with the fact that the NDP legislation had removed Home Care from OHIP, the government now had the tools it needed to shift onto consumers costs that formerly had been publicly paid for. With the movement of more publicly insured services out of hospitals into the community, the effect of these actions by successive governments was to passively privatize not only services formerly under Home Care, but also, potentially, services that would have been covered under the Canada Health Act had they remained within hospital walls.

By failing to replace the NDP's Bill 173 as the legislative framework for the new CCACs, the Conservative government gained important advantages. First, it was able to establish the CCACs quickly. New legislation would have had to be moved through a complex and probably lengthy process open to public and political scrutiny with the potential for mobilizing opposition to the government's initiative. Second, the Conservative government gained additional 'wiggle room,' which it attempted to use to cap public entitlements (Office of the Provincial Auditor General of Ontario, 1998a,b).

For instance, in response to a consumer who sought to appeal a decision of his local CCAC, provincial government lawyers argued that there was no right of appeal. CCACs, they argued, were 'creatures of government policy' and thus were not covered under the Long-Term Care Act (Bill 173), which specified a basket of mandatory services and includes a patient's bill of rights as well as a statutory appeal mechanism. Although the province's quasi-judicial Health Services Appeal Board subsequently ruled against the government, finding that the CCACs were obliged to meet legislative requirements, the government first ignored this ruling, then subsequently introduced provincial regulations imposing maximum allowable hours of service available through the CCACs and thus not subject to appeal at that level (Care Watch Ontario, 1999; Health Services Appeal Board, 1999; Williams et al., 2001).

In August 1996 the premier announced the appointment of Cam Jackson as minister without portfolio with responsibility for seniors issues, removing this function from the Ministry of Citizenship, Culture and Recreation (MCCR). While the MOH would retain the budget and policy-setting functions for LTC, Jackson was responsible for overseeing the implementation of the CCACs (Government of Ontario Premier's Office, 1996). However, Jackson was not part of the Harris inner circle. Indeed, many viewed his appointment as a minister without portfolio rather than as a full-fledged cabinet minister as the price Jackson had to pay for having run an energetic campaign against Mike Harris for the leadership of the party (P).

A few respondents believed that Jackson's appointment was designed to ease the workload of the minister of health by taking over the implementation of LTC and also to ensure that the initial momentum and visibility were sustained (P, P, G). Hospital restructuring had begun, and the ministry was also in the middle of contentious negotiations with physicians. Indeed, on 9 December 1996 Health Minister Jim Wilson had to step down temporarily after one of his aides breached confidentiality provisions by disclosing billing information about a physician. Although eventually cleared of personal involvement by Information and Privacy Commissioner Tom Wright in a 20 February 1997 report, Wilson was obviously not in a position to devote the time needed to LTC restructuring (Wright, 1997). Neither was his temporary replacement as minister of health, David Johnston, who continued to bear heavy responsibilities as chair of Management Board. Whatever its other merits, this move created, once again, an institutional wedge between the policy maker and budget holder for LTC services and the implementers of the reform. Yet again, restricted access to the decision maker allowed implementation of the Conservative vision to move forward with few obstacles. In addition, Jackson was given responsibility only for seniors' issues, while disability issues remained under MCCR. This action narrowed the scope of conflict and turned LTC again into a seniors' reform.

7.3.5 Assessment of CCACs

Although the CCACs were not yet up and running at the time of our interviews, stakeholders were willing to speculate about how they believed the model would work.

7.3.5.1 Consumers

Seniors saw the model as a government-run program, rather than one that was community driven. Some focused on the perceived diminution in sensitivity to local issues arising from the larger catchment areas associated with the smaller number of organizations. For example, in Toronto there were going to be six CCACs, as opposed to sixteen MSAs. They were concerned that the system would be more fragmented because the community support services would be outside the CCACs. They also recognized that their worry that Bill 173 left too many details to be worked out in the regulations gave a similar freedom to the Conservative government to move on its very different agenda.

The disability groups were less concerned about FP provision or market mechanisms. From their perspective, the new model would enhance consumer choice and independence in decision making. Since the government would continue the direct-funding pilot projects, the most vocal disability groups were content. The one concern they voiced was whether the Bill of Rights under Bill 173 and an effective complaints procedure would be implemented.

For their part, some ethnocultural communities feared that their agencies, although no longer threatened by the MSA model, would not be as successful at winning contracts because of the nature of the services they provided. Similarly, they believed that the Progressive Conservatives, with their focus on the bottom line, were not interested in supporting diversity. Each CCAC would be allowed to determine whether and how these issues would be addressed.

Those supporting the CCAC model, such as FP providers, contended that consumers wanted to get on with reform, noting that this time a different set of consumers represented at the consultations were airing their views.

P: They [consumers] said, 'Let's get on with it. You know, we can't go back to more consulting, more reviewing, any of that, because we're just stalling' ... You had a very broad spectrum there, of consumers' groups, which I've never seen in the room before. During the MSA stuff, when you talked to consumers or consumers being represented, it was Jane Leitch through the Seniors' Alliance group. And there are those who believe that ... they were a puppet for Consultant A's group who was funded to promote a policy that the government wanted.

7.3.5.2 Labour

Organized labour favouring NFP service provision saw the Conservative model as a threat. They argued that NFPs would not be able to compete with FPs in a public market based on quality and price, particularly since quality was so ill defined. They were afraid that eventually the delivery dimension of LTC community-based services would switch from largely NFP to FP. Lurking beneath the surface of this concern was fear of an eventual takeover by U.S. nationals and the inevitable Americanization of health care in Canada.

P: [We're very frustrated] with the fact that the choice for the provider will be based on cost and quality. Because we don't think that quality will continue to be a key force, but rather, cost will be. Also a concern that, while initially, let's say in a community you have VON. You have several small FP companies, and maybe they're pretty well equal. They're sitting ducks for an American company coming in and undercutting the whole lot and then getting that contract because with free trade, and so on, we don't have anything that would prevent that.

P: There is a real danger that care will be provided by the lowest bidder, the way that the proposals are set up and the contracts will be applied. Although they say that quality of care will receive equal attention as the amount of money that agencies are asking for. I don't believe in the long run that that's going to have as much hold, as much sway as cost. So I do think that there's a real danger that our quality of care is going to hit the tubes.

The other issue and sort of related to that also, is that there are some very large concerns, very large organizations, very large companies who are coming in and underbidding like crazy and are able to and willing to take a loss for the first three or four years in order to get their foot in the door, get contracts, and then slowly, you know, the price will increase.

The cost to the Ontario public will increase. ... Also concerned too that FP entities are going to be providing probably a lion's share of the care, just because of the way it's structured.

We have heard, and other work I'm doing and have been doing, is the American health care companies see Canada as the unopened oyster and home care as the foot to get into the door. And we're already seeing it in long-term care facilities [that] are being bought up by, in Peterborough, Omnicare – Huge American corporation who has just bought up six nursing homes. And this is supposed to be an area they're losing money [in]. Then why are these American corporations so interested in buying up our nursing homes here? And a lot of people say that they're getting a foot in the door to provide the other home care services. And I think that this home care, without these kinds of protections that [are] in the MSA, we're going to move into an FP Americanized health care system with user fees. And this is the way it's going to be done. And the CCACs provide no protection against it.

For one labour organization, the CCAC model, on its own, would not have been so ominous. Given the decisions that this government were taking in other sectors, however, they viewed it as 'yet another nail in our tradition of public health care' (C).

P: When we were doing the MSA stuff, we ... didn't have this commission [Health Services Restructuring Commission] running around the province closing hospitals. We didn't have deregulation of the removal of standards in long-term care facilities. We didn't have the user fees for drugs for seniors and low-income families. We didn't have the sell-off of ambulance services to American firms. You know, it might have been more innocuous ... except that they stripped away those two significant pieces of the legislation [80-20 rule and labour adjustment]. It might have just been seen as 'same as, different name' with a slightly different spin, and they're not going to have the direct service providers. But given the context and the shifting ground in all the other areas of the health sector, it's a little more ominous, I think.

The labour movement saw that workers, their compensation packages, and work standards were going to be the elements in the contracting process that would be manipulated to produce a competitive bid.

P: Contracting out workers in competition with each other and therefore their wages and benefits become ... cards that are kind of dealt on the table and go to the lowest bidder. And often what they're bidding with is the quality of somebody's work. Workers are constantly hearing that they have to be more flexible. Those workers, [who] are more flexible, they'll get your work if you're not more flexible. They can do it cheaper ... It means you don't have a contract language that protects you from a two-hour week this week and a fifty-hour week next week, you know. We know what they're doing to employment standards. [You don't have] a contract that says, or a health and safety legislation that says one-person lifts are not safe and you can refuse to do that work. And ... you de regulate a work environment to make it so-called flexible.

7.3.5.3 NFP Providers

Provider agencies, not surprisingly, were split in their support of the Conservative model along FP and NFP lines. Inherent in this split was the difference in the values they held, which was reflected in the ways that they conducted their programs. For example, NFPs put more emphasis on responsiveness to community needs and workers' well-being than on the ability to satisfy shareholders. There was a view that the Conservative model would ultimately erode the values underlying NFP service provision.

P: I find this [PC model] is cut-throat ... There's clearly conflict in values between the NFPs and the FPs. Well, they'd [FPs] like to think that that isn't the case, but there still is a bottom line; there still is profit going to the owners of the organizations. And that's got to come out of service, or off the backs of the workers ... And I think, the winners at the end of the day – and there are some NFPs who have decided to take on the sort of the business mantra. So it's leading to conflict, too. I think the people have had some value dissonance within their own organization because they're again weighing survival versus staying solid to our values ... I think at the end of the day, what it means for everyone is less service for people and less quality service.

NFP providers also believed that the government was naive in thinking that managed competition would be more cost effective. Recalling that their model was a federation of existing agencies, they saw the CCAC as an additional level of bureaucracy. Moreover, they believed that, contrary to the notions of efficiency, there were considerable costs in managed competition that were not considered or talked about.

P: I've argued there's a cost to have managed competition and we need to know that. And that conversation has never really been had. And there's a reason, and that's because of the whole politics. So it's clear to me that's what the whole agenda is behind it is to really have the commercial sector play a role. Because if it was to really create a more cost-effective system, people would be looking at what [we've] talked about. Because it doesn't take anyone a great deal of difficulty to know that that's [CCAC] an infrastructure layer in the system that's redundant.

Echoing the labour movement, the privatization (meaning commercialization) of the sector was seen as the real danger of the CCAC model. Managed competition would eliminate the NFP sector, leave Ontario open to U.S. nationals, and ultimately result in increased prices and costs to Ontarians that would not be reversible. In this scenario, indigenous NFP and FP agencies would lose out.

P: If you want to go the one next step after that, after we're [NFPs] gone, and after all the mergers and acquisitions have come in, so that commercial organizations are basically now in control of our community-based services ... We've got multi-service, multi-national, and there's maybe two or three of them, that have literally bootlegged our entire community-based services – guess what they're going to do? Push the prices up. And what's going to happen? Regardless of the stripes of the government of the day, what is going to happen is the same exact thing as with nursing homes right now ... The government isn't able to move on them because if they kicked them out they'll have to take over. But imagine, you know, ten years out. We might have to buy back the long-term care system from three multinational corporations, one in Belgium, and one in Japan, and one in America. And the government's going to look at it and say, 'We're stuck with this because we can't afford to buy that back. Our NFP partners are gone.' Too bad. There's nobody out there.

P: Strangely enough, this has been shared to me by Canadian FP agencies. They are very concerned that a lot of multinational private companies are coming up from the States to undercut, because it is going to be competitive and they can undercut at the beginning. They'll have backing from their own companies ... and will come in at very cheap rates. And both the FPs and NFPs will be lost ... And if we were to look to south of the border and visited several of the various agencies around, the quality of standards and the quality of service that is provided to the seniors is not what I would say would be the quality in Canada [we want] ... And I worry about even the FP agencies that are here and have struggled and worked and built up their own businesses and will be losing their businesses.

One critic in government echoed these concerns. For this interviewee, Canada did not have the market base to sustain agencies without CCAC contracts in a managed competition environment. Moreover, the FP motive in driving down costs from his perspective would erode quality and safety by encouraging the substitution of health care workers with less-qualified, lower-skilled, and cheaper workers. Ironically, once again, the NDP legislation made provisions for exactly this scenario.

G: What they're saying is that they believe that we have an adequate size, first of all a population and secondly potential provider agencies who could, even without the government contracts, stay alive and provide the service. That won't happen. We don't have an adequate sector base for an organization that doesn't get the contract to stay in business. We're just too small.

They haven't defined quality. What you get is what you pay for. And they are going to, under the tendering process, get the lowest bid. Now what that means is that there may be lower qualifications for nursing care. And we're seeing that happening in our hospitals now where the R.N.s are the ones being displaced and it's the nurse's aides who are less qualified, have a different function, but now are taking on more and more responsibility in the hospital structure. That is clearly going to happen in Home Care ... because so much of the cost of any health care delivery is the human resources cost. And what you will also find are general health workers, or whatever it's called, which are people who basically have extremely little training; they'll be delivering a lot of care.

One respondent from an NFP organization, while believing that the NFPs could and would successfully adjust to managed competition, stated that one of the beneficial aspects inherent in a NFP environment, the cooperative spirit, would deteriorate. Information that up to now had been shared freely to improve services was now a strategic resource that had to be well managed in a competitive environment.

P: They recognized that they have to change a lot of their perception of how they operate – a simple thing like openness. This happens to be a fairly open organization. It recognizes, however, that if it's competing with other people, it cannot do the equivalent of revealing trade secrets or trade strategies. It might have got up at an annual meeting, two years ago, and said, 'This is what we plan to do for the future.' They're now saying, 'Can we afford to do that, because our competition's going to be at our annual meeting? Do we want them to know what our game plan is?' So I think there'll be a real change in how non-profits perceive their role. I mean they've always been competitive, but it's been a different kind of competition. It hasn't been so much a bottom line, we can do it cheaper competition.

Indeed the competitive environment was viewed as being responsible for dissolving the coalition of the four NFP organizations that had formed at the beginning of this government mandate.

P: [I: Does the group of four still exist?] I would say its life probably ended pretty much when we finished the transitional support [period]. Because now that that's finished, we're now into a competitive model, and everyone's competing for market share.

One respondent believed that NFPs, through the elimination of waste and inefficiency, were up to the task of becoming more competitive. He described strategies that could be employed to keep these organizations viable; strategies that might go against their value of developing services to meet needs rather than to generate profits or lower bids.

P: They will go in two directions in the course of becoming competitive. One is they'll try to produce the lowest-cost product for the public dollar. They'll do it by controlling wages within their organizations, by trying to cut other kinds of administrative overhead within their organizations. Many of the really big non-profit services are administratively heavy. So, I think that those are ways they'll try to cut their costs. And I think they'll be largely successful in that regard. I think they'll try to bid on things where they know they can be low cost and will worry less about providing the things that they'd like to provide, [that] they feel in their hearts they ought to provide, or that they can't be competitive at. And I think the second thing they'll do is they'll try to go after the non-government dollar market much more than they have over the last twenty years. We non-profits have gotten pretty comfortable sucking at the public trough.

When the public trough gets smaller, they'll see if there are any other troughs out there ... Those could be through insurance companies, it could be through user-pay, it could be through appealing to markets that aren't even in the province.

7.3.5.4 FP Providers

The FP organizations that had promoted the managed competition model thought, not surprisingly, that the values underpinning NFP and FP agencies were not as different as the non-profit providers alleged; that lack of business acuity, not competition, threatened the viability of an organization; and that Canada was not under siege by the Americans.

P: The quality of the service had nothing to with the tax status of the organization. It had to do with management. Good managers produce good care; bad managers produce bad care. It had nothing to do with profits. The next question is, 'What is profit?' ... Profit is simply a cost. It's got a name, 'profit,' but it's simply a cost of an organization being able to stay in business for their future and to continue what they're doing ... They [NFP organizations] have inefficiencies versus profit.

P: If you're a company, you're foolish to put all your money, all your service into one contract. You've got to diversify ... Agencies who haven't thought through a business plan, good business strategy, are not economically viable, and that's because they're mismanaging themselves.

P: I've personally watched – this is many years ago in the nursing home sector – the largest American company providing nursing home care would come into Canada and be gone in less than a year because they didn't understand the environment. They thought it was another America ... I watched them do this ... They didn't understand the governmental level of administration of the system. And it was not an experience they enjoyed. And they got out as fast as they could ... Because Canada is different. Canada is a public health care system that's publicly administered.

The CCAC model represented a considerable ideological shift away from NDP values. Market principles of competition and efficiency became pre-eminent. Equity and security for consumers and labour were trumped by equality between FP and NFP providers ('even playing field') and security for all providers, once they would no longer be forced to amalgamate into MSAs. While the NDP spoke of consumer empowerment in terms of consultation and authority in decision making, the Conservative government spoke of consumer voice in terms of consumer satisfaction, as expressed through competition among providers. No longer were special-interest consumers (ethnocultural, persons with disabilities, and seniors) or labour allowed to represent their interests directly on CCAC boards. These interests were to be expressed by the general board membership.

Advocates of the CCAC model insisted that consumer choice would increase, since CCACs had to contract, where possible, with more than one agency for particular service contracts. In reality, however, choice of provider agency would rest less with the consumer than with the CCAC and would depend upon which agencies had been successful in the competitive process. Consumers had argued earlier that choice of the individual provider was more important than choice of provider agency. Managed competition could further threaten this notion of choice for consumers; should the provider agency whose worker the consumer preferred not be successful in the next round of competition, the only way the consumer could continue to choose that provider would be to change agencies or privately purchase those services. Persons with disabilities continued to be allowed to opt out of the LTC model through direct funding. Direct funding for persons with disabilities was very much in keeping with a conservative agenda where the consumer/client has control and money follows the client. Ethnocultural consumers were notionally allowed choice if their preferred agency were successful in gaining a CCAC contract.

Labour was the big loser in this model. Since wages are the largest component of service costs in this labour-intensive field, managed competition, with its emphasis on lowest costs, threatened to erode existing compensation packages and working conditions and to undermine the power of the unions. With provider agencies' no longer being transferred to MSAs and the privilege unionized workers received under Bill 173 no longer in force, the union movement was denied the growth they had been promised by the NDP in the community sector to compensate for ongoing losses within hospitals.

While all existing provider agencies would now have the opportunity to remain in business, the new managed competition process was thought to advantage FP over NFP agencies. In a competition based on 'best quality at the best price,' where quality is ill defined and where most of the costs of agencies are salaries, it was believed that price would win out. FP organizations were believed to have a competitive edge on the price dimension, since they tended to pay poorer salary and benefit packages to their workers than NFP agencies. Moreover, while NFP agencies were subject to pay equity legislation that would force many to increase wages in this predominately female and historically underpaid field, many FP competitors were not subject to the same requirement. In addition, it was thought that larger FP organizations, having the infrastructure and experience to respond to RFPs, would enjoy an additional advantage. Since it was was doubtful that agencies unable to win a contract would be able to stay viable until the next competition, the balance in the LTC market could shift over time to commercial agencies and, in an era of global markets and trade agreements, to American multinationals.

7.4 Government Interests in the Development of the CCAC Model

Respondents from government did not disagree with the assessments of the interest groups. The Conservatives were guided by their *Common Sense* document, which emphasized their desire for less government, more competition and market mechanisms, adherence to the bottom line, involvement of the commercial sector, and more distance between themselves and the NDP. For many, the reform now took on a 'market liberal' ideological bent, in contrast to the more socialist leaning evident under the NDP. The Conservative government's interests and the ideology underpinning them were, to these respondents, transparent.

G: I think that this government needed to distance itself enormously from the NDP. I think that it needed to send a strong signal to the business community that the health care system in Ontario was open for business.

G: [Their interests] are (a) not to do the NDP model, and (b) to encourage the private sector to take over the provision of these services.

P: So it became clear that in my judgment we were just talking another shift in ideology. And I don't think there was much clarity to what that really looked like other than it wouldn't – the structure would not be MSAs. So I think the next step to that was, if not MSAs, then what kind of a structure accommodates the private sector? And that brought in the ideology ... They wanted to transfer or re-invent, something a bit different than Home Care and that's where the CCACs were created with placement and Home Care coming together and the opportunity for the private sector to compete for all of the services. So in essence, there was almost a deregulation, if you want to use that term, of home care services in the community. Because previously under the Home Care Programs the mandate was always that the Home Care Programs could and should provide the services, or they could purchase the services ... With this new model ... the market becomes open and you compete for the work. And that whole conflict of interest, arm's length, governance piece is actually quite foreign in the NFP or hospital sector. We really don't worry about conflict of interest and what is the profit of health care. I mean that's just not a language of any other sector of the health system. In the community that language has now come about, and I think, because of the whole role for the private sector in this service delivery component.

C: They're trying to get more private sector business involved.

C: Privatization – they don't believe in providing any services. Everything must be on a business basis, which means it has to make money ... They want to do away with public services.

P: Ideologically it's [CCACs and managed competition] quite compatible with their direction – privatization of services and a cheapening of services ... Much less interest and emphasis on the role of government in the provision of services. I mean they don't really believe in a social security net in the way I think that Ontarians have been used to.

G: A couple of things. One is that they wanted something that didn't look like it was designed by the NDP. I think they wanted something that would allow private enterprise to play on a competitive basis.

C: I think it's [Conservative agenda in LTC] two things: one is money. I mean whatever they do, it's always money first, to save money first. I think the second thing is they want to make it, – the private sector has been pushing them to privatize as much as they can of health. I think they have contributors who they owe big time. They're trying to get the government out of doing things.

P: Well, I think it's the same model that's behind all of their fundamental philosophy of this particular so-called Common Sense Revolution.

They're more in the business of getting government out of delivering services than they are of anything else. And this tax thing is actually, you know, giving taxes to people is really, everything they've done, deregulating anything, not just in health care, environment, whatever it is. There's the deregulation moves, the privatization moves, the open for competition – is to get government out of the business of delivering service and leave it open to market. And I think we're just going to see it full force here in home care.

The government's decision to move community support services outside the realm of the CCAC's responsibility was seen as yet another way of focusing on the bottom line, a way of keeping tight control over spending and reducing government's responsibility in the future.

Meanwhile, the federal Liberals were receiving policy advice about LTC. In October 1994 the federal government established the National Forum on Health (National Forum on Health, 1997), which travelled across Canada consulting Canadians, commissioned papers, and geared up to advise the government on ways to improve the health care system and the health of Canadians. One of the issues that was being explored was the changing nature of care, the shifting locus of care from hospitals to the community, and the potential de-insuring of formerly insured health services. It was anticipated that one of the forum's recommendations would be to establish a publicly funded federal-provincial Home Care Program within or alongside Medicare. One respondent believed that the Ontario government did not include community support services under the CCACs for this reason, to ensure that Ontario would not be liable for publicly providing a wider range of services under Home Care, should such a program be established.

P: If the federal government comes up with a national home care funding program, you know, if they actually decide to include drugs and home care in the Canada Health Act provision, then those [community support services] are services that they don't want to have included.

For another respondent (G), the government did not need to control access to community support services as much as it did to professional, homemaking, and personal support services. The latter services, which were to be purchased by the CCACs, were far more costly.

Many respondents believed that unlike the situations under the two earlier governments, the locus of policy development under this government was highly centralized in order to ensure that its agenda, as articulated in *The Common Sense Revolution*, was pushed through quickly. Once again, institutional arrangements were put in place to promote government interests and ultimately the ideology underlying them.

G: The government seems to be run out of the Premier's Office by a handful of people, and they tend to direct what is going on. I don't see the ministers playing the same role as under the previous three governments ... It's a way that a lot of governments work when they want to make sure that their agenda is going to get through without any hitches and without any sidelines. If you have a government that wants to be really focused and they have certain things they want to have done, if you start to let other people have their ideas, your agenda can be derailed. And that happened in [the NDP] government ... So if they are focused entirely on privatization, cutting the deficit, and bringing in tax reforms, if you have ministers that are given a full reign to do what they want to do and start consulting and going out. And their bureaucrats have been working on issues for the last ten or fifteen years ... If central control is taken away, then they're just not going to be able to get their agenda done.

C: Decisions are not made by policy people, not made by bureaucrats, not made even in some cases by ministers. They're coming out of a central point – from the premier's office.

P: [The Premier's Office] because they were determined to make the CSR into a real agenda ... And someone sits and ticks off boxes as each thing gets done. And that person sits in the Premier's Office.

A variation on this theme was articulated by one respondent, who believed that reform was not centrally controlled but was being developed in the minister of health's office.

G: My suspicion is that because Jim [Wilson] was clearly on the record as knowing what he opposed and what he would do, that he is in fact probably driving this one. Because they moved fairly quickly, even though in almost all policy aspects this government is driven in the Premier's Office. I said earlier that most premiers would question the wisdom of putting a critic in as minister. And I suspect Mr Harris has had cause to question putting Jim in as health minister for that very reason.

There are hostages out there, things that you said in opposition that you now have to follow through on. But he came to office with a clear sense of direction and the ministry has been following that.

The almost unanimous view was that, under this new regime, Ontario had indeed gone to market. Conservative ideology – more market provision (preferably FP provision) of services, less government, cost cutting, and a removal of the vestiges of an NDP model – was underlying the government's interest in LTC reform. Policy was more centrally controlled and driven to ensure that this agenda moved forward.

7.5 Societal Interests

Although the policy interests of stakeholder groups did not change, previous commonalities were no longer sufficient to maintain alliances. Underlying differences among allied groups, which had been submerged under the NDP, resurfaced. The government's highly structured consultation and institutional barriers to ministerial access left little time or opportunity for groups to influence the reform. Alliances shattered as distrust grew and groups repositioned themselves under the new order. Other groups merely faded away.

7.5.1 Changing Structure of Societal Groups

Without their special status and government resources and with a clear message from the Conservatives that the MSA model was out, consumers had very little to say under this government. In addition, seniors' groups were particularly susceptible to turnover among their leadership as formerly vibrant seniors aged.

P: They're [SCCA] still there, but they certainly don't have the linkages they had before. They were seen as a very strong NDP group, [and] had a very adversarial relationship with, particularly, Jim Wilson when he was in opposition through the Standing Committee hearings. And they taught me, you always be nice to people.

O: The members of the SCCA still stay in touch with each other but they are not as active as they once were. There have been some deaths in the leadership group. Sad that they would die or get ill before they could see any change from all their efforts.

As the Conservative agenda across many diverse policy sectors was implemented in full force (e.g., downsizing of hospitals and the civil service and cutbacks in the broader public sector), the labour movement was fighting many other battles and was spread too thin.

Most of the input of interests for the CCAC reform accordingly came from provider organizations. While the FP and NFP agencies were united in their opposition to the MSAs, once the Conservatives came to power, the commonality that these groups shared started to fall apart. As it turned out, their shared interests under the NDP lay in opposing what they did not want; there was considerably more disagreement about what each did want. When the Conservative consultation asked for alternatives to the MSA, the different factions in the Group for LTC Reform started to meet separately to develop models, which, not surprisingly, diverged from one another. With the shift in government ideology and direction in this policy sector, the balance of power between the FP and NFP organizations transferred to the former. The FP organizations saw that their time had come. This respondent describes the shift.

P: When it came time to try and do something constructive as opposed to destructive in terms of objecting – the Conservative government had come into power and there was already a divisiveness in the group [Group for LTC Reform] – the commercials [FPs] were pulling further away from the NFPs. Originally the NFPs had held all the power, because the NDP did not favour the commercial sector. So I think the commercials found it very helpful [under the NDP government] to be part of a group that was this involved, and it gave them relationships and some respectability they didn't have. That shoe switched ... OHHCPA [the FP providers association] got together under the very capable direction of Vida Mazza and started to develop their model. Their model in many ways is very much similar to the one that the Home Care Program Association developed and, in part, probably because Vida had been the president of the Home Care Program Association so she knew that system. And it was really almost what you see as the CCAC. The NFP group which was VON, St Eliz., OCSA, and Red Cross got together and spent a lot of time trying to come up with an alternative model.

Some organizations described the way in which NFPs, sensing the change in the ideological wind, started to meet quietly apart from the other organizations in the Group for LTC Reform.

P: At the same time, there was a 'group of four,' [as] they were called, within the Long-Term Care Reform Group who had put together some thoughts about what they might propose [to the PC consultation]. But they had not let the rest of us know. But we found out. And at one of our meetings of the Group for Long Term-Care Reform, it became clear they were meeting in the hallway ... I thought we had agreed we'd all be proposing one approach and we were [not] going to go off and do our own thing. But it became clear that they were going off to do their own thing. And at that meeting I remember very clearly talking about hidden agendas. And it was the OHA [Ontario Hospital Association] who cottoned on to this ... And we questioned them. And they said, 'No, there's no model. We've just put some thoughts together.' But in a group that [had] worked so hard together, and all of a sudden a smaller group was going off, doing things that they weren't prepared to share with us. [It] felt like they were going off to present, to develop something to present to this government. And there we'd be sitting without a counter-proposal. So this all happened very quickly because we had a sixty-day time frame ... The group of four said, 'Don't worry, we'll look after you' ... The break up of the group came essentially with that chasm where you saw a subgroup going off to do, serve its own interest without informing the rest of the group. So the rest of the group said ... 'If they're going to put forward a proposal, we're certainly going to have to protect our interest and put forward a proposal.'

P: The four NFP service providers got together without anyone's knowledge to develop its own proposal. We caught wind of it ... and asked for an accounting of what was going on, given that we had committed to working as a group. And then we heard that the four went off to do their own thing. And they essentially said, 'Well, trust us. We can't reveal everything to you right now but trust us, and we'll make sure your interests are served in our proposal' ... So we developed our own proposal. We felt we had to. We had been left with no choice but to do that.

P: The government was asking about alternatives to MSA. But we didn't know at the time, and we know now, that some of the more major non-profits got together and went to government with something else, long before we did.

P: I remember ... saying, 'We need to talk. You know. We've got to come up with something as an alternative.' Because we didn't have anything. I felt that what the group was doing was just a sham. All they were doing was opposing Bill 173, and we knew the NDP weren't going to be elected, but as soon as someone else gets elected they're going to say, 'Okay, now what's your model?' And we knew there wasn't anything ... The commercial sector had lobbied really hard during the election campaign and had helped finance their election campaigns too, so now you know, was payoff time, and that's the way politics works. So we knew that there was going to be a lot of pressure. We had to come up with an alternative. So we met over the summer and then came up with this partnership model ... So we had agreed by prior decision that each of our four organizations, when we presented at these hearings, would present not necessarily a final model but the beginning of that model. And it actually got refined a little bit as it went along, because I think the very first time it was presented by [one of the organizations], the first plan was that no 'FPs' would be allowed on the board of this partnership organization. And it got lambasted by other people in the room.

One respondent from an NFP agency indicated that even within the informal coalition of NFP groups there was dissent between the professional service providers and the support service providers. In the end, however, the feeling was that it was better to submit one model from their side than multiple ones.

P: We really felt strongly that the future particularly was going to be more of a commercial/NFP tension, that it was going to be that old sort of, health and community and social services, but we weren't successful in selling that. Anyway, it wasn't one of the happier moments in my career. We had an opportunity and we threw it away ... We were told it would be unacceptable to submit ... two NFP models. It was one or none.

With distrust rampant among the members of the Group for LTC Reform, organizations began to take sides.

P: You've got Home Care, that is, the Public Health Units, and the FPs lined up to support the model [CCAC]. On the other side you've got the NFPs lined up against the model. The sector's essentially split.

The government effectively changed the power balance among societal groups in this policy community. It marginalized groups that had been powerful under the NDP by removing the resources formerly provided by that government, by limiting consultation, and by creating multiple battle fronts. The Conservative ideology bred distrust among former provider allies and, along with the highly constrained consultation, led to the splitting of groups. As societal groups withdrew into their own corners of interests, the government was in full control of the agenda.

7.5.2 Interests Advanced by Societal Groups at the Consultation

The societal groups were now realigned into four camps. Consumers and labour, the favoured interests under the NDP government, still wanted the MSA model. Municipalities and the Public Health Units wanted to consolidate their power by expanding the status quo and taking over the management of those Home Care Programs not currently under their control. The FP providers and Home Care staff wanted a case/care management split, a competitive purchaser/provider split, and governing boards without providers. These features would give the FP providers unfettered access to the home care market, give the Home Care staff a continuing role to play in the new system, and serve as a bulwark against the Public Health Units draining Home Care resources for their own purposes. Finally, the NFPs wanted a partnership or federation of provider organizations that would be directly funded by government and where care and case management were performed by these organizations. They did not want others performing their assessments or managing their cases, nor did they want to have to compete with the FPs for contracts.

G: One model was very close to the one they [government] chose. It was the Community Care Access Centre, obviously, that was supported by the Ontario Home Health Care Providers Association. And [it] had sort of a parallel ... in the submission that was made by the Home Care programs themselves, but not the sponsors [municipalities, Public Health Units] of Home Care. Obviously it was couched very carefully because they [Home Care staff] didn't want to tell their bosses [Public Health Units] that they wanted a different model. But obviously it was also a case management model. So that was one model.

You had a second model that was principally put forward by the municipalities and boards of health, that said that the current method of running Home Care was perfectly fine. And if there were any problems with it the municipalities could look after it, and that municipalities should have the first right of refusal in terms of the system. And of the thirty they ran, that they probably want to continue to run, and that in the other eight areas of the province that would give them an option of taking over those too if they wished to.

And then you had a third group of people who came in and said that they wanted, thank you very much – these are the consumer groups and the labour groups – they came in and said, 'Gee, we want the MSA. We know you've ruled it out but we still think that's the one we want.'

And then you had a fourth group, which was the major non-profit providers, who came in and said, 'No, we don't think we should have a model that separates out case management from care management. We think that in fact, the system should be run by a partnership arrangement among the service providers and that they should be funded directly by government rather than through an intermediate agency such as Home Care or the CCAC. And that they could work together to develop efficiencies by integrating the functions of case management and care management and eliminating some of the duplications involved at the separate care, case management level. And so that was the fourth model on the table. And considering those four models, as you know, which one won.

Another government interviewee expanded on the interests of the various groups and described the process of reaching a solution.

G: [The municipalities and the Association of Local Health Professionals] 'didn't want to lose Home Care Programs nor the administrative dollars that went with that. [The NFP sector] had no doubt they could provide the highest quality. In fact they argued that their quality of service would be way and above most of the providers because their wages were higher, that their staff were less transitory, had more stability. They had training. They did research. They did a lot that commercial agencies, they claimed, didn't do. So they said, we have no problem providing you with the highest quality at the highest dollar. But we can't do it at the best price because we know the commercial agencies can undercut us ... the concern about the Wal-Mart of health care. [The FP agencies] realized that the charitable organizations had been able to do things over the years that somebody in business for themselves simply can't do. They don't have the fat to do it ... They felt that the non-profits could be more competitive. And they were willing to concede that the non-profits might need a chance to become competitive. So negotiations occurred ... And what was finally decided on was a three-year period of decreasing protections for current service providers. And so it guarantees 90 per cent, 80 per cent, 70 per cent of volume. In other words, VON, who says, 'We've been in business for a hundred and some odd years,' or whatever, weren't going to just go bankrupt overnight. It also meant that new commercial agencies couldn't just move in from the get-go and take over the whole market. That there would be a gradual effect ... To have it more of an evolutionary effect than revolutionary.

While NFP and FP providers would not disagree with the above depictions, their own words highlight some nuances. One NFP provider said it was very difficult arguing for the primacy of NFP provision for its own sake in the context of a 'managed competition' environment. NFP providers sought to argue that NFP had nobler motives than making profits and hence would require fewer safeguards against conflicts of interest. Such statements were unconvincing to decision makers, particularly in a climate where efficiency arguments ruled supreme over equity and security. Their arguments would have to be phrased in the new discourse to get an audience.

P: They [the NFPs] had to either argue it two ways: to say NFPs are better so just use us; or they would [have] to say, well, because we don't need this arm's-length relationship and because we are NFP, we could govern and we could deliver ... And a few of us in a softer way started to put together this federation model where everyone would be positioned in a partnership, and each one may or may not deliver the services, and we may out-source some of them. Now, of course, it wasn't going to fly ... and this government was not going to have NFP preference. Now if it was a Liberal government, this partnership model would have been, I think, a potential opportunity. But it was clear to me that wasn't going to fly. So the best attempt was to try to influence the OHHCPA's [Ontario Home Health Care Providers' Association] model. So much of our argument was ... that you don't need the home care case manager, and that that's a cost in the system ... that's where the duplication and added cost is. That any professional going into the home is making an assessment determining the care treatment, and in essence should be the resource manager, because they are there functioning in that role in the hospital system.

An NFP provider indicated that, unlike the commercial agencies, worker protection had been one of his group's main concerns. They had negotiated the protection of volume in the transition period not so much out of self-interest as to protect workers.

P: Because when you have competition which drives price down, and you have all your money going to pay the workers, you know, what's going to be driven out? So we really wanted to make sure that where there was competition, the compensation to the worker was moved outside and you competed on another piece. And we had come up with a very simple mathematical model ... and it just allowed competition on what was overhead ... It's not quite the way it ended up.

Similarly, the protection of workers and efficiency arguments were used as the justification to rethink managed competition, leaving the door open for a model that combined both case management and care functions.

P: And the argument of the managed competition is simply – it really is exploiting the workers who are non-unionized, in the short term to be paid as low as possible with no benefits. So your leverage of how to get more out of the system is really to lower the worker pay. Or our argument was really look at the system. Look at some of the duplications and functions and figure out another approach.

When government agreed to the three-year transition period of protected home care volumes, not surprisingly the FPs wanted a much shorter period. The sooner they could compete on an even playing field, the quicker they could increase their share of the market. However, one NFP provider indicated that it was clear that the longer transition period would benefit the FPs as much as the NFPs.

P: They did recognize that it [a shorter period] wasn't in the best interest of them either. They probably didn't admit that to the government, but privately I'm sure [they] could realize that they couldn't pick up the volume that quickly ... if the whole of the non-profit sector failed, especially in nursing, and they had to pick up the business, they couldn't handle it, couldn't handle that large an increase [in volume].

The volunteer community support sector within the NFP sector was more concerned about having to compete for contracts having had no experience in this area or resources to engage in competition. They were relieved that support services were excluded from the mandate of the CCAC, and would be directly funded by government.

P: They haven't had to do business with Home Care in the past. They haven't had the same kind of familiarity with them. And I guess [they] were a little bit concerned about losing out and so losing a contract.

There were a number of overriding issues for the commercial agencies that made their model incompatible with the one proposed by the NFPs. The lack of separation of case management and care provision functions and the purchasing of services through informal agreements under the old Home Care governance structure, they argued, had led to the misuse of funds.

P: You [shouldn't] be on the board making decisions about who gets contracts or be privy to information that would give you an advantage in the contract. So there would be no conflict of interest. That was a key principle as well for us. There were decisions made, for instance, under Public Health around purchasing items through the Home Care Programs' budget that were unnecessary for home care. Hundreds of thousands of dollars were spent on automated equipment that was placed in the Public Health Units. We're talking about lots of money that was diverted from the mission of that Home Care Program to purchase [things] for the Public Health Units ... So that was one key principle: get the board straightened out.

The commercial agencies wanted to separate the case management and care functions, so that staff of the CCACs would perform only assessments, eligibility determination, and quality control. The provision of all care should be purchased from outside providers. They believed that when the two functions were combined in a single organization, it led to conflict of interest situations.

P: When the Home Care Program made decisions it sometimes favoured the provider, the therapist, rather than the client. So when [a] case manager had complaints from clients saying, 'I don't know when my therapist is coming', the Home Care Program wouldn't say, 'Oh, we'll fix that.' They'd say, 'Too bad! Our therapists' needs come before yours.' So we felt we've got to get rid of that. If we're really going to move to an accountable, customer-focused system, we've got to get the providers out of there.

Lastly, they needed a structure that allowed them to provide service on at least an equal footing with the NFP sector.

P: We wanted the opportunity to compete in a fair and competitive environment. So we promoted – we felt that to get there, we needed to have some sort of structure. That was the request for [a] proposal process where you'd bid on a contract based on the quality that you could provide at the best cost.

For their part, the staff of the old Home Care Programs advocated their retaining brokerage and case management. As such, they would easily slide into place in the new organizations (P).

In the end, for most of the societal interests, especially providers, fatigue and a desire to move on took over, and this fatigue provided the government with greater opportunity to pursue its agenda. One provider captured this sentiment.

P: I think everybody was so profoundly tired and we had all got to the point where we simply said, 'Just give us some kind of opportunity to stay alive and we'll be happy.' And I think they [the government] capitalized on that emotional sense that all of the providers had – it was like, you know, I don't have any more time to worry about the detail of things.

With the viability and independence of provider groups no longer threatened by the amalgamated model of the MSA, interests of provider organizations split, and the Group for LTC Reform fell apart. Any opposition to the increase of FP provision and market mechanisms was effectively silenced under the Conservative agenda; the interests of consumers and labour groups were simply ruled out of order. The NFPs' efforts to forestall the inevitable failed. Managed competition came to Ontario.

7.6 Influence of Interests

What influence did interests have on policy making by the PC government? Did societal interests influence government, or did the interests of particular groups merely line up with the plans government had already formed? Our respondents differed in their analyses. There was considerable agreement that only certain groups had had direct access to the Conservative government policy makers – in particular, the FP providers.

There also was agreement that groups that had supported the NDP (particularly the SCCA and labour) had had little say under the Conservatives. There was disagreement, however, as to whether those groups were influencing government, or whether they were helpful to government because they reinforced the Conservatives' own policy objectives.

C: They did include the Senior Citizens' Alliance [in their consultation], but they didn't give them the same platform that the NDP gave them because it was an NDP group, or [was] perceived to have power within the NDP, so they wouldn't give them the same voice.

Having spent all their resources (under the PCs they were no longer funded) and energies promoting the MSA, the SCCA was more or less beaten down. As one government official said, 'Haven't heard from the alliance at all' (G).

The disability community were less involved with the Conservative position. They were concerned with allocation rather than financing or delivery mechanisms, and these concerns had been addressed. Their objective of direct funding and control over the hiring and managing of their own providers represented a market-based allocation approach (i.e., money follows clients) and was more in keeping with Conservative ideology. Therefore, there was less need to mobilize and be active in this policy arena (C).

LTC was no longer a high-priority area for labour; other issues took precedence. The Conservatives were bent on undoing many of the protections for labour in all sectors that the NDP had introduced. Unions now had to fight for their interests on many fronts and with relatively little success (Cameron and White, 2000). They had to resort to mounting mass demonstrations through their Days of Action, which failed to stop a determined government. The Conservatives also discontinued the funding previously provided by the NDP for labour's policy work.

P: The funding ran out ... The person who was, quote, assigned to it [government relations staff] is doing WCB [Worker Compensation Board], doing health and safety. There's huge amounts of legislation on that right now, running campaigns. [The staff member] has been pulled in to do the Days of Action. They need another body to do the work ... The WCB and the health and safety stuff are huge changes that are happening to all workers, not just healthcare workers. It includes health care workers, but the changes that are coming down on that are just enormous. And I don't think it was a decision of choosing one over the other. The person who got assigned to, to add health to their list was already overwhelmed.

P: We don't have an opportunity to just sit and talk about mutual interests. And they're [the PC government] profoundly anti-union. And they're driven to privatize, you know, to put as much of the delivery of health care into the private sector as possible. So we don't really have a starting point because those are fairly important things for us.

While ideology silenced the consumer and labour voice, it responded to the provider voices. However, not all providers were given the same audience with this government. It was widely believed by respondents, including those from the FP organizations, that the FP agencies were most influential in reform.

C: The private providers are playing a big role in the back room. And they're certainly the people who are playing a role in the regulation issues, the Red Tape Commission.

P: Private owners of private entities. I think that's who is mostly speaking to this government ... Business has a very strong ear of government. They certainly had access where I think a lot of other people haven't.

P: The FPs got whatever they want.

P: I believe the FP sector has a huge influence.

P: FPs – and they, what was interesting is, they've become the equivalent of the Seniors' Alliance, I think, with the NDP ... They seemed to have had a fair bit of access with the government ... They seem to have assumed a new ascendance.

P: Certainly it was pretty clear that the commercial group had the ear of the government. It was clear to me. I mean, I was absolutely convinced that it was going that way. So how do we influence that?

The old Home Care Programs were also seen as influential with the Conservatives. Because the Home Care Programs along with the Placement Coordination Agencies in all parts of the province, with the exception of Metropolitan Toronto, were going to become CCACs, the Ontario Home Care Programs Association (OHCPA) was in favour of this model. The case managers would transfer to the new agencies. The direct providers (e.g., rehabilitation therapists) would be employed by the CCAC during the three-year transition period, by which time they were to become private contractors bidding for service contracts.

A number of groups believed that the Ontario Home Health Care Providers Association and the Ontario Nursing Home Association (ONHA) (FP facilities) were particularly influential. According to one respondent, the ONHA had targeted Mike Harris about ten years before and had provided financial support (P).

P: Oh they're certainly listening very strongly to the nursing homes, the private nursing home association [ONHA]. I also know they're listening very closely to the private Home [Health] Care Providers Association [OHHCPA]. I know both the executive directors in those organizations ... have the ear of the minister quite closely.

One respondent, who concurred with this view, also understood that the Conservatives were able to move their agenda forward quickly and decisively precisely because the societal groups in this policy community were not cohesive and, therefore, were not an organized force to be reckoned with.

P: There was a sense at the time, very strong, that the interest group, that the FPs were very strong in support of the Conservatives through their campaign. And that to a large extent moving to the managed competition in the community sector versus anywhere else in the health system was a payback to the privates who had underwritten the costs of some of the campaign or were very strongly in support of the Conservatives. They [government] owed it to them. And it would be easier to implement it in the community, because after all it was pretty fragmented. There weren't power players like hospitals, CEOs, you know, committed to the NFP and boards where the money really was. That this would be a good place to get an inroad. You know, it's sort of fragmented and they could very surreptitiously sort of move in and win contracts and gain market share and grow and change.

One respondent indicated that because of the beliefs of this government and the preferred access they gave to the FP sector, his organization changed its approach in hopes that speaking the same language would allow it to 'fool the government' (P).

P: How we changed from the NDP to this government. I think that when you're speaking to this government, you need to ensure that there's a cost-effectiveness comment. You know, that you have to take on the issue of cost effectiveness. What we've tried to do is broaden this government's conception of cost effectiveness by talking about the concept in broader terms, like investing in people's health is an investment, really is definitely cost effective as opposed to the alternative. You don't talk a lot about equity and equal access. You don't emphasize that to the same degree. Our central message hasn't changed but the way it's packaged certainly has.

Those who believed that the relationship was not one of influence suggested that the Conservatives' ideological beliefs in market, market mechanisms, and adherence to the bottom line predetermined the shape of the reform.

G: I'll bet they didn't pay attention to anybody. I believe that the Tories had a set point of view about introducing a managed care approach to long-term care and that's what they did.

P: They are not interested, I mean the sand and gravel lobby would be saying the same thing [that they had no access to government], I would suspect ... They care about cost. That their entire – what they call the Common Sense Revolution is about getting the cost out of running Ontario. And so anything else that you want to talk to them about except new and different ideas to get costs out, they're not interested. So it's even the next plateau from being locked out. It's – they don't want to know ... They've said , 'we're not even going to listen to people, because we know what they're going to say. Change is tough. We're going to have to just do it for people, and they'll thank us hopefully afterwards. Pray to God we get a second term, and by the end of the second term, people will see that there's significant benefit being derived from all this.'

7.7 Conclusions

Before the Conservative government assumed power, it was clear to the LTC policy community how it intended to reform this sector. Through the publication of *The Common Sense Revolution*, the party's ideology was evident: less government, more market mechanisms, a focus on efficiency and cost reduction, disempowerment of unions, and empowerment of the FP sector. The first act in this policy field was to halt the implementation of Bill 173, which went against its agenda of competition and FP provision, namely, the MSAs, the 80-20 rule, and the labour adjustment strategy. Ironically, the NDP legislation allowed the Conservatives to develop a model that would have been anathema to the previous government.

The Conservatives established institutional structures and constraints that would make it difficult to derail their agenda. They organized a quick and highly focused consultation, which foreclosed any discussion about MSAs and impeded the ability of societal groups to organize their thoughts or resources. They distanced the minister of health from both the consultation and the implementation of the CCACs by giving responsibility for the former to Helen Johns, Jim Wilson's parliamentary assistant, and for the latter to Cam Jackson, minister without portfolio responsible for seniors issues. Finally, they centralized policy decision making in the Premier's Office.

The coalitions and alliances that the NDP had either directly fostered, indirectly created through the bringing together of disparate interests to fight a common enemy, or inadvertently given birth to through the Social Contract quickly unravelled. The thin veneer of common interests broke down as groups attempted to influence the reform. Labour and seniors were silenced because of their previous associations and because their interests were antithetical to those of the government. If this government was influenced by any group at all, it would have been the FP providers, which either had provided campaign support or had a common agenda.

The CCAC model differed from the earlier models in the opportunity it provided the FP sector to increase their market share. Managed competition moved allocation to the market end of the continuum, disadvantaging NFP agencies. The only way for them to compete in this environment was to become more like the FPs. In their efforts to stay viable, they were adopting strategies typically associated with commercial enterprises. Whether or not agencies would be able to survive if they lost a contract bid to compete again was in doubt. Through the mechanism of competition, one of the Harris government's achievements in this sector has been to further fragment an already loosely connected sector.

One trend that has already become evident is the creation of a new dynamic of expectations. Home care clearly exists at the interface between medical and social. The reform rhetoric created an expectation that all but the very sickest individuals could remain within the community, as long as sufficient supports were available. It did not create a consensus as to the boundaries between services that should be 'socialized' and paid for collectively and those that would remain an individual responsibility. Despite increased spending for home care, the CCACs are widely seen to have inadequate resources to meet the demands placed upon them, particularly as hospitals have restructured and have shortened their average length of stay as a matter of public policy. In particular, limitations on the number of publicly funded hours of care that can be provided through CCACs are having the effect of moving those inadequately served in one of two directions: either back to hospitals and other institutions that will provide publicly financed care (albeit often at higher cost), or towards private payment for the additional services. Ironically, while professing the merits of small government, the state has become increasingly directive towards those providing services paid for by government. However, there is relatively little regulation of privately paid for care. The restructuring of the health care system, the shifting of care into the community and outside the constraints of the Canada Health Act, the de-insuring of Home Care by removing it from the OHIP budget, and the opening of the community sector to competition and more FP provision, particularly by American multinationals, are likely to have major consequences for Canadian health care in the years to come.

CHAPTER EIGHT

Moving towards Home: Policy Change and Policy Stasis beyond the Medicare Mainstream

8.1 Reforming Community-Based Long-Term Care in Ontario

The period between 1985 and 1996 in Ontario was characterized by marked volatility in government policy in the field of community-based long-term care (LTC). Three successive governments proposed five different reform initiatives. While each reform was cloaked in the rhetoric of improved access and quality, as well as consumer independence and choice, the five initiatives integrated different, and sometimes contradictory, decisions about how community-based services should be funded and delivered and how resources should be allocated by public government to private providers, both for-profit (FP) and not-for-profit (NFP). While the first three initiatives were essentially incremental variations on a brokerage theme, the next two marked major shifts in policy direction, veering from the command-and-control centralized Multi-Service Agencies (MSAs) of the socialist-leaning Rae New Democratic Party (NDP) government, which called for services to be delivered by unionized state employees, to the Community Care Access Centres (CCACs) of the Harris Progressive Conservatives (PCs), who institutionalized the logic of 'managed competition' between FP and NFP providers and the idea that the state should fund but not directly provide services.

In this concluding chapter we consider the substantive and theoretical implications of our historical-institutional examination of this twisting pathway of policy development. Looking first at the content of policy, we begin by reviewing similarities and differences in the design decisions about financing, delivery, and allocation involved in the successive reform 'models' put forward by successive provincial governments. In doing so we confront key questions about the public/private mix and the role of public governments in the provision of community-based care. We also raise questions about the extent to which governments may centralize or diffuse decision-making around how allocation decisions are made.

We then shift our attention to policy process, particularly to the important and interconnected roles played by ideas, interests, and institutions. Here, we emphasize the relative lack of 'constraint' placed on governments in determining LTC policy. Community-based LTC integrates a range of personal and social support services that go well beyond conventional ideas of acute health care. There is minimal agreement on the rights of individuals or the role of the state in providing such care, and hence there are fewer ideological constraints on deciding what governments should provide and how they should provide it. In community-based LTC the state faced a policy community characterized by relatively few established institutions and by many diverse, fractured, and relatively powerless interests. Finally, in contrast to the mainstream of Canada's physicians and hospital system, in which policy making is constrained by the conditions of the Canada Health Act and the terms of federal-provincial fiscal arrangements as well as the strong institutionalized interests of the medical profession, community-based LTC falls beyond most such institutional constraints. Thus, in this field at least, the state can be characterized as 'strong,' with considerable latitude to design reforms consistent with its ideological predilections. As we have seen in the previous chapters, governments took advantage of this latitude over the course of the successive policy initiatives we have described.

Finally, we consider implications for the future of the post-war state. Here, we focus on the extent to which the ongoing shift from the Medicare 'mainstream' to Medicare's 'margins,' including community-based LTC, entails not only a shift in the site of care, but an erosion of the post-war state's role in health care. While the mainstream of hospital and physician services continues, for the most part, to resist political and ideological forces aimed at 'reducing,' 'rethinking,' or otherwise shrinking the state's role, community-based LTC more closely resembles other policy fields such as education, social welfare, and housing. Indeed, as we have documented in previous chapters, in Ontario, the logic of competitive market forces has now been established as a means of gaining efficiencies that adherents of neo-conservative market ideologies do not think the public state can attain. At the same time, the state's role has been circumscribed by capped budgets and restricted service eligibility criteria. As long as these policies remain in place, they not only limit the role of public government in the delivery and funding of care in the near term, but also appear to limit possibilities for the state's future expansion into the field of community-based care. However, the realities 'on the ground' suggest that community-based LTC will only grow in importance, fuelled by both an increased demand from technological changes and an ageing population and decreased supply in proximate policy fields as government shifts more care from the Medicare mainstream to the community. Accordingly, it is likely that this policy debate will reopen under subsequent governments, and the design decisions described in this study will be revisited.

8.2 Summary: Policy Content and Process under Successive Governments

As we have seen, the successive reform initiatives proposed by the Liberal, NDP, and Progressive Conservative governments of Ontario, while justified in similar rhetoric and aimed at ostensibly similar goals, integrated quite different design decisions about financing, delivery, and allocation. These decisions, particularly during the later NDP and PC periods, were more than simply technical variations on a theme; they reflected fundamentally different perspectives on the balance between public and private roles and responsibilities. We now review each of the successive reform initiatives in turn, focusing on the extent to which the design decisions they incorporated shifted the public/private balance and the way in which the policy process unfolded.

8.2.1 One-Stop Shopping/Access (Liberal, 1987)

The two Liberal government mandates marked a period of measured incremental change in the LTC policy sector. Spurred by concerns about an ageing population and the potential call on future spending given the prevailing mode of caring for seniors in institutions, the new government agreed with their Conservative predecessors that keeping seniors in the community for as long as possible appeared to be more cost effective. Moreover, they recognized that social supports were at least as important as health care in meeting the policy goal of preventing seniors from deteriorating to the extent that they would require institutionalization. This approach was in keeping with the growing awareness of the importance of prevention and wellness, as opposed to focusing only upon curative medicine, and with the recognition that 'health' was more than the absence of disease. Community care, home care, health care, as well as social supports, therefore, were going to be important in the new approach.

In Ontario, however, those community-based services that did exist were fragmented, uncoordinated, and difficult to access. Most (80 per cent) of the provincial budget for community services was spent on home health care, even though the majority of care was provided by either the volunteer social support sector or families. Although reform of this sector was considered necessary if its emphasis on health care was to change to social services, and if access and efficiency were to improve, One-Stop Shopping/Access could be viewed more as an incremental consolidation of existing public and private roles than as a radical change in policy direction.

8.2.1.1 One-Stop Shopping/Access: Financing

When the provincial Liberals began the reform processes charted in this book, in-home professional and homemaking services were fully funded by the provincial Home Care Program and the Integrated Homemaker Program. The first Liberal reform model did not change the status quo, which left these services as entitlements as long as they were deemed necessary by a physician. Community support services were partially covered within the Ministry of Community and Social Services (MCSS); this category of 'non-medical' services, albeit important, was outside universal entitlements and was financed by a mix of public and private resources (with the publicly financed portion often being means tested). This arrangement would remain largely unchanged, although the amount of money budgeted for these programs would be increased.

In terms of eligibility, One-Stop Shopping/Access was primarily intended to serve the needs of the elderly; the Liberal reform did not exclude other needs groups such as the disabled, however, to the extent that they were also eligible for the Home Care and Integrated Home-maker programs.

8.2.1.2 One-Stop Shopping/Access: Delivery

The One-Stop Shopping/Access model also retained the existing mix of NFP and FP providers. The primary expansion of the public role was as a coordinator of access, and even that role would be occupied not by government per se, but by a new group of quasi-governmental local agencies, which would provide comprehensive functional assessments, provide some services under their direct control, or arrange for the provision of necessary services. It was intended that such local agencies would be able to rationalize and integrate existing services. For example, the case management component of the Home Care and Integrated Homemaker programs was to be fully integrated with the comprehensive case management approach.

8.2.1.3 One-Stop Shopping/Access: Allocation

The One-Stop Shopping/Access model was widely characterized as a 'brokerage' model. While the local coordinating agency would provide some services directly (e.g., assessment), most services would continue to be provided by 'third party' private agencies with which the new organizations would 'broker' public funding. Although 'brokerage' remained undefined, it was anticipated that the process would be more cooperative than competitive. Thus, instead of the individual client attempting to negotiate services with multiple providers, a single agency would contract for needed services. Anticipated advantages included improved access, cost-efficiencies (since it was thought that a single agency would have greater bargaining power than any individual), and enhanced quality assurance and accountability. While the government was therefore not directly responsible for the services individuals received, it took a greater role in managing the marketplace. This was not really a change to a purchaser/provider split, since the government had not been a direct provider of services except through local public health units. However, an additional layer, the one-stop agency, was added between the provincial purchaser and the providers. In theory, this model did not look substantially different from the CCAC approach eventually adopted by the Harris PC government. In practice, however, the two models differed in their respective ethos, one based on cooperation and NFP preference and the other on competition; their implications are discussed below.

8.2.1.4 One-Stop Shopping/Access: Policy Process

The Liberals' main policy interests were to de-medicalize the community sector and to integrate and coordinate access to these services. One mechanism used to advance those goals was modification of institutional structures both within and outside government. Inside government, they channelled the process for reform away from the Ministry of Health (MOH), and gave the lead for reform to the Office for Senior Citizens' Affairs (OSCA). They also sought to facilitate integration of services at the community level by setting up a dual-reporting relationship. The assistant deputy ministers (ADMs) responsible for LTC community services in both MOH and MCSS reported to the two deputy ministers. Integration and coordination of services at the community level was to be achieved through the new one-stop agencies.

One-Stop Shopping/Access was little more than tinkering with the existing system. Furthering this incrementalist approach, the Liberals cautiously introduced pilot projects to test out the new model and allowed the flexibility for each model to be developed according to the needs of the particular community.

8.2.2 Service Access Organizations (Liberal, 1990)

The second Liberal model involved the establishment of Service Access Organizations (SAOs). While in many ways similar to One-Stop Shopping/Access, the SAO reform contained the potential for an important contradiction: it was designed to incrementally extend public coverage, but at the same time it would remove the funding of home and community care from the universal entitlements of Medicare, eliminating a major constraint on coverage decisions by future governments.

8.2.2.1 Service Access Organizations: Financing
Under the SAO model, public funding would also cover the administration of these local agencies, the costs of service coordination and facility placement, and the costs of formal in-home services. In addition, government was going to increase public funding for community support services to 60 per cent, and eventually to 70 per cent, of their budgets. There would be no consumer charges for medical treatment (usually provided by nurses or therapists) or for personal support and care services (assistance with bathing, eating, and toileting). Charges for cleaning, cooking, laundry, shopping, home maintenance, and meals services would be based on ability to pay, but this would be assessed on income, not on assets.

The new model contained the potential both to expand and to contract coverage. It explicitly covered services both to seniors *and* to persons with disabilities, thus shifting from a user focus to a program focus. This direction was supported by the disability community, who favoured the shift by the province from a medical model to a population health model. The disability community also recognized that seniors were increasingly stressing autonomy and independence, which implied that their policy goals might be congruent. At the same time, however, fearing the fiscal pressures of an ageing society, the province now attempted to set limits on its obligation by creating regional funding envelopes for all services. This meant that home care funding would eventually be 'pulled' from OHIP entitlements – where funding had proved politically difficult to control – to new budgets, which would be capped. The logic of capped budgets would, in effect, translate into restrictions on entitlements. Eventually, the home care budget would indeed be combined with the budgets for LTC facilities and community support services under one capped envelope. With this new model, the Liberal government had signalled important changes in the institutional framework of home and community care; although public coverage would, in principle, be extended to encompass additional needs groups and services, even medically necessary care delivered in the community by persons other than physicians would formally be removed from the protection of Medicare's 'mainstream.' The creation of a single, capped budget would allow for the allocation and reallocation of resources to reflect the changing needs of community; it would also provide governments greater flexibility in controlling or capping budgets and, in this way, shift the balance between public and private.

8.2.2.2 Service Access Organizations: Delivery

On the delivery side, the SAO reform involved few changes. Services would continue to be provided by the mix of NFP and FP providers. The SAO, like One-Stop Access, would act as a single point of access, referral, assessment, and service coordination, as well as purchaser of in-home professional and homemaking services. It would also control entry into LTC institutions. Community support services would continue to be accessed directly by consumers or by referral from the SAO. Sponsoring agencies for service access could be existing or new organizations, but to avoid conflicts of interest, current direct providers of service could not also assume the SAO function.

8.2.2.3 Service Access Organizations: Allocation

Allocation mechanisms would also remain essentially unchanged. Funding for community support services would come directly from government. SAOs would purchase in-home professional and homemaking services from budgets received from government. Although the nature of the contracting process for in-home services was not made clear, government sources indicated that it would continue more or less on the same informal, cooperative basis. For both in-home and community support services there would be a purchaser/provider split, and funds would be channelled through a mediating agency (SAO) for in-home services.

8.2.2.4 Service Access Organizations: Policy Process

Although they obtained a majority for their second mandate, by 1989, when the Liberals introduced the SAO model, they were becoming aware of an impending recession. As a result, they knew that they would have to make hard and unpopular decisions in the near future. They hoped that by calling an early election, they could take advantage of their current popularity and then ride through the recession. Hence, their second LTC model was as cautious as their first: again incremental changes were proposed, while hard actions, such as the transfer of home care from the OHIP budget to a capped envelope, were left to some unspecified future date in their next mandate.

The series of reports released by the Premier's Council on Health Strategy refocused emphasis on the broader determinants of health and the importance of health promotion and disease prevention, in a move away from illness and cure. To further institutionalize the de-medicalization of the sector, MCSS was given the lead for reform, and a single LTC division was created, the ADM of which reported to the deputy ministers of both MOH and MCSS. In keeping with the Premier's Council on Health Strategy recommendation on decentralization and local authorities, fourteen local Area Offices were created to administer the sector.

Societal interests during the Liberal period were highly fragmented. Home Care and NFP professional agencies were perceived to dominate. The NFP support agencies, however, recognized the need to pool their resources to gain a greater influence in the policy community. By the end of the second Liberal mandate, they had formed the Ontario Community Support Association (OCSA) and with it had created a capability to anticipate and respond more coherently to policy issues. Advocacy groups for seniors, persons with disabilities, and the ethnocultural community had not yet mobilized, and they remained primarily as single, disparate voices. The large health associations, such as the Ontario Medical Association (OMA) and the Ontario Hospital Association (OHA), either felt they had little interest in LTC reform or were otherwise occupied with issues of greater immediate importance to their memberships. Given the gradual and minimal approach of the government, there was little in the LTC reforms proposed by the Liberals that would mobilize societal inter-

ests. As a result, the shape of the policy community remained fragmented, and the relative power balance of groups within it was not
altered to any great extent during this period.

8.2.3 Service Coordination Agency (NDP, 1991)

The first NDP model, the Service Coordination Agency (SCA) was also
incremental; it did not depart significantly from the SAO model. The
SCA was described as retaining the substance of the earlier model under
different names; tellingly, the NDP document was printed on recycled
paper (Baranek, Deber, and Williams, 1999; Deber and Williams, 1995).
However, the NDP, for their own ideological reasons continued to 'push'
home and community care out of the Medicare 'mainstream' while somewhat expanding eligibility for those services.

8.2.3.1 Service Coordination Agency: Financing
The model was intended to consolidate the Home Care Program, Placement and Coordination Services Program, Integrated Homemaker Program, Attendant Outreach Program, and the Homemakers and Nurses
Services Program into an integrated Health and Personal Support Program, which would be fully funded by government. This change was
motivated by the NDP's distrust of 'professional dominance.' Access to
non-professional services would no longer depend on the receipt of professional services, which had been under the 'gatekeeping' control of
physician referral. Community support services would be expanded with
consistent eligibility criteria and user fees, and priority would be given
to underserviced areas. While each area of the province would have flexibility in developing its own services, the government would establish
criteria to determine a basic level of mandatory services.

Diminishing the need for municipal contributions, public funding for
community support services would increase from 70 to 100 per cent of
their approved budget, less revenue from other sources. However, these
services continued to include a co-payment made by the consumer. As
in the Liberal SAO model, both the elderly and persons with disabilities
were eligible to receive services.

8.2.3.2 Service Coordination Agency: Delivery
Forty SCAs would be established across the province to replace and consolidate services provided by the Home Care and the Placement Coordination Services programs. Personal health and support services would

be accessed through the SCA, while community support services could be accessed directly by potential clients.

Reflecting basic NDP ideology, preference for funding and contracts in this model were to be given to NFP providers. Moreover, government was to extend pay equity requirements to all providers in the community, increase homemakers' wages, and assist displaced hospital workers in accessing jobs in the expanded community sector.

8.2.3.3 Service Coordination Agency: Allocation
Allocation resembled the Liberal SAO model; the SCA would broker funding for personal health and support services, while community support services would continue to be funded directly by government. However, the government also introduced direct-funding pilot projects, which fall at the 'market' end of the allocation continuum, for persons with disabilities who wished to purchase their own attendant care.

8.2.3.4 Service Coordination Agency: Policy Process
The election of the NDP majority government in 1990 was a first in Ontario history and a surprise to everyone, including many of their own candidates. Not well prepared to govern, the New Democrats first produced an LTC model very similar to that developed by their predecessors, no doubt because the bureaucracy had been allowed to continue to develop reform. Grafted on were some elements more in keeping with NDP beliefs: increased funding for community support organizations from 70 to 100 per cent of an agency's approved budget after deducting revenue from other sources; concessions to workers; and a preference for not-for-profit delivery.

Within government, the lead agency for the LTC reform was switched from MCSS to MOH in 1992, with the amalgamated LTC division now reporting only to the minister of health. This move, which undermined the efforts to de-medicalize LTC, was probably sparked more by the relative strength of the minister of health, Frances Lankin, compared with the new minister of community and support services, Marion Boyd, than by a careful analysis of the governance implications. LTC was a 'signature priority' of the NDP government, and Frances Lankin was believed to be more able to get the job done. Having amalgamated the cultures of these two ministries in one division, the NDP felt that the government had successfully weakened the medical model enough to make it safe to situate LTC back within the Ministry of Health. This shift would also make it simpler to re-medicalize LTC under subsequent governments, however, and would allow even medically necessary care to be removed from the list of entitlements.

The process used by the NDP involved elaborate public consultations. While this process bought the New Democrats some time to formulate their own unique approach, it did so at the expense of vastly increasing the 'scope of conflict' and raising what proved to be incompatible expectations within the policy community (Deber and Williams, 1995).

8.2.4 Multi-Service Agencies (NDP, 1993)

The introduction of the MSA model marked an important watershed in LTC policy development. Government abandoned the 'brokerage' models in favour of direct service provision by a government agency whose employees were likely to be unionized. This was also the first reform model to be enshrined in legislation; before losing power in the provincial election of 1995, the NDP passed Bill 173, which established MSAs. Although the MSAs later were repudiated by the PC government of Mike Harris and replaced by CCACs, Bill 173 was retained as the institutional framework for home and community care in Ontario. While expanding the scope of services and eligibility, this bill formally removed home and community care from the universal entitlements of the Medicare mainstream, which would provide even more policy flexibility to subsequent governments.

8.2.4.1 Multi-Service Agencies: Financing
For the first time, community support services were explicitly included in the basket of services to be paid for from the public purse through the MSA. Such services would not be free to all users: co-payments would be required, albeit assessed on the basis of income, not assets. The MSA would also provide fully funded health and personal support services. Full funding of all services to all eligible persons was not guaranteed, however, since the new Community Services Funding Envelope was to be located outside the provincial health insurance plan, under which care was an entitlement, thus giving government greater flexibility to increase or decrease funding and services.

8.2.4.2 Multi-Service Agencies: Delivery
The MSA also departed from the earlier 'purchaser-provider' split models by moving delivery of community-based services to the staff of the publicly funded, NFP MSAs. MSAs would not be allowed to spend more

than 20 per cent (originally 10 per cent) of their budgets to purchase services external to the agency (the 80-20 rule). This element of the reform would effectively shut out not only private commercial providers, but also private NFP providers, including those supported by various ethnocultural and faith communities. Moreover, through Bill 173, this control would be further consolidated by concentrating power over the MSAs in the office of the minister of health: the minister would determine not only MSA budgets, but which agencies would become (or continue as) MSAs. The NDP proposal thus effectively consolidated the government's direct control over both the funding and the delivery of home and community care. By creating an environment friendly to labour, the government went a long way towards ensuring that care was likely to be delivered in the future by a unionized workforce.

8.2.4.3 Multi-Service Agencies: Allocation

The MSAs were given responsibility for budgets and service provision, with the province retaining veto power over policy decisions. This reform moved allocation towards the central planning end of the allocation spectrum. Although the MSA, which was funded by government, was not a government agency per se, the distinction between purchaser and provider was blurred. Neither was it clear whether the limited potential for purchase of services from external providers would be based on informal brokerage or would introduce the market allocation mechanism of competitive contracts.

8.2.4.4 Multi-Service Agencies: Policy Process

To guard against resistance from the bureaucracy, the NDP drafted the MSA model in the minister of health's office rather than within the ministry. Reflecting the party's political ideology and policy interest, the model enhanced the position of organized labour and of community support services. It centralized delivery under one administrative structure and gave the minister of health considerable powers over the new model agency.

To arrive at the model, the NDP conducted a massive public consultation and funded key interest groups (the SCCA, OCSA, and the Ontario Federation of Labour) to provide a counterweight to the more established provider interests. This process was in keeping with NDP beliefs in participatory democracy and community empowerment as well as their ties to the social support sector and labour. Moreover, preference in the consultations was given to consumers and front-line workers. These actions, however, were viewed with considerable scepticism by most groups in the policy community. Indeed, many came to see these favoured groups as puppets mouthing the government's mantra.

Policy development during the NDP period was heavily constrained by the economic position of the province. The deficit was rising, government revenues were reduced by the recession that had begun by 1992, and Ontario's formerly excellent credit rating was downgraded. Unlike other provincial governments, including the later Harris Conservative government, the New Democrats did not make spending cuts early enough in their mandate. Had they done so, they might have had enough time to try to build support for the necessity of the cuts and possibly given themselves the ability to increase spending on priority policies towards the end of their mandate. In contrast, Saskatchewan's NDP government, under the leadership of Roy Romanow, had been faced with the unwelcome discovery that the previous government had left them a deficit of $850 million, rather than the $265 million they had been led to expect. Its response was to appoint a royal commission to look into the economic state of the province; the inquiry helped to convince the public that urgent and drastic actions were required and left it able to innovate once the fiscal affairs of the province were in better repair (Blakeney and Borins, 1998).

The Ontario New Democrats instead tried the approach of a 'Keynesian deficit' in their first budget, hoping to spend their way out of the recession but, in the process, incurring a $10 billion deficit. Like other governments who had tried this path, they quickly discovered they could not maintain such a level of spending without exploding the deficit. In 1993 they belatedly introduced an Expenditure Control Plan, which both raised taxes and reduced government expenditures. In an effort to protect publicly funded jobs, they coupled this plan with what they termed the Social Contract, according to which labour was expected to trade off wages for employment security. Although the government's intent was to preserve jobs, the Social Contract forced employees to take unpaid days off, which meant breaching existing negotiated agreements. It was hoped that both measures would save the province $6 billion in that fiscal year. Both sets of actions alienated the unions. (Employers who needed to maintain services also found their costs increasing, since they had to fill the gaps with workers paid at overtime rates.) The labour movement did not forgive the NDP for the Social Contract and withdrew support during the 1995 election. The attempt to appease labour by concessions in Bill 173 did not molify the unions but did awaken other opposition and turned formerly supportive groups, such as OCSA, against the legislation.

In the end, the New Democrats were just able to push their legislation through before facing the electorate. It had been slowed considerably by the processes that reflected their beliefs in community empowerment, participatory democracy, and the preservation of jobs; in the end it resulted in broadening the scope of conflict. The Social Contract process brought together 'sector' tables and provided an avenue for societal interests to coalesce, which further delayed passage of the legislation. Despite this opposition, the NDP was able to legislate a model that gave promise of increasing public, as opposed to private, financing and delivery and a top-down, command-and-control allocation mechanism. It was a Pyrrhic victory. There was no opportunity to implement their reforms before the election was called. With no administrative structures in place, the Harris Conservatives were given broad latitude to interpret the legislation in a way more to their liking.

8.2.5 Community Care Access Centres (PC, 1996)

The 1995 victory of the market-oriented Progressive Conservative government of Mike Harris produced a second major shift in policy direction.

8.2.5.1 Community Care Access Centres: Financing

The Harris reform, introduced as a priority of the new government early in its term, established forty-three CCACs across Ontario. In contrast to the MSAs, these new organizations would not provide services other than case management and placement into facilities. They would be given the mandate and funding to determine service eligibility and to purchase professional services (nursing, rehabilitation therapy, medical supplies, etc.), homemaking services (housecleaning, laundry, shopping, etc.), and personal support services (physical assistance with those activities of daily living a person cannot perform independently because of a permanent disability or illness). Social support services were no longer part of the mix.

The CCAC reform marked an important ideological break from the previous models, particularly the MSA, by emphasizing market competition. At the same time, it incorporated those features of the MSA model that allowed government to limit its obligations. The CCAC model clearly removed LTC as an entitlement; CCACs would work within capped budget envelopes determined by the province. Although professional and personal support services arranged by CCACs would involve no user fee if the CCAC chose to provide them from its capped budget, there was no guarantee that any services would be available; potential clients were entitled to be assessed for services but not to receive them (Baranek, Deber, and Williams, 1999; Williams et al., 1999; Williams et al., 2001). Although the PC reform appeared to expand eligibility to the elderly, adults with physical disabilities, and people of any age requiring health services at home or at school, over time this reform would reduce access to service for many individuals by introducing stricter eligibility criteria and service limits at the same time as needs for home and community care were expanding as a result of hospital closures and bed reductions.

8.2.5.2 Community Care Access Centres: Delivery

In another key departure from the NDP reform proposal, the CCACs would fund but not provide home and community services; services would continue to be provided by private agencies under contract with CCACs. Also in contrast to the NDP emphasis on non-profit provision, the CCAC model introduced market competition between not-for-profit and for-profit providers. Not only was competition permitted, it was encouraged as a means of maximizing quality while minimizing costs. This was consistent with the Harris Conservatives' ideologically rooted beliefs that market forces were a superior means of ensuring the 'highest quality, best price' and that FP providers, precisely because of their competitive nature, were better equipped to achieve such objectives than NFPs, which, from some viewpoints, were often not run in a businesslike fashion. In a sector where labour was the highest source of costs, it was also believed that the non-unionized FP providers would be better able to be competitive by reducing the wages of workers. Little attention was given to whether labour supply would be sufficient to staff these providers at the rate government wished to pay.

8.2.5.3 Community Care Access Centres: Allocation

The major innovation of CCAC reform was in allocation. Funding for professional, homemaking and personal support services would be provided by government to CCACs through envelope funding. But rather than providing these services directly, CCACs would purchase them from both FP and NFP agencies through a process of 'managed competition,' which would shift allocation towards the market allocation end of the continuum. After an initial three-year transition period during which the market shares of existing providers would be protected in decreasing amounts, contracts were to be awarded based on a competitive RFP (request for proposal) process, which meant that, in effect, providers would submit bids for service contracts. As a result, all existing service providers would have 90 per cent of their 1995–96 Home Care Program volume protected in year one, 80 per cent in year two, and 70 per cent in year three. Thereafter, the NFPs and the FPs would have to compete on an even playing field. Out-of-country agencies would be permitted to bid for contracts. The three-year transition period was intended to allow all providers, especially the NFP agencies, to reach a common level in terms of competition based on best quality / best price. Quality, however, was tied to structural and process criteria rather than to outcomes (Williams et al., 1999). Existing agencies were bound by certain constraints (particularly those arising from pay equity) that did not apply to newly formed provider organizations.

Community support services were once again outside the reform, although many could continue to be funded directly by government through other programs. The direct funding of pilot projects for persons with disabilities would also continue.

On the surface, the Conservative CCAC model was similar to the Liberal SAO model, but with key differences. Unlike the earlier model, a competitive process replaced the informal brokerage method of allocation. In a sector where cooperation formerly had ensured the sharing of best practices, under the PCs' competitive model, information and best practices became proprietary rights and moved the provision of care into Starr's conception of 'private' and 'closed' (Starr, 1989). Moreover, because quality is harder to define in care sectors, cost would be the key variable determining successful bids (Baranek, Deber, and Williams, 1999; Williams et al., 1999). The reform had the strong potential to make major changes to the FP/NFP balance to the sector; whether they were 'overdue reform' or 'destabilization' has proved a source of dispute.

8.2.5.4 Community Care Access Centres: Policy Process

The Conservatives were clear before they were elected that their agenda was going to be retrenchment, less government, and more market mechanisms. Even as the government, their ideology was very much infused with an anti-government brush. Within LTC, their policy interests were to dismantle the pieces of Bill 173 they found ideologically offensive – the MSAs, the labour adjustment policies, and the 80-20 rule for external purchase – and bring the LTC sector to market. Every action they took was to speed the implementation of their vision for reform of this sector and to eliminate or put up barriers to special interest lobby groups, which could slow the process down.

The Conservatives conducted a quick and highly circumscribed consultation, controlling both who was invited to participate and the agenda for discussion. Within months of assuming office, they announced the implementation of CCACs. They centralized policy decision making within the political arm of government to ensure that policies reflected the spirit and letter of the *The Common Sense Revolution*, to the extent that most respondents we interviewed believed policy was being formulated in the Premier's Office rather than within the component ministries.

On the whole, in keeping with their anti-political – and what some would believe their anti-democratic – ideology, the PCs successfully insulated themselves from the pressure of many interest groups. Within LTC they were able to create a barrier between societal interests and the minister of health's office by giving responsibility for the consultation to a parliamentary assistant and by giving implementation of reform to a minister without portfolio. The withdrawal of funding support from government and the reduced access to government decreased the ability of all groups, including those formerly favoured under the NDP (SCCA, OCSA, and organized labour) to have an impact. Moreover, organized labour perceived that lobbying against the actions of this government in other policy sectors had higher priority, which diverted their attention away from the reform of LTC. The coalition of providers that had formed under the NDP mandate, the Group for LTC, dissolved under the pressure of competing against one another for contracts. Although the government did have the support of some groups, namely, the FP providers, opposing interests were not able to mobilize an effective counter-attack.

The legacy of the Harris government's reforms is still being played out. Their reform, aided by institutional structures they introduced, was designed to shift financing and delivery to the private, market side of the public-private divide and to direct allocation to the market end, with its emphasis on competition, price, and difficult-to-define quality. In the epilogue (section 8.4), we will address the likelihood that this policy direction will prove more sustainable than the earlier efforts.

8.2.6 Summary of the Reform Models

In table 8.1 we summarize the differences across the models in financing, delivery, and allocation. While there are some differences in financing, most of the key differences lie in the allocation and delivery dimensions. In the long run, however, it is a change in the financing of services that may have the biggest impact on the consumer. The transfer of the Home Care Program budget out of OHIP under Bill 173 was made under the NDP government ostensibly for the purposes of integrating budgets and hence services. A consequence was that this provision allowed the more market-driven Conservative government to limit and contract the provision of publicly funded community care. Actions by the Conservative government that occurred after the period of time covered in this research have, in actuality, placed stricter eligibility restrictions on home care and instituted service limits, moving it further away from a fully insured service based on need. Consumers who have used up their allowable allotment will either have to do without or have to pay for these services in private commercial markets.

On the delivery dimension, the Liberal models left the balance between the private NFP and private FP providers in place, the NDP models heavily favoured NFP delivery (with the MSA model approaching a quasi-public agency) and protected and promoted the interests of organized labour, while the Conservative model favoured FP agencies and attempted to de-unionize the sector.

Allocation moved from a moderate position in the centrally planned end of the continuum under the Liberals, to extreme planning under the NDP, and then back to the extreme market allocation end under the Conservatives.

8.3 Ideas, Interests, and Institutions

How can one account for the relatively wide swings in policy models for the LTC community-based sector? The initial models indeed represented incremental policy change, but the MSA and CCAC models did not do so. At a time when governments were responding to the calls of a neo-conservative agenda and the invocations to reinvent themselves by scaling back, deregulating, and privatizing services, the NDP government proposed a model that concentrated control and services under a quasi-public agency. The Progressive Conservatives then implemented a model that, although similar in some ways to the one proposed by the Liberals a decade before, incorporated a definite pro-market twist. The wide swings in LTC policy were in marked contrast to the path of medical services policy, which showed remarkable stability over that same period (Hutchison, Abelson, and Lavis, 2001)

8.3.1 Ideas

The various reforms highlighted and incorporated divergent ideas about the roles of the public state and private markets. What was a pub-

TABLE 8.1
Summary of Key Policy Design Decisions in Long-Term Care Reform

Government and Date	Model	Financing	Delivery	Allocation
Liberal (1987)	One-Stop Shopping/Access	*Who:* Persons over age 65 *Public-private funding:* a) Fully provincially funded services: in-home services (professional, homemaking), functional assessments, placement services b) Public/private financing: community support services	Existing mix of FP and NFP providers; One-Stop Access would provide information for all services, coordinate access to, deliver or purchase in-home services for, and coordinate access to institutions	New agency to broker (informal contracts and purchase of service agreements); in-home services from external providers; direct provincial funding for community support services; cooperative model; purhaser/provider split
Liberal (1990)	Service Access Organization (SAO)	*Who:* Persons over 65 and disability population *Public-private Funding:* a) Fully provincially funded services: in-home services; b) Public/private financing: community support services (co-payments based on income rather than assets) c) Regional funding envelope d) Capped budget for home care	Existing mix of FP and NFP providers; SAO would provide information for all services, coordinate access to, deliver or purchase in-home services, and coordinate access to institutions	SAO broker in-home services from external providers; direct provincial funding for community support services; cooperative model; purchaser/provider split
NDP (1991)	Service Coordination Agency (SCA)	Same as SAO, except community support services receive 100% of approved budget after revenues.	Same as SAO, except community NFP provider preference	Same as SAO

TABLE 8.1 (concluded)

Government and Date	Model	Financing	Delivery	Allocation
NDP (1993)	Multi-Service Agency (MSA)	*Who*: Elderly and disability population *Public-private funding*: a) Fully provincially funded: in-home services, case management, placement b) Public/private financing: co-payments for community support services based on income c) MSAs must provide a defined basket of services that include community support services d) Home care/support services in single capped budget	Single NFP agency (MSA) to provide *all* care; up to 20% of MSA budget for purchase of external service from FP and NFP agencies	Regional planning; government allocates all funding for both in-home and community support services to MSAs, who pay salaried employees; cooperative model; no purchaser/provider split. Persons with disabilities funded directly to purchase their own services; market model; purchaser/provider split
PC (1996)	Community Care Access Centre (CCAC)	*Who*: Elderly and disability population *Public-private funding*: a) In-home services provincially funded b) Public/private financing: community support services c) Capped budget for home care	Mix of FP and NFP providers, but managed competition contract process will likely give preference to FP agencies	Government provides CCACs with budget to contract in-home services from external providers through competitive process; competitive market model; purchaser/provider split. Government funds community support service agencies directly; cooperative model; purchaser/provider split

lic responsibility? What should be left to private interests? Clearly, vulnerable populations had greater needs for medical and social supports than their healthier counterparts. Although particular groups, such as the elderly or those with disabilities, were more likely to have such needs, there were no clear boundaries separating those who did or did not need help. Neither were there clear guidelines as to when such requirements should be socialized and when they should be left to individuals and their families. A similar set of divergent ideas underlies debates about the extent to which the state should assist a host of potentially vulnerable groups with other needs. Should parents be helped by publicly financed day care? Should family caregivers receive payments or tax credits for staying at home? Should such assistance be extended to stay-at-home parents? In most industrialized societies, needs designated as 'medical' have been 'privileged' and society has been willing to assist with the bills. Needs designated as 'social' evoke far less agreement. Thrown into the mix is the evidence that the precursor of good health, the prevention of further deterioration of disease and poor health, is often in the social domain. Should a prudent government subsidize preventive services to avoid more costly medical ones further down the road? These disputes accordingly interacted with questions about the relative roles of medical versus social models of care. These conflicting positions were then played out in the varied design decisions about entitlements for services: who would be eligible, what services would be incorporated into the 'basket,' as well as questions about the place for co-payments.

At one end of the spectrum there appeared to be agreement, even by the advocates of retrenching the state, that medical services should continue to be publicly funded. One simple rubric was that services that would have been paid for within a hospital should continue to be paid for if an individual was being treated at home. Most of the reform plans, accordingly. continued to incorporate home nursing and key rehabilitation services. Using similar logic, both the Kirby report (Standing Senate Committee on Social Affairs Science and Technology, 2002) and the Romanow report (Commission on the Future of Health Care in Canada, 2002) have made similar judgments and recommended funding home care for those recently discharged from hospital and those needing palliative care at the end of life. At the other end of the spectrum were activities usually performed by family members and/or volunteers: transportation, friendly visiting, and delivery of prepared meals. In none of the reform plans was full payment for these services envisioned, although in the MSA model many of them would have been provided by paid workers. In the middle, and clearly reflecting the divergent ideas, was homemaking. Whose responsibility was personal care and cleaning? Lines were drawn differently in different models. Assistance with bathing, for instance, was considered closer to the 'medical' realm, and was often covered. Assistance with meal preparation or cleaning was seen as closer to the sorts of activities of daily living that fewer believed should be socialized and therefore was more likely to drop out of the basket. Both the written material and the interviews highlighted significant differences in views on the public subsidization of non-professional services and non-professional providers.

Ideas also undergirded the debate about delivery. What was the role for FP versus NFP providers? For unionized workers? For volunteers? Were volunteers 'scab labour' or part of 'civil society'? How important was it to ensure 'good jobs at good wages,' as opposed to 'efficiency'? How important was it to ensure standardized, uniform levels of services, or was there room for flexibility? Each side selected loaded, value-laden terms to advance its agenda.

Allocation mechanisms also reflected a set of ideas about the relative merits of planning versus competition. Would the market yield the best results? In competition, would important policy goals be neglected? How important was stability? Again, the varied models reflected varied ideas.

8.3.2 Interests

The ability of the state to control the policy agenda was strongly influenced by the nature of the policy community. Both consumers and providers were fragmented, and there were few interests that could either organize to maximize their voice or maintain their mutual interests long enough to control policy development (Williams, et al., 1999). Lacking strong ideological and political consensus about what government should do and facing a policy community characterized by hard-to-mobilize consumers and multiple, mostly small providers, governments had great latitude not only to dictate policy content, but also to control the policy process.

8.3.3 Institutions

An additional factor, which greatly contributed to the volatility of the policy field, was a relative lack of institutional constraints. This is in marked contrast to the mainstream of Medicare, which has shown relative structural and institutional stability. For example, despite over thirty years' advocacy of reform of primary care delivery, little has yet happened. Indeed, early in its mandate, the Harris government declared its intention to change the way primary care was delivered. The 'omnibus legislation' (Bill 26, 1995) might have paved the way for reform; it expanded the role of nurse practitioners, permitted Ontario residents to enrol in primary care groups, and allowed for the establishment of population-based capitation (as opposed to fee-for-service) payment mechanisms. In 1998 the government established fourteen pilot Primary Care Networks in seven Ontario communities, and in 2001 it created the arm's-length Ontario Family Health Network (OFHN), with a mandate to persuade 80 per cent of Ontario physicians to participate in reform by 2004. This goal looks increasingly unattainable. Indeed, flexing its considerable political muscle, the Ontario Medical Association (OMA) did not vote to allow the OFHN even to begin offering template agreements to family physicians in northern and rural Ontario until November 2001. Not until January 2002 did it allow an agreement to be offered to family physicians across the province, and organized groups of family physicians continue to resist reform as an unwarranted intrusion into their professional autonomy. As of February 2003 only 106 of Ontario's 24,000 physicians (half of whom are family practitioners) had enrolled in the Family Health Network, and primary care reform continues to founder.

One clear factor contributing to the stability of the Medicare mainstream is the dominance of collegial mechanisms and medical influence (Deber and Williams, 2003; Hutchison, Abelson, and Lavis, 2001; Tuohy, 1999a,b). The Canada Health Act (CHA) and the control of the federal government through fiscal transfers as well as broad public support introduced an institutional stability to our system not experienced in the United States or Britain; Canadian Medicare has been distinguished by extensive accommodations or 'implicit bargains' between public government and the private medical profession involving government's asserting the right to make health policy in the public interest, while allowing the medical profession to retain a substantial degree of clinical autonomy and control over the delivery of publicly funded services (Stevenson and Williams, 1985; Stevenson, Williams, and Vayda, 1988; Williams et al., 1995).

This stability was evident during the economic slowdown of the early 1990s. Although events during this period gave rise to the creation of internal markets in health care in Britain and to merged markets of health insurance and health care delivery in the United States, in Canada the system remained relatively unchanged. Stability *within* the medical mainstream, however, has not always translated into the stability of the larger health care arena. Hospital budget constraints have resulted in shorter lengths of stay, while technological advancements have allowed for more care to be provided outside hospitals. In consequence, care has shifted from hospital to home and community; from a policy standpoint, this means that care has increasingly moved from the protection of the CHA to an arena of greater volatility. At Medicare's 'margins' far greater variation across and within provinces is thus becoming evident. Not only is more care shifting from the public to the private sector in both financing and delivery of health services, some analysts have noted that it is moving from open arenas of decision making, accountability, and scrutiny to the closed board rooms of private business (Fuller, 1998). From the standpoint of the policy process, changes in the nature and site of care also move decision making into a different policy community with a different internal logic.

Policy communities are shaped by three sets of structures: the autonomy and capacity of state agencies; the organizational development of sectoral interests; and the relationships or networks that develop between the state and societal actors (Coleman and Skogstad, 1990a,b). The Medicare mainstream policy community is dominated by a strong societal actor representing organized medicine and by powerful interests representing hospitals. In contrast, in the LTC community-based sector, societal interests were diverse, loosely connected agencies and advocacy groups, largely without stable funding, large sources of revenue, administrative bureaucracies, or shared interests. They faced a knowledgeable professional bureaucracy within government. Without a strong force like a medical or hospital association as a counterbalance in the sub-government, the state was able to push forward its own agenda. Societal interests occasionally appeared to have influence, but one might argue that they were privileged only if their agendas were in concert with those of the state. Indeed, the implications of the shifts in the consultation process – the two extremes being the NDP and the PC processes – imply that even the involvement of societal actors was at the sufferance of (and in the manner defined by) the provincial governments of the day. This is further evidence that such a policy network consisted of a strong government and a weak, fragmented set of societal interests.

As noted, existing state institutions, such as the CHA and its associated fiscal penalties, did not apply in the community-based LTC sector. Even the passage of the New Democrats' MSA model in Bill 173 failed to constrain the Harris Conservative government; it was able to implement the radically different CCAC market model within the context of that legislation. In part, this flexibility arose from the governmental practice – long characteristic of health-related legislation in Ontario – of writing legislation broadly and leaving details to be implemented through regulation. The main impact of the NDP legislation thus was ironic: by transferring the Home Care Program budget out of OHIP, with the intent of integrating budgets and removing them from the sphere of medical dominance, it also removed them from the institutional logic and universal entitlements of the Medicare mainstream.

Constrained by the institution of Medicare and by the interests embedded in it, Ontario governments, regardless of political stripe, have moved to shift more and more care (both services and needs groups) outside the mainstream and into the margins, where governments have more freedom to act. In so doing, they have set the stage for change in the state's role in the field of health care as a whole. Precisely because they are at the margins of this role, policy sub-fields like home and community care are politically more volatile and are more open to the logic of commercial private markets. Thus, while Medicare remains resilient, it covers a declining proportion of health care, and the role of the state accordingly diminishes. Indeed, the areas of Canadian health care experiencing the fastest growth are those beyond universal entitlements, including prescription drugs and home care (Canadian Institute for Health Information and Statistics Canada, 2001).

8.4 Epilogue: Reining in the Community Care Access Centres

Since these chapters were written, the policy trade-offs have reasserted themselves, casting doubt on the stability of the CCAC model as first implemented and re-emphasizing the fundamentally different political dynamics that operate in the field of community-based LTC, particularly compared with the hospital and physician mainstream. Accordingly, the future of Ontario's forty-three Community Care Access Centres currently is murky. As detailed throughout this book, among the stated objectives of all the community-based long-term care reform initiatives proposed by successive provincial governments was the provision to consumers of one-stop access to high-quality, community-based services that responded to their needs.

If such welfarist, consumer-centred goals had constituted the 'top line' of justification for reform, however, the 'bottom line' continued to be government's need to find ways to control rapidly escalating health care costs. They were expected to escalate even more rapidly as the population aged and as new and more expensive technologies allowed people to live longer (albeit often with higher levels of need). Furthermore, costs would be harder to manage as the public, along with the organized health care professions, continued to exert massive political pressure on governments at all levels to stem the perceived erosion of publicly funded Medicare resulting in large part from those government funding constraints.

These goals of service improvement and cost containment were likely to clash. Certainly, a major design characteristic of the CCAC reform was the establishment of global funding envelopes, which the CCACs would use to purchase services for eligible consumers who required them. These envelopes would be set unilaterally by the province, with some adjustments based on population needs, and CCACs would have no access to additional funds. In principle, at least, the reform therefore could almost certainly achieve the goal of cost-containment, even if other goals, such as cost efficiency, improved service quality, or consumer independence, were not achieved. Under the market-oriented Harris Progressive Conservative government, cost containment, if not cost reduction, became all the more pressing as the government engaged in a series of personal and corporate tax cuts that significantly reduced its total revenues even as the federal government continued to baulk at full restoration of the cuts it had made to the health and social care transfers to the provinces during the mid-1990s.

Ontario's CCACs quickly found themselves at the centre of these conflicting forces. Their funding envelopes were based on historical (i.e., pre-hospital restructuring) home care budgets. These budgets were now expected to meet rising service demands, including pressure to serve the growing number of post-acute-care patients discharged 'quicker and sicker' from hospitals. This task proved difficult for many CCACs across the province, and they began to run significant operating deficits. As CCAC executive directors and boards became more vocal in their calls for increased provincial funding, the province responded in several ways.

One approach was to enact regulations that placed eligibility restrictions and service maxima on home care, restricting the flexibility of individual CCACs and their case managers. Regardless of assessed need, there is now a provincially set maximum number of hours that can be provided by the CCACs. Priority is given to the 'acute' patients, rather than individuals with chronic needs originally believed to be the targets of the program. Those who have used up their allowable allotment are expected to do without additional services or to pay for these services privately. The province also clarified the priority to be given to various potential client groups. As a result, the main consumers of home and community care are no longer seniors or the disabled with long-term needs, but people of all ages with acute-care requirements. An unintended consequence is that, lacking other options, frail seniors who require but cannot receive home care are falling back into the institutional sector – putting renewed pressure on hospital emergency rooms, becoming 'bed blockers' in acute-care settings, and becoming candidates for nursing home beds. The policy direction of decades – encouraging home care to promote wellness and discourage institutionalization – has thus been effectively reversed.

The province also provided selective 'budget enhancements' and then bailed out CCACs in fiscal difficulty. When these measures failed to stem increasing costs and budget overruns, the province launched a two-prong political offensive against the CCACs. According to the government, CCACs had been provided with sufficient resources to meet service needs; by definition, therefore, the problem must have been that some CCACs were poorly managed and inefficient.

In June 2001 the provincial government announced that all CCAC budgets would be frozen at 2000–1 levels and that CCACs could no longer run operating deficits. While some CCACs had anticipated this announcement and already had made significant service cuts, the impact on the seventeen CCACs across the province still running budget deficits was 'devastating.' Squeezed between increasing service demands and now even more limited funding, the only option for these CCACs was to implement cuts. While strategies varied across the province, common outcomes were staff layoffs, even tighter eligibility requirements, and reduced service levels. Non-medical services appear to have been the most drastically affected: CCACs and community service agencies reported significantly reduced volumes of homemaking and personal support. In the absence of systematic evaluation, it is difficult to judge whether these services had contributed to the health and well-being of those receiving them, or whether these constraints yielded desirable efficiencies or even increased independence. Hollander (2001; Hollander and Tessaro, 2001) suggests that cuts to 'lower level,' non-medical, community-based services, while saving money in the short run, may actually cost the health system more over the longer term as individuals turn to more costly medical care and institutionalization. A study in Saskatchewan was more sceptical (Saskatchewan Health Services Utilization and Research Commission, 2000).

From a policy process standpoint, however, these government attempts to control CCAC spending led to an unprecedented political alliance between the organizations representing not-for-profit (NFP) community service agencies (OCSA) and for-profit providers (Ontario Home Health Care Providers Association [OHHCPA]). They contended that instability in CCAC funding, together with the use of increasing proportions of this funding in administrative overheads, had eroded the stability of the home and community care sector as a whole (OHHCPA and OCSA, 2001). Failure to win CCAC contracts has chased some long-time providers, particularly the Victorian Order of Nurses, out of home care provision throughout much of the province. The reductions in volume even for agencies that won contracts have added further strains, including the demise of VHA Home Healthcare (Hamilton), formerly a main provider of homemaking services to that community. As noted, however, outcomes for individual consumers remain unclear.

The second prong of the government's political offensive against the CCACs took the form of a direct provincial takeover of CCAC governance. As described earlier, since their inception, CCACs had been governed by volunteer community boards that exerted overall control over CCAC operations and hired executive directors (EDs). As some CCACs (and their EDs) became more vocal in their criticism of government funding shortfalls and service reductions, however, the government took the radical step of replacing all existing CCAC boards and EDs with boards and EDs hand-picked by the government and appointed through order-in-council. Similar tactics were later used to take over those school boards refusing to make sufficient cuts to balance their budgets.

The speed of the government takeover was remarkable and reinforces the findings about the relative weakness of the policy community that it faced. On 7 November 2001 the Harris government introduced Bill 130, the Community Care Access Corporations Act (Government of Ontario, 2001); this act was passed into law with little debate or public response before the provincial Parliament recessed for Christmas. Perhaps not surprisingly, given that the legislation in effect fired current CCAC boards and EDs and left it to government to appoint replacements (but also left open the possibility that it might reappoint those now holding positions should the government deem them politically acceptable), there was little critical response from the CCACs, and a number actually expressed support on their Web sites for the government's unilateral actions. As one ED noted privately, the main objective of the legislation was to 'muzzle' CCACs politically; that objective was clearly met. Of the forty-one CCAC EDs in place prior to 1 January 2002 (two CCACs had been administered by hospitals), seven were fired outright; several others were reappointed to different CCACs where, presumably, they had not built coalitions with their boards or communities.

8.4.1 Romanow and the Future of Medicare

A second major development with a potential impact on community-based LTC was created by government reactions to the November 2002 release of the long-anticipated report of the Commission on the Future of Health Care in Canada (2002). Led by the former Saskatchewan NDP premier, Roy Romanow, this high-profile commission was established by a federal government increasingly concerned about public perceptions of the erosion of Canadian Medicare and the universal access to health care that it provided Canadians. The commission's mandate was to make recommendations about options for Medicare's future, including those proposed by adherents of free-market ideologies, which could lead to a growing reliance on private commercial funding and delivery of health care. Over the course of eighteen months, the group reviewed available evidence, commissioned numerous research papers and reports, and held broad-based public consultations across the country.

In its report the Romanow Commission came down strongly in support of universal Medicare, which was characterized as a public good, a national symbol, and a defining aspect of Canadian citizenship. Rejecting arguments that Medicare was 'unsustainable,' the Commissioners also rejected, on both economic and ethical grounds, what they described as 'radical' private-market approaches to financing insured services, including the establishment of a parallel private commercial health care system. Instead, they argued strongly not only for maintaining universal coverage for hospital and physician care, but for incrementally extending coverage to certain services and sectors identified as having become increasingly important as more care was moved out of hospitals. An expanded 'basket' of insured services would clarify the coverage of diagnostic procedures such as MRIs, 'catastrophic' drug expenditures, rehabilitation services provided under provincial workers' compensation programs, and home care. Other recommendations were made about modifying health care delivery, particularly encouraging primary-care reform and better electronic health records. However, the home care recommendations were limited. Rather than proposing full coverage for a comprehensive home care program, home care was defined in relatively narrow terms. It was recommended that approximately $980 million per year in additional federal funding be spent to 'kick-start' expanded provincial home care programs in three priority areas: home mental health case management and intervention ($568 million), post-acute rehabilitation and medical care ($323 million), and palliative care ($89 million). With the exception of the mental health recommendations, this definition was restricted to the acute-care substitution functions; coverage for the maintenance and nursing-home substitution functions was noticeably absent, as was inclusion of social supports. Although it may be argued that the Romanow recommendations are an initial first step in expanding government funding of home care services, history and our analysis would indicate that future public coverage of clients with chronic conditions will be hard to achieve in this sector.

While initial reaction, particularly from Alberta, Ontario, and Quebec, questioned federal authority to steer provincial health care priorities at all, at the same time claiming that the amounts of new money recommended by Romanow were insufficient to restore the federal funding 'share' to mid-1990s levels, a new health care financing agreement was reached at the First Ministers' meeting held in January 2003 (First Ministers, 2003). This agreement provides the provinces with considerable new federal funding, although less than the provinces would like. Despite the relatively few strings attached, both sides have agreed about the necessity of improving accountability for how public money is spent. Details are being worked out; they offer a faint possibility that additional institutional constraints may indeed be placed upon provincial freedom of action in these proximate policy fields.

The question is, then, what are the prospects for community-based long-term care in Ontario in the wake of this agreement? On the one hand, by emphasizing that the 'new money' should be tied, at least in part, to the extension of universal coverage to certain home care services, CCACs may achieve restored funding and modify current service caps. Before the cuts began, however, Ontario had one of the most expansive home care programs in Canada; even at present, it provides a far higher level of service than is available in some other provinces. It is highly unlikely that the provinces will agree to a level of care above that currently provided by Ontario. In addition, for the most part the June

2001 budget caps cut homemaking and personal support services. They may serve an important preventive and maintenance function, but they clearly lie outside the limits recommended by the Romanow and Kirby reports and echoed in the federal-provincial accord. If anything, this focus would suggest the increasing 'medicalization' of publicly funded services, which in turn could also mean a further erosion of the LTC and preventive function of the CCACs.

Further threatening the CCAC model were the recommendations of a second, parallel federal inquiry by the Standing Senate Committee on Social Affairs, Science and Technology (the Kirby Committee). From its comprehensive investigation of possible reforms to the federal-provincial institutions, funding mechanisms, and operations of Medicare recommendations emerged for expanded coverage for post-acute (as well as palliative) home care (Standing Senate Committee on Social Affairs Science and Technology, 2002). Unlike Romanow, however, who left aside the issue of who would be the holder of the purse of new home care funding, Kirby was clear: new funding should be directed first to hospitals. According to Kirby's logic, this would allow hospitals to benefit from shorter in-patient stays, increase their uptake of post-acute home care services, encourage vertical integration of hospitals and home care, and prevent the shifting of hospital costs to the home.

If implemented in Ontario, the Kirby recommendations would have important implications for CCACs. On the one hand, it is again acknowledged that more post-acute-care needs are now located in the community as a result of restructuring initiatives that have reduced hospital beds and average lengths of stay. The committee members also recognize the need to overcome institutional barriers (both funding and legislation), which continue to demarcate a clear line between hospital and home care and stand in the way of greater integration of acute and post-acute care. However, in shifting post-acute care to hospitals, their recommendations would likely also reduce the role of CCACs. Ironically, the fact that CCACs already have shifted the focus of their activities to short-term services for those patients discharged from acute hospitals would make it easier to eliminate the CCAC bureaucracies. The issue with which the reform began – how to care for the frail elderly and others needing supports at home – would be ignored. Moreover, the older infrastructure that had managed those cases was already subsumed into the CCAC structures. The Kirby recommendations, if implemented, therefore eventually would lead to a requirement to reinvent new structures to manage these functions.

Another policy initiative in a proximate sector, however, is likely to further complicate home care in Ontario. In May 1998 the Harris PC government announced its intention to spend more than $1 billion to create 20,000 new LTC beds in private facilities by 2006 and to upgrade an additional 16,000 existing beds; most of these beds have been awarded to FP providers. In subsequent economic analyses it has been suggested that that number might be excessive (Coyte and Baranek, 2001; Coyte et al., 2002), and government may yet revisit the precise numbers. Nonetheless, because the private sector has made heavy investments in upgrading existing facilities and building new ones, there is considerable pressure on government to fill these beds. Anecdotal evidence suggests that CCAC case managers are now more aggressively counselling seniors requiring LTC at home to seek admission instead to a facility. If true, this trend would effectively reverse the long-standing policy direction, repeated in each of the LTC reform initiatives, of reducing institutionalization by increasing access to community-based care. Although initially slated to come on-stream by 2006, much of this expanded institutional capacity is now likely to be fully operational by the end of 2004.

At the same time, the province has moved to streamline placement coordination by restricting patient choice. Whereas previously seniors could have their names placed on waiting lists for up to five facilities of their choice and could defer admission if admission was not yet required when a bed became available, the new rules allowed seniors to be on waiting lists of no more than three facilities and specified that they would lose their place on the waiting list if they did not accept admission when it was offered. In addition, these waiting lists now included patients in hospitals deemed to be eligible for a facility placement. Such designation thus has financial consequences, since to discourage 'bed blocking,' patients in acute-care hospitals are required to pay the daily LTC facility accommodation rate of approximately $45.00 as soon as they are designated as nursing home eligible, whether or not they are eventually placed in a facility.

Combined with a history of antagonistic relations with the provincial government and increasing criticism from both FP and NFP providers, these pressures may point to a changing, and perhaps reduced, future role for Ontario's CCACs. Whether or not such change takes place, it is clear how easily it could occur. CCACs are not 'safe'; as we have shown, in this policy field, when governments choose to act, they may do so with few constraints.

8.5 Whither the State in Health Care?

The final chapters are yet to be written in the saga of home and community care policy in Ontario. Nevertheless, the history of policy development over the past decade suggests important possibilities not only for policy content and process, but for the future role of the state in health care.

Throughout we have suggested that, in spite of mounting political pressures, Medicare's 'mainstream' of hospital and physician services remains remarkably resilient. As always, Medicare faces ongoing challenges to its sustainability, and public discontent with waiting lists and perceived access barriers has been rising. NFP delivery has been challenged by the emergence of FP private clinics that perform hospital services; comprehensiveness has been eroded by delisting of certain insured services provided by physicians (Fuller, 1998; Taft and Steward, 2000; Williams et al., 2001). To this point, however, such erosion has been mostly at the margins, and virtually all physician and hospital services continue to be publicly funded by provincial health insurance plans, including those 'core' services provided by FP clinics (Canadian Institute for Health Information and Statistics Canada, 2001).

The stability of the Medicare mainstream is in large part due to Medicare itself and to the Canada Health Act, its institutional base, which set clear limits on the role that private financing can play in the provision of medically necessary hospital and physician services; public Medicare effectively prohibits their purchase in privately insured markets. Indeed, Medicare itself constitutes an institutional bulwark against the reintroduction of private, commercial insurance markets, which in the pre-Medicare period had failed to provide adequate coverage for medical services to more than half of Canadians and had proved remarkably costly. Economic analysis done for the original Royal Commission on Health Services concluded that for every dollar paid by subscribers to private commercial insurance companies in the pre-Medicare period, only 65 cents was returned as medical services (Berry, 1964; Canada Royal Commission on Health Services, 1964). In both the Kirby and Romanow reports, examining the future of Canada's health care system, a strong argument is made for continuation of full public financing for 'medically necessary' services; public opinion strongly concurs.

Nevertheless, the saga of LTC reform and the testimony given to these panels suggest that in spite of mainstream Medicare's apparent resilience, the state's role in health care and universal entitlements to care

are eroding. The erosion is particularly evident as one moves beyond the 'mainstream' of medically necessary hospital and physician services to a broader definition of health care. These broader services are often delivered outside hospitals by providers other than physicians, and they are intended not simply to cure illness, but also to promote personal autonomy and independence, to maintain functional ability, and to prevent or delay institutionalization. Under current legislation and federal-provincial funding arrangements, provinces may agree to provide public coverage for services outside Medicare's mainstream; however, they have no obligation to do so. Indeed, once in home and community, even medically necessary services previously provided in hospitals under universal coverage may or may not be covered. This is crucial precisely because, as a result of technological advances and health care restructuring initiatives, more and more care is moving beyond hospitals and doctors' offices and thus beyond Medicare's institutionalized entitlements. While such a shift in the site of care has long been advocated by health care reformers as a means of redressing the historical dominance of physicians and hospitals, empowering individuals and communities, and shifting more resources to health promotion, the outcome has also been to shift care beyond Medicare's protection. Indeed, the push to restructure hospitals has dramatically reduced beds, admissions, and average length of stay across the country, in an effort to reserve hospitalization for those requiring that intensity of care (Canadian Institute for Health Information and Statistics Canada, 2002). Ontario's reforms of home and community care have 'de-institutionalized' and 'de-medicalized' both mainstream services and needs groups by placing them beyond universal coverage. Indeed, the home and community care sector may act as a safety valve for increasing costs in the Medicare mainstream. In the less politically mobilized and more factioned terrain of home and community, there are relatively few constraints on shifting health care from the collective logic of public entitlements to the competitive logic of private markets (Williams et al., 2001).

Meanwhile, the attempts to de-medicalize and de-institutionalize care for clients with chronic needs (the frail elderly and persons with disabilities) have reversed. Home care is now dominated by those who require acute-care services, and clients with chronic needs are provided with a reduced level of service or no service, or are encouraged to enter LTC facilities.

These observations bring us full circle to our initial comments: ongoing health care restructuring initiatives in Ontario and in other provinces that shift growing proportions of care from hospital to home and community are significant, not only because they change the site of much care, but because they have critical implications for the role of the state.

Like other elements of post-war states, health systems are, in essence, redistributive mechanisms; thus, shifts from the logic of public entitlements to the logic of private markets have significant implications for the social distribution of the costs of illness, for social equity, and for illness itself. This impact is considerable: in spite of highly publicized cuts in federal transfers to the provinces and provincial attempts to control costs, health care spending still accounts for almost 10 per cent of Canada's GDP, more than 33 per cent of all provincial government spending, and up to 45 per cent of all provincial program spending if debt service is excluded. What happens in health care affects all other programs and elements of the post-war state as well as the economy and society more generally.

Because Medicare marked a shift in the locus of care not only from home to hospital in the post-war period but from private to public responsibilities for health care, a shift back to home and community may mark an important watershed for the role of the post-war state. Medicare emerged historically as a response to the perceived failure of private, commercial markets to provide Canadians with needed access to health care. Now, it exists as an anomaly within a more general shift towards state retrenchment and private markets. To adherents of neo-conservative, free-market ideologies, Medicare is seen as a leading example of the failure of the post-war state to ensure access to health care on a cost-efficient, sustainable basis. Although public opinion polls suggest that this rhetoric is not well accepted by Canadians (Mendelsohn, 2002), public anxiety as to the 'sustainability' of the system has increased. It is thus worth noting the possible discrepancy between the rhetoric of improved access, universality, and client and community empowerment that has accompanied recent reforms of home and community care in Ontario and the forthright statements by that same political regime to reduce the state's role in favour of market forces, even as it continues to voice support for the principles of the Canada Health Act.

These developments emphasize the importance of addressing health care not simply as a single policy field, but as a set of proximate policy sub-fields each with its own distinctive policy dynamic. Of course – and this is a key point – the dynamics of policy change in proximate policy sub-fields is not independent. Constrained by the institution of Medicare and the interests it embeds, all Ontario governments, regardless of political stripe, have moved to shift more and more care (both services and needs groups) outside the mainstream and into the margins, where they have more freedom to act. In so doing, they have set the stage for change in the state's role in the field of health care as a whole. Precisely because they are 'at the margins' of this role, policy sub-fields like home and community care are more volatile politically and more open to the logic of commercial private markets. Thus, although Medicare remains resilient, it covers a declining proportion of health care, and the role of the state accordingly diminishes. Medicare, the most visible landmark of Canadian health care, spans only hospital and physician services; sub-fields – such as home and community care along with rehabilitation services, pharmaceuticals, health promotion, and public health – are key to the health and well-being of individuals and the population as a whole, but they operate within distinct policy arenas. Indeed, the areas of Canadian health care experiencing the fastest growth are those beyond universal entitlements, including prescription drugs and home care (Canadian Institute for Health Information and Statistics Canada, 2001).

In deconstructing health care in our analysis we gain considerable advantages. For instance, we can begin to account for the fact that states may appear to be both simultaneously strong and weak. The Canada Health Act and its precursor legislation established a legitimate role for the state in health care, contributed to the crystallization of an idea of health care based on post-war curative technology, and reinforced the political power of the organized medical profession to resist state reforms perceived as threatening its economic and clinical freedom (Williams et al., 2002; Williams et al., 1995). Such power has effectively restricted attempts to include physicians under regional health care reforms in all provinces without exception, and the profession continues to block efforts, even in Ontario, to introduce primary-care reforms designed to change the way medical practice is organized and funded (Williams et al., 2002). The state is thus relatively weak when it tries to deal with the 'mainstream' of Medicare. Outside the mainstream, however, in the proximate policy sub-field of home and community care, the state has proved to be remarkably capable of achieving reforms deemed important. The results are evident: while no Ontario government has yet been able to change the way in which primary care physicians practise, successive governments have moulded home and community care to their own political and ideological agendas.

In the case of home and community care, the state was an active and, in important ways, dominant actor. Through the course of Ontario's series of reform initiatives, the province took a lead role in shaping not only policy options, but the internal dynamics of the policy community. As we have suggested in this volume, the state was able to take such a 'strong' role because neither institutions, ideas, nor interests greatly constrained its freedom of action. The Peterson Liberal, Rae NDP, and Harris Conservative governments were new-to-power majority governments within an institutional structure facilitating action; there were relatively few blocking points in the Ontario legislature. Thus, when the party in power had a clear agenda, they had the tools to implement it.

The Rae government chose to implement its plans in ways that would give it maximum flexibility, but that also allowed its successors to radically alter how such services would be financed and delivered. Home care was transferred from the Ontario Health Insurance Plan (OHIP) to its own legislation. Most key design decisions were placed within the regulations rather than within the legislation, thereby enabling subsequent governments to make many alterations without legislative scrutiny. In consequence, yet another potential obstacle to change was removed.

Here, it is helpful to note the concept of 'contingency' introduced by Weir (1992). This concept draws attention to the fact that there are multiple, sometimes overlapping policy fields, and that events originating in one field can impact on another. While much neo-institutional literature tends to be focussed within the boundaries of a single policy field, Weir suggests that it is also necessary to consider developments in proximate fields. Even neo-conservative governments committed ideologically to doing so are unable to sustain full frontal attacks against Medicare, the key element of the post-war state, in the face of public opinion and powerful vested interests. Health care, however, defined beyond Medicare's hospital and physician doctor mainstream, can and does experience massive change in the role of the state.

Moving beyond the protection of Medicare may, indeed, open these policy fields to global forces (Baranek, Deber, and Williams, 1999; Redden, 1999; Williams et al., 2001). As more and more care is shifted beyond the bounds of universal government health insurance and into commercialized markets, there is increasing concern that care previously exempt from global trade agreements, such as the General Agreement on Trade in Services (GATS) and the North American Free Trade Agreement (NAFTA), may now fall under their auspices (Canadian Health Services Research Foundation, 2002). Although such agreements do not prevent a government from re-entering a field with a commercial presence, it appears that private investors are entitled to claim compensation for harm to their property (market share or goodwill), which under the terms and conditions of NAFTA is likely to be substantially more generous than under domestic law (Appleton, 1999). Moreover, under NAFTA foreign corporations (but not their domestic counterparts) have the right to make claims against any Canadian government (including provincial and local levels) on the basis of any legislation, policy, or practice and to have such claims adjudicated by an international tribunal. In community-based LTC in Ontario, government policy reforms have deliberately promoted the expansion of FP enterprises as a means of increasing competition with NFP and driving down costs; such shifts may prove difficult and potentially expensive to reverse. As Paul Starr (1982) observed in his groundbreaking analysis of American medicine two decades ago, the 'coming of the corporations' was likely not only to erode the state's ability to achieve health care reform, but to ensure that the logic of economic markets trumped the logic of public entitlements on a permanent basis.

This is a story without an end. Government may have implemented a policy reform, but a large and growing number of elderly and disabled are requiring services, and the resources allocated are inadequate to provide the level and quality they and their families demand. Staff shortages are growing, particularly as managed competition controls wages within the sector, while the expansion of other facilities (particularly the promised 20,000 new nursing-home beds) attracts away staff at higher wages. Still there is no consensus on ideas, interests remain fragmented, and the institutional structures around LTC give enormous policy latitude to the government in power. The particular design decisions made by the Conservative government appear no more stable than those inherent in the previous four reform models. Whichever party holds power, additional reforms appear inevitable; their direction, however, does not.

References

Advocacy Centre for the Elderly (ACE) (1994) 'Submission to the Standing Committee on Social Development. Bill 173 The Long Term Care Act, 1994.' 15 September.

Akande, Z. (1991) 'Statement to the Legislature on the Redirection of Long-Term Care Services.' Minister of Community and Social Services. 11 June. Available at http://www.ont/a.on.ca./hansard/house_debates/38.part session 1/a045.htm.

Alzheimer Ontario (1994) 'Long Term Care: Towards Success or Failure? Submission to the Standing Committee on Social Development. Bill 173 An Act respecting Long-Term Care.' August.

Appleton, B. (1999) 'International Agreements and National Health Plans: NAFTA.' In *Market Limits in Health Reform: Public Success, Private Failure*. Ed. D. Drache and T. Sullivan. London: Routledge.

ARA Consulting Group (1995) 'Alternatives to the MSA: A Summary of Discussions with Key Groups Representing LTC Consumers, Providers and Workers.' Prepared for the Long-Term Care Division, Policy Branch, Ministry of Health. 26 September.

Armstrong, P., and H. Armstrong (2003) *Wasting Away: The Undermining of Canadian Health Care*. 2d ed. Toronto: Oxford University Press.

Armstrong, W. (2000) *The Consumer Experience with Cataract Surgery and Private Clinics in Alberta: Canada's Canary in the Mine Shaft*. Report published by the Consumers' Association of Canada (Alberta). January.

Arrow, K.J. (1973) *Theoretical Issues in Health Insurance*. Colchester, U.K: University of Essex.

Association of Municipalities of Ontario (AMO) (1994) 'Bill 173 – The Long Term Care Act. AMO's Presentation to the Standing Committee on Social Development.' 24 August.

Auditor General of Canada (1999) 'Federal Support of Health Care Delivery.'
    Report of the Auditor General of Canada, chap. 29. November. Available at
    http://www.oag-bvg.gc.ca.
Baranek, P., R.B. Deber, and A.P. Williams (1999) 'Policy Trade-Offs in "Home
    Care": The Ontario Example.' *Canadian Public Administration* 42, 69–92.
Baumann, A., L. O'Brien-Pallas, M. Armstrong-Stassen, J. Blythe, R. Bourbon-
    nais, S. Cameron, D.I. Doran, M. Kerr, L.M. Hall, M. Vezina, M. Butt, and
    L. Ryan (2001) 'Commitment and Care: The Benefits of a Healthy Work-
    place for Nurses, Their Patients and the System.' CHSRF Policy Synthesis.
    Available at http://www.chsrf.ca/docs/finrpts/pscomcaree.pdf [Feb 18,
    2002].
Beer, C. (1990) 'Charles Beer, Minister of Community and Social Services,
    Releases Plan for LTC.' News release. MCSS. 30 May.
Béland, F., and D. Arweiler (1996a) 'Conceptual Framework for Development of
    Long-Term Care Policy. 1. Constitutive Elements.' *Canadian Journal on Aging*
    15, 649–81.
– (1996b) 'Conceptual Framework for Development of Long-Term Care Policy.
    2. Conceptual Model.' *Canadian Journal on Aging* 15, 682–97.
Bendick, M., Jr (1989) 'Privatizing the Delivery of Social Welfare Services: An
    Ideal to Be Taken Seriously.' In *Privatization and the Welfare State*. Ed. S.B.
    Kamerman and A.J. Kahn. Princeton, N.J.: Princeton University Press.
Berg, B. (1998) *Qualitative Research Methods for the Social Sciences*. 3d ed. Washing-
    ton, D.C.: Congressional Quarterly Press.
Berry, C.H. (1964) *Voluntary Medical Insurance and Prepayment*. Royal Commission
    on Health Services. Ottawa: Queen's Printer.
Blakeney, A., and S. Borins (1998) *Political Management in Canada*. 2d ed. Tor-
    onto: University of Toronto Press.
British Columbia Royal Commission on Health Care and Costs (1991) *Closer to
    Home: The Report of the British Columbia Royal Commission on Health Care and
    Costs*. Vols 1 and 2. Victoria, B.C.: British Columbia Royal Commission on
    Health Care and Costs.
Brooks, S. (2000) *Canadian Democracy: An Introduction*. 3d ed. Toronto: Oxford
    University Press.
Browne, P.L. (2000) *Unsafe Practices: Restructuring and Privatization in Ontario
    Health Care*. Ottawa: Canadian Centre for Policy Alternatives.
Cameron, D.R., and G. White (2000) *Cycling into Saigon: The Conservative Transi-
    tion in Ontario*. Vancouver: UBC Press.
Canada Royal Commission on Health Services (1964) *Canada Royal Commission
    on Health Services*. Vol. 1. Ottawa: Queen's Printer
Canadian Centre for Policy Alternatives (CCPA) (2000) *Health Care, Limited: The*

Privatization of Medicare. A Synthesis Report Prepared by the CCPA for the Council of Canadians, with Guidance from CCPA Research Associates Pat Armstrong, Hugh Armstrong, and Colleen Fuller and in collaboration with the Canadian Health Coalition. November. Available at http://www.policyalternatives.ca/publications/health_care_ltd.p df.

Canadian Health Services Research Foundation (2002) 'Globalization and Canada's Healthcare System.' Material prepared for the Commission on the Future of Health Care in Canada, Issue/Survey Paper. July.

Canadian Home Care Association (1998) 'Portrait of Canada: An Overview of Public Home Care Programs.' Background information prepared for the National Conference on Home Care. February.

Canadian Institute for Health Information (2000) 'Hospital Discharges, Age-Standardized Discharge Rates, Patient Days and Average Length of Stay, Canada and Provinces/Territories, 1994/95–1998/99.' Hospital Morbidity Database. Available at http://www.cihi.ca.

Canadian Institute for Health Information and Statistics Canada (2001) 'Health Care in Canada.' Available at http://www.cihi.ca.

– (2002) *Health Care in Canada 2002.* Ottawa: Canadian Institute for Health Information.

Canadian Pensioners Concerned, Ontario Division (1994) 'Presentation to Standing Committee on Social Development on Bill 173 An Act Respecting Long-Term Care.' 24 August.

Canadian Red Cross Society, Ontario Division (CRCS) (1994) 'Fact Sheet #1: Bill 173.' Fact sheet based on the submission to the Standing Committee on Social Development. 14 August.

Care Watch Ontario (1999) 'Does Long Term Care Have Any Legal Status in Ontario?' *Who Cares? A Newsletter about Community Care,* Spring, 1.

Catholic Women's League of Canada (CWL), Ontario Provincial Council (1994) 'Presentation by the Ontario Provincial Council of the Catholic Women's League of Canada to the Standing Committee on Social Development.' 4 October.

Chappell, N.L. (1994) 'Home Care Research: What Does It Tell Us? *Gerontologist* 34, 116–20.

Chessie, K. (2000) 'No Evidence Found that Preventive Home Care Improves Seniors' Health Outcomes: Study.' *A Closer Look.* Saskatoon: Saskatchewan Health Services Utilization and Research Commission. Summer. Available at http://www.hsurc.sk.ca/publications/pdfs/summercloserlook.pdf.

Citizens for Independence in Living and Breathing (1994) 'Brief to: Standing Committee on Social Reform.' 4 October.

Coalition of Consumer and Provider Groups (1994a) 'Coalition of Consumer

and Provider Groups Demand Changes to Long Term Care Bill.' Press
release. Toronto. 25 October.

- (1994b) 'Statement to the Media re: Bill 173 – An Act Respecting Long Term
Care.' 25 October.

- (1994c) 'Workers Not Treated Equally by Long Term Care Legislation.'
Media release. Toronto. 16 November.

Coleman, W.D., and G. Skogstad (1990a) 'Conclusion.' In *Policy Communities and
Public Policy in Canada: A Structural Approach.* Ed. W.D. Coleman and G.
Skogstad. Toronto: Copp Clark Pitman.

- eds (1990b) *Policy Communities and Public Policy in Canada: A Structural
Approach.* Toronto: Copp Clark Pitman.

Commission on the Future of Health Care in Canada (Roy J. Romanow, Commissioner) (2002) *Building on Values: The Future of Health Care in Canada: Final
Report.* Ottawa: Queen's Printer.

Coyte, P.C., and P.M. Baranek (2001) 'Identifying the Assumptions Used by Various Jurisdictions to Forecast Demands for Home and Facility-Based Care for
the Elderly.' Report to the Ontario Ministry of Health and Long-Term Care,
prepared under grant 02709 to the University of Toronto, March 2001. Available at http://www.hcerc.utoronto.ca/research.html#Reports.

Coyte, P.C., and W. Young (1997a) 'Applied Home Care Research.' *International
Journal of Health Care Quality Assurance,* 10, 1–5.

- (1997b) Reinvestment In and Use Of Home Care Services. Technical Report
No. 97-05-TR. Institute for Clinical Evaluative Sciences. Toronto. November.

Coyte, P C., A. Laporte, P. Baranek, and W.S. Croson (2002) 'Forecasting Facility
and In-Home Long-Term Care for the Elderly in Ontario: The Impact of
Improving Health and Changing Preference.' Hospital Management
Research Unit Report to the Ontario Ministry of Health and Long-Term l
Care, April 2002. Available at http://www.hcerc.utoronto.ca/
research.html#Reports.

Crowley, B.L., D. Zitner, and N. Faraday-Smith (2002) 'Operating in the Dark:
The Gathering Crisis in Canada's Health Care System.' Atlantic Institute for
Market Studies (AIMS). Available at http://www.aims.ca.

Culyer, A.J., and B. Jönsson, eds. (1986) *Public and Private Health Services: Complementarities and Conflicts.* New York: Basil Blackwell.

Daw, J. (1995) 'Check Your Health Coverage Next Trip.' *Toronto Star,* 15 October, E8.

Deber, R.B. (1991) 'Philosophical Underpinnings of Canada's Health Care System.' *Canada-U.S. Outlook* 2, 20–45.

- (2000a) 'Getting What We Pay For: Myths and Realities about Financing Canada's Health Care System.' *Health Law in Canada* 21, 9–56.

- (2000b) 'Who Wants to Pay for Health Care?' *Canadian Medical Association Journal*, 163, 43–4.
- (2002) 'Delivering Health Care Services: Public, Not-for-Profit, or Private?' Commission on the Future of Health Care in Canada, Discussion Paper No. 17. August.
- ed. (1992) *Case Studies in Canadian Health Policy and Management*. Vol. 1. Ottawa: Canadian Hospital Association Press.
Deber, R.B., and A.P. Williams (1995) 'Policy, Payment and Participation: Long-Term Care Reform in Ontario.' *Canadian Journal on Aging* 14, 294–318.
- (2003) 'Government, Politics, and Stakeholders in the United States and Canada.' In *Government Relations in The Health Care Industry*. Ed. P. Leatt and J. Mapa. Westport, Conn.: Praeger Publishers.
Deber, R.B., A.P. Williams, P. Baranek, and K.M. Duvalko (1995) 'The Public-Private Mix in Health Care: Report to the Task Force on the Funding and Delivery of Medical Care in Ontario.' Ontario Ministry of Health. Toronto. November.
Deber, R.B., L. Narine, P. Baranek, N. Sharpe, K.M. Duvalko, R. Zlotnik-Shaul, P. Coyte, G.H. Pink, and A.P. Williams (1998) 'The Public-Private Mix in Health Care.' In *Striking a Balance: Health Care Systems in Canada and Elsewhere*. Ed. National Forum on Health. Vol. 4. Sainte-Foy, Que.: Éditions Multi-Mondes.
Devereaux, P.J., P.T.L. Choi, C. Lacchetti, B. Weaver, H.J. Schünemann, T. Haines, J.N. Lavis, B.J.B. Grant, D.R.S. Haslam, M. Bhandari, T. Sullivan, D.J. Cook, S.D. Walter, M. Meade, H. Khan, N. Bhatnagar, and G.H. Guyatt, (2002) 'A Systematic Review and Meta-Analysis of Studies Comparing Mortality Rates of Private for-Profit and Private Not-for-Profit Hospitals.' *Canadian Medical Association Journal* 166, 1399–406.
Doern, G.B., and R.W. Phidd (1992) *Canadian Public Policy: Ideas, Structure, Process*. 2d ed. Toronto: Nelson Canada.
Donelan, K., R.J. Blendon, C. Schoen, K. Davis, and K. Binns (1999) 'The Cost of Health System Change: Public Discontent in Five Nations.' *Health Affairs* 18, 206–16.
Dumont-Lemasson, M., C. Donovan, M. Wylie, and Federal-Provincial-Territorial Advisory Committee on Health Services Working Group on Continuing Care (1999) 'Provincial and Territorial Home Care Programs: A Synthesis for Canada.' Minister of Public Works and Government Services Canada. Ottawa. June.
Ekos Research Associates Inc. (1998). 'Rethinking Government IV.' Presentation to the National Conference on Home Care. Halifax, 9 March.
- (2001) 'Rethinking Government: Exploring Changing Relationships among

Individuals, Government and Business.' Research study begun in 1994. Information available upon subscription. http://www.ekos.com/studies/government.asp.

Evans, J.R. (1987) *Toward a Shared Direction for Health in Ontario.* Report of Ontario Health Review Panel. Toronto: Ontario Ministry of Health.

Evans, R.G. (1984) *Strained Mercy: The Economics of Canadian Health Care.* Toronto: Butterworths.

Evans, R.G., M.L. Barer, G.L. Stoddart, and V. Bhatia (1993a) 'It's Not the Money, It's the Principle: Why User Charges for Some Services and Not Others.' University of British Columbia Centre for Health Services and Policy Research, HPRU, 1993: 16D. December 1993. Available at http://www.chspr.ubc.ca//hpru/pdf/hpru93_16D.pdf.

– (1993b) 'Who Are the Zombie Masters, and What Do They Want?' University of British Columbia Centre for Health Services and Policy Research, HPRU, 1993: 13D. December 1993. Available at http://www.chspr.ubc.ca//hpru/pdf/hpru93_13D.pdf

Fassbender, K. (2001). 'Substudy 3: Cost Implications of Informal Supports.' National Evaluation of the Cost-Effectiveness of Home Care, Victoria, B.C. April. Available at http://www.homecarestudy.com.

Federal, Provincial and Territorial Working Group on Home Care (1990) 'Report on Home Care.' Health and Welfare Canada, Health Services and Promotion Branch.

First Ministers (2003) '2003 First Ministers' Accord on Health Care Renewal.' 5 February. Available at http://www.hc-sc.gc.ca/english/hca2003/accord.html.

Foot, D.K., and D. Stoffman (1998) *Boom, Bust, and Echo 2000: Profiting from the Demographic Shift in the New Millennium.* Toronto: Macfarlane Walter & Ross.

– (2000) 'The Toronto That Will Be.' *Toronto Life,* January, 84–90.

Fuller, C. (1998) *Caring for Profit: How Corporations Are Taking Over Canada's Health Care System.* Vancouver: New Star Books.

Government of Canada (1984) Canada Health Act (Bill C-3). S.C. 1984, 32–3 Elizabeth II (R.S.C. 1985, c. 6; R.S.C. 1989, c. C-6).

Government of Ontario (1990a) Health Insurance Act. R.S.O. 1990, c. H.6. Amended by 1992, c. 32, s. 15; 1993, c. 2, s. 12; 1993, c. 10, s. 53; 1993, c. 32, s. 2; 1994, c 17, ss. 68–74; 1996, c. 1, Sched. H, ss. 1–35; 1996, c. 21, s. 51; 1997, c. 16, s. 7; 1998, c. 18, Sched. G, s. 54; 1999, c. 10, ss. 1, 2; 2000, c. 26, Sched. H, s. 1; 2000, c. 42, Sched., ss. 17–19; 2001, c. 8, ss. 32, 33; 2002, c. 18, Sched. I, s. 8.

– (1990b) Ministry of Community and Social Services Act. R.S.O.1990, c. M20. Amended by 1993, c. 2, ss. 23, 24; 1994, c. 27, s. 67; 1997, c. 25, s. 4 (4).

– (1993) 'Jobs and Services: A Social Contract for the Ontario Public Sector. Proposals.' 23 April.

- (1994) Long-Term Care Act, 1994. S.O. 1994, c. 26. (Bill 173 An Act respecting Long-Term Care. 3d Session, 35th Legislature, Ontario 43 Elizabeth II.) Available at http://www.e_laws.gov.on.ca/DBLaws/Statutes/English/941 26_e.htm.
- (2001) Community Care Access Corporations Act, 2001, S.O. 2001, c. 33. Amended by 2001, c. 33, s. 23. (Bill 130 An Act respecting Community Care Access Corporations. 2d Session, 37th Legislature, Ontario 50 Elizabeth II).
- Premier's Office (1996) 'Premier Fine-Tunes Cabinet.' Press release, 16 August.
Grier, R. (1994a) 'Remarks on Long-Term Care Reform.' Remarks by The Hon. Ruth Grier, Ontario Minister of Health, to District Health Councils' Conference. Toronto. 11 January.
- (1994b) 'Statement to the Legislature Re: Long-Term Care Community Services Legislation.' Ontario Minister of Health. Toronto. 6 June.
Group for Long Term Care Reform (1995a) 'Letter to Ad Hoc Group Members Re: Membership in the Group for Long Term Care Reform.' Letter from E. Lynn Moore (chair) to membership, 16 February.
- (1995b) 'Terms of Reference.' February.
Hall, L. McG., D.I. Doran, G.R. Baker, G.H. Pink, S. Sidani, L. O'Brien-Pallas, and G.J. Donner (2001) 'A Study of the Impact of Nursing Staff Mix Models and Organizational Change Strategies on Patient, System and Nurse Outcomes: A Summary Report of the Nursing Staff Mix Outcomes Study.' Faculty of Nursing, University of Toronto.
Hall, P. (1992) 'The Movement from Keynesianism to Monetarism: Institutional Analysis and British Economic Policy in the 1970s.' In *Structuring Politics: Historical Institutionalism in Comparative Analysis*. Ed. S. Steinmo, K. Thelen, and F. Longstreth. Cambridge: Cambridge University Press.
Harris, Mike (1995) 'Premier Halts Multi-Service Agencies.' News release. Toronto. 12 July.
Havens, B. (1995). 'Long-Term Care Diversity with the Care Continuum.' *Canadian Journal on Aging* 14, 245–62.
Health Services Appeal Board (1999) 'Order, in the Matter of Ian Strathern and Community Care Access Centre Niagara and Douglas Jackson.' File I.C. 6149. 6 January.
Health Services Restructuring Commission (1997) 'A Vision of Ontario's Health Services System.' January. Available at http://192.75.156.24/vision.htm.
- (1998) 'Change and Transition: Planning Guidelines and Implementation Strategies for Home Care, Long Term Care, Mental Health, Rehabilitation, and Sub-Acute Care.' April. Available at http://192.75.156.24/puple_sf_0498. doc.

Heiber, S., and R.B. Deber (1987) 'Banning Extra-Billing in Canada: Just What the Doctor Didn't Order.' *Canadian Public Policy* 13, 62–74.

Himmelstein, D. Woolhandler, S., and I. Hellander (2001) *Bleeding the Patient: The Consequences of Corporate Health Care.* Monroe, Maine: Common Courage Press.

Himmelstein, D.U., S. Woolhandler, I. Hellander, and S.M. Wolfe (1999) 'Quality of Care in Investor-Owned vs. Not-for-Profit HMOs.' *Journal of the American Medical Association* 282, 159–63.

Hirschman, A.O. (1970) *Exit, Voice and Loyalty: Responses to Decline in Firms, Organizations, and States.* Cambridge, Mass.: Harvard University Press.

Hollander, M.J. (1994) 'The Costs and Cost-Effectiveness of Continuing Care Services in Canada.' Queen's–University of Ottawa Economics Working Paper No. 94-10. Ottawa.

– (2001) 'Substudy 1: Final Report of the Study on the Comparative Cost Analysis of Home Care and Residential Care Services.' National Evaluation of the Cost-Effectiveness of Home Care. Victoria, B.C. April. Available at http://www.homecarestudy.com.

Hollander, M.J., and P. Baranek (1997) 'Long Term Care Services.' In *A Critical Review and Analysis of Health Care Related Models of Resource Allocation and Reimbursement in the Ontario Context.* Ed. M.J. Hollander, R.B. Deber, and P. Jacobs. Victoria, B.C.: Canadian Policy Network, Health Network.

Hollander, M.J., and M.J. Prince (2002) 'Analysis of Interfaces Along the Continuum of Care: Final Report: "The Third Way": A Framework for Organizing Health Related Services for Individuals with Ongoing Care Needs and their Families.' Home Care / Pharmaceuticals Division, Policy and Communications Branch, Health Canada. Ottawa.

Hollander, M.J., and Angela Tessaro (2001) 'Evaluation of the Maintenance and Preventive Function of Home Care.' Final Report. Prepared for the Home Care / Pharmaceuticals Division, Policy and Communications Branch, Health Canada by Hollander Analytical Services. Victoria B.C. March. Available at http://www.hollanderanalytical.com/downloads/preventivehomecare report.pdf

Hollander, M.J., R.B. Deber, and P.Jacobs, eds (1998) *A Critical Review of Models of Resource Allocation and Reimbursement in Health Care: A Report Prepared for the Ontario Ministry of Health.* Victoria, B.C.: Canadian Policy Research Networks.

Hollander, M.J., N. Chappell, B. Havens, C. McWilliam, and J.A. Miller (2002) 'Substudy 5: Study of the Costs and Outcomes of Home Care and Residential Long Term Care Services.' National Evaluation of the Cost- Effectiveness of Home Care. Victoria, B.C. February. Available at http://www.homecarestudy.com.

Hospital Report Research Collaborative (2001) 'Hospital Report 2001: Acute Care.' Canadian Institute for Health Information. Ottawa.

Hutchison, B., J. Abelson, and J. Lavis (2001) 'Primary Care in Canada: So Much Innovation, So Little Change.' *Health Affairs* 20, 116–31.

Immergut, E. (1992) 'The Rules of the Game: The Logic of Health Policy-Making in France, Switzerland, and Sweden.' In *Structuring Politics: Historical Institutionalism in Comparative Analysis.* Ed. S. Steinmo, K. Thelen, and F. Longstreth. New York: Cambridge University Press.

Jackson, R.A. (1994) 'Home Care: The Cornerstone of Health Renewal in Nova Scotia.' *Leadership in Health Services* 4, 5–14.

Jacobs, P. (2001) 'Substudy 9: Costs of Acute Care and Home Care Services.' National Evaluation of the Cost-Effectiveness of Home Care. Victoria, B.C. April. Available at http://www.homecarestudy.com

Jacobs, P., E. Hall, I. Henderson, and D. Nichols (1995) 'Episodic Acute Care Costs: Linking Inpatient and Home Care.' *Canadian Journal of Public Health* 86, 205.

Johnson, J.B., and R.A. Joslyn (1995) *Political Science Research Methods.* 3d ed. Washington, D.C.: Congressional Quarterly Press.

Kamerman, S.B., and A.J. Kahn, eds (1989) *Privatization and the Welfare State.* Princeton, N.J.: Princeton University Press.

Kellow, A.J. (1988) 'Promoting Elegance in Policy Theory: Simplifying Lowi's Arenas of Power.' *Policy Studies Journal* 16, 713–24.

Knapp, M. (1986) 'The Relative Cost-Effectiveness of Public, Voluntary and Private Providers of Residential Child Care.' In *Public and Private Health Services: Complementarities and Conflict.* Ed. A.J. Culyer and B. Jönsson. Oxford: Basil Blackwell.

Lalonde, M. (1974) *A New Perspective on the Health of Canadians: A Working Document.* Ottawa: Information Canada.

Lankin, F. (1992a) 'Remarks to the Ontario Community Support Association.' Ontario Minister of Health, Report on the Long-Term Care Consultation. 25 May.

– (1992b) 'Remarks to the Senior Citizens' Alliance for Long-Term Care.' 6 July.

– (1992c) 'Statement to the Legislature re: Long-Term Care.' Ontario Minister of Health. 26 November. Available at http://hansardindex.ontla.on.ca/hansardeissue/35_2/1086 a.htm

– (1992d) 'Statement to the Legislature re: Long-Term Care.' 2 December. Available at http://hansardindex.ontla.on.ca/hansardeissue/35_2/1089 a.htm.

Leitch, J. (1991) Personal communication to Frances Lankin, Marion Boyd, Elaine Ziemba (chair). SCCA. 22 June.

Liberal Party of Ontario (1990) 'Working for Ontario: The Peterson Team.'
    News release. MCSS. 30 May.
Lomas, J., and A.-P. Contandriopoulos (1994) 'Regulating Limits to Medicine:
    Towards Harmony in Public- and Self-Regulation.' In *Why Are Some People
    Healthy and Others Not? The Determinants of Health of Populations.* Ed. R.G. Evans,
    M. Barer, and T. Marmor. New York: Aldine De Gruyter.
MacDonnell, S. (2001) 'A Commitment to Care: Community Support Services
    for Seniors.' Allocations and Community Services Department, United Way of
    Greater Toronto. November.
Maioni, A. (1997) 'Parting at the Crossroads: The Development of Health Insur-
    ance in Canada and the United States.' *Comparative Politics* 29, 411– 32.
– (1998) *Parting at the Crossroads: The Emergence of Health Insurance in the United
    States and Canada.* Princeton, N.J.: Princeton University Press.
Manzer, R. (1994) *Public Schools and Political Ideas: Canadian Educational Policy in
    Historical Perspective.* Toronto: University of Toronto Press.
McFetridge, D.G. (1997) 'The Economics of Privatization.' C.D. Howe Institute
    Benefactors Lecture. Toronto. 22 October.
McLean, I., ed. (1996) *The Concise Oxford Dictionary of Politics.* Oxford: Oxford
    University Press.
Mendelsohn, M. (2002) 'Canadians' Thoughts on Their Health Care System:
    Preserving the Canadian Model through Innovation.' Paper prepared for the
    Commission on the Future of Health Care in Canada. June.
Multicultural Alliance for Seniors and Aging (1994) 'Brief on Bill 173 presented
    to the Standing Committee on Social Development.' Presented by Dr D. Ore-
    opoulous, president, and Dr J. Wong, vice-president, on behalf of the Multi-
    cultural Alliance for Seniors and Aging. 13 September.
National Forum on Health (1997) *Canada Health Action: Building on the Legacy:
    The Final Report of the National Forum on Health.* Vol. 1. Ottawa: National Forum
    on Health.
Naylor, C.D. (1986) *Private Practice, Public Payment: Canadian Medicine and the Pol-
    itics of Health Insurance 1911–1966.* Kingston, Ont.: McGill-Queen's University
    Press.
Nickoloff, B., B. Quinn, H. Zulys, and R.B. Deber (1994) 'To Be or Not To Be:
    Coordinating and Integrating Services for the Elderly.' Paper for Case Studies
    in Health Policy. HAD5765. University of Toronto (course director, Raisa
    Deber).
O'Brien-Pallas, L., and A. Baumann (1999) 'The State of Nursing Practice in
    Ontario: The Issues, Challenges and Needs.' Nursing Effectiveness, Utiliza-
    tion and Outcomes Research Unit, College of Nursing, University of Toronto.
O'Brien-Pallas, L., A. Baumann, and J. Lochhaas-Gerlach (1998) 'Health

Human Resources: A Preliminary Analysis of Nursing Personnel in Ontario.'
Report prepared for Ontario Ministry of Health and Long Term Care Nurs-
ing Task Force. Nursing Effectiveness, Utilization and Outcomes Research
Unit, Faculty of Nursing, University of Toronto.

Office of the Auditor General of New Brunswick (1998) '1998 Auditor General's
Report.' Chapter 14: 'Special Report for the Public Accounts Committee,
Evergreen and Wackenhut Leases.' Available at http://www.gnb.ca.

Office of the Auditor General of Nova Scotia (1997) '1997 Auditor General's
Report.' Chapter 8: 'Education and Culture: Public-Private Partnerships for
School Construction.' Available at http://www.gov.ns.ca/audg/1997ag.htm.

– (1998) '1998 Auditor General's Report.' Chapter 7: 'Education and Culture:
Public-Private Partnerships for School Construction Follow-up Review.' Available at http://www.gov.ns.ca/audg/1998ag.htm.

– (1999) '1999 Auditor General's Report.' Chapter 5: 'Education: Public-Private
Partnerships (P3s) for School Construction – Follow-up Review.' Available at
http://www.gov.ns.ca.

Office of the Provincial Auditor General of Ontario (1998a) '1998 Annual
Report.' Available at http://www.gov.on.ca/opa/english/r98t.htm.

– (1998b) *1998 Annual Report of the Provincial Auditor General of Ontario to the Legislative Assembly.* Toronto: Queen's Printer for Ontario.

– (1999) '1999 Annual Report.' Available at http://www.gov.on.ca/opa/
english/r99t.htm.

– (2000) 'Special Report on Accountability and Value for Money.' Chapter 4:
'Follow-up of Recommendations in the 1998 Annual Report.' Available at
http://www.gov.on.ca.

Ontario Association for Volunteer Administration, Ontario Association of Directors of Volunteers in Healthcare Services, and Volunteer Ontario (1994)
'Brief Presented to the Standing Committee on Social Development Hearings
on Bill 173 An Act Respecting Long Term Care.' 4 October.

Ontario Association of Residents' Councils (1994) 'Letter from Peter J. Kehoe to
the Honourable Bob Rae, Premier, Province of Ontario, Re: Bill 173, The
Long-Term Care Act.' 29 September.

Ontario Coalition of Senior Citizens' Organizations (OCSCO) (1994) 'Presentation to the Standing Committee on Social Development: Bill 173 – An Act
Respecting Long Term Care.' 16 August.

Ontario Community Support Association (OCSA) (1994) 'Presentation Notes to
the Standing Committee on Social Development Regarding Bill 173 "An Act
Respecting Long-Term Care."' 17 August.

Ontario Federation of Labour (OFL) (1994) 'Submission by Julie Davis, Secre-
tary-Treasurer, Ontario Federation of Labour to the Standing Committee on

Social Development Regarding the Long-Term Care Act, 1994 (Bill 173).'
3 October.

Ontario Home Care Programs Association (OHCPA) (1994) 'Submission to the
Standing Committee on Social Development Regarding Bill 173, "An Act
Respecting Long-Term Care."' 15 September.

Ontario Home Health Care Providers' Association (OHHCPA) (1994) 'Submission to the Standing Committee on Social Development: Bill 173 – An Act
Respecting Long Term Care. Government of Ontario.' 17 August.

– (2001) 'Private Sector Delivery of Home Health Care in Ontario.' Hamilton,
June. Available at http://www.ohhcpa.on.ca/docs.

Ontario Home Health Care Providers' Association (OHHCPA) and Ontario
Community Support Association (OCSA) (2001) 'Building a High Performance Home and Community Care System in Ontario.' 31 October. Available
at http://www.homecareontario.ca/docs/papers/OHHCPA_OCSApaper.
pdf.

Ontario Hospital Association (OHA) and Council of Chronic Hospitals of
Ontario (CCHO) (1994) 'A Joint Presentation by the Ontario Hospital Association and the Council of Chronic Hospitals of Ontario to the Ontario Legislature's Standing Committee on Social Development Regarding Bill 173, the
Long-Term Care Act.' Speaking notes for remarks by Isabelle Laurent, chair-
elect, Ontario Hospital Association. 12 September.

Ontario March of Dimes (1994) 'Submission to the Standing Committee on
Social Development on Bill 173.' August.

Ontario Minister of Finance (1993) 'Ontario's Expenditure Control Plan.' April.

Ontario Minister of Health (1992) 'Expanded Homemaker Services, New Palliative Care Policy to Improve Long-Term Care.' News release. 2 December.

– (1994) 'Compendium – Long-Term Care Act, 1994: An Act Respecting Long-
Term Care.' 6 June.

Ontario Ministry of Community and Social Services (MCSS) (1989) 'Looking
Ahead: Trends and Implications in the Social Environment.' May.

Ontario Ministry of Community and Social Services (MCSS), Ontario Ministry of
Health (MOH), and Ontario Ministry of Citizenship (MC) (1991) *Redirection
of Long-Term Care and Support Services in Ontario: A Public Consultation Paper.*
Toronto: Queen's Printer for Ontario.

Ontario Ministry of Community and Social Services (MCSS), Ontario Ministry of
Health (MOH), Ontario Office for Senior Citizens' Affairs (OSCA), and
Ontario Office for Disabled Persons (ODP) (1990) *Strategies for Change: Comprehensive Reform of Ontario's Long-Term Care Services.* Toronto: Queen's Printer
for Ontario.

Ontario Ministry of Finance (1993) 'Ontario Budget.' May.

Ontario Ministry of Health (MOH) (1994a) 'Grier Tables Legislation for Long-Term Care Expansion.' News release. Toronto. 6 June.

- (1994b) 'Redirection of Long-Term Care and Support Services in Ontario: Questions and Answers.' January.
- (1995a) 'Halting MSA Development: Qs and Suggested As.' 10 July.
- (1995b) 'Request for Proposals. Discussions with Key Groups Representing Long- Term Care Users, Providers, and Workers.' 14 July.
- (1996a) 'Backgrounder: Community Care Access Centres.' 25 January.
- (1996b) 'Community Care Access Centre: Job Description for Board Members.' 21 March.
- (1996c) 'Community Care Access Centres: Board Orientation.' Long-Term Care Division. June.
- (1996d) 'Government Unveils Plan for Speedy Long-Term Care Reform.' News release. 25 January.
- (1997) Personal communication to the authors.

Ontario Ministry of Health, Long-Term Care Policy Branch (1993) 'Draft Manual for Community-Based Services Provided by Multi-Service Agencies.'

Ontario Ministry of Health (MOH) and Ontario Ministry of Community and Social Services (MCSS) (1992) Compendium. Bill 101 Long-Term Care Statute Law Amendment Act, 1992. First reading 26 November. Second reading, 2 December.

Ontario Ministry of Health (MOH), Ontario Ministry of Community and Social Services (MCSS), and Ontario Ministry of Citizenship (MC) (1993a) *Partnerships in Long-Term Care: A New Way to Plan, Manage and Deliver Services and Community Support: A Policy Framework*. Toronto: Queen's Printer for Ontario. April.

- (1993b) *Building Partnerships in Long-Term Care: A New Way to Plan, Manage and Deliver Services and Community Support: A Local Planning Framework*. Toronto: Queen's Printer for Ontario. May.
- (1993c). *Partnerships in Long-Term Care: A New Way to Plan, Manage and Deliver Services and Community Support: An Implementation Framework*. Toronto: Queen's Printer for Ontario. June.
- (1993d) *Partnerships in Long-Term Care: A New Way to Plan, Manage and Deliver Services and Community Support: Guidelines for the Establishment of Multi-Service Agencies*. Toronto: Queen's Printer for Ontario. September.

Ontario Ministry of Health (MOH), Long-Term Care Division, and Ontario Ministry of Community and Social Services (MCSS) (1992a) 'Redirection of Long-Term Care and Support Services in Ontario.' Consultation with Provincial Associations. May.

- (1992b) 'Results from the Consultation on the Redirection of Long-Term

Care and Support Services in Ontario.' A report from the Government of Ontario. 27 May.

– (1993) 'Community-Based Services Provided by Multi-Service Agencies.' Long- Term Care Policy Branch, Draft. 20 August.

Ontario Ministry of Treasury and Economics (1992) '1992 Ontario Budget: Managing Health Care Resources.' Supplementary Paper. May.

Ontario Nurses' Association (ONA) (1994) 'Submission by the Ontario Nurses' Association to the Standing Committee on Social Development on Bill 173 – Long Term Care Act, 1994.' 3 October.

Ontario Office for Senior Citizens' Affairs (OSCA) (1985) 'Ministers Consultation Meetings: Summary of Comments and Suggestions on Programs and Services for Senior Citizens in Ontario.'

– (1987a) 'Minister for Senior Citizens' Affairs Announces One-Stop Access Sites.' News release. 11 June.

– (1987b) 'One-Stop Access.' Backgrounder. 11 June.

– (1987c). 'One-Stop Shopping or an Integrated Approach to Community Health and Social Services.' Consultation Tour. Slide Presentation. Winter.

Ontario Public Service Employees Union (OPSEU) (1994) 'Bill 173: The Rhetoric and the Reality. A Presentation to the Standing Committee on Social Development by the Ontario Public Service Employees Union.' 16 August.

Ontario Task Force on Aging (1981) 'The Elderly in Ontario: An Agenda for the '80s.' Secretariat for Social Development. Government of Ontario. December.

Organisation for Economic Co-operation and Development (OECD) (1987) *Financing and Delivering Health Care: A Comparative Analysis of OECD Countries.* Paris: OECD.

– (1990) *Health Care Systems in Transition: The Search for Efficiency.* Paris: OECD.

– (2000): 'A Comparative Analysis of 29 Countries.' OECD Health Data. Compact Disc. Paris: OECD.

Osborne, D.E., and T. Gaebler (1992) *Reinventing Government: How the Entrepreneurial Spirit is Transforming the Public Sector.* Reading, Mass.: Addison-Wesley.

Pal, L.A. (1992) *Public Policy Analysis: An Introduction.* 2nd ed. Scarborough, Ont.: Nelson Canada.

Podborski, S. (1987) *Health Promotion Matters in Ontario: A Report of the Minister's Advisory Group on Health Promotion.* Toronto: Ontario Ministry of Health.

Poullier, J. (1986) 'Levels and Trends in the Public-Private Mix in Industrialized Countries' Health Systems.' In *Public and Private Health Services: Complementarities and Conflicts.* Ed. A.J. Culyer and B. Jonsson. Oxford: Basil Blackwell.

Preker, A.S., A. Harding, and P. Travis (2000) '"Make or Buy" Decisions in the Production of Health Care Goods and Services: New Insights from Institutional Economics and Organizational Theory.' *Bulletin of the World Health Organization* 78, 779–89.

Premier's Advisory Council on Health for Alberta (2001) 'A Framework for Reform.' Report of the Premier's Advisory Council on Health. December.

Premier's Council on Health Strategy (1989a) *From Vision to Action: Report of the Health Care System Committee.* Toronto: Queen's Printer for Ontario.

– (1989b) *A Vision of Health – Health Goals for Ontario.* Toronto: Queen's Printer for Ontario.

– (1991a) *Achieving the Vision: Health and Human Resources.* Health Care System Committee. Toronto: Queen's Printer for Ontario.

– (1991b) *Local Decision Making for Health And Social Services: Report of the Integration and Coordination Committee.* Toronto: Queen's Printer for Ontario.

– (1991c) *Nurturing Health – A Framework on the Determinants of Health.* Toronto: Queen's Printer for Ontario.

– (1991d) 'Towards a Strategic Framework for Optimizing Health, 1987–1991.' Government of Ontario. Toronto.

– (1991e) 'Towards Health Outcomes: Goals 2 and 4: Objectives and Targets.' Health Goals Committee. Government of Ontario. Toronto.

Progressive Conservative Party of Ontario (1994) *The Common Sense Revolution.* Toronto. May.

Pross, A.P. (1992) *Group Politics and Public Policy.* 2d ed. Toronto: Oxford University Press.

– ed. (1975) *Pressure Group Behaviour in Canadian Politics.* Toronto: McGraw-Hill Ryerson.

Qualitative Solutions and Research Pty Ltd (1997) 'QSR NUD*IST4: User Guide 1997.' Australia.

Rachlis, M.M. (2000) 'The Hidden Costs of Privatization: An International Comparison of Community Care.' Part II in *Without Foundation: How Medicare Is Undermined by Gaps and Privatization in Community and Continuing Care.* Ed. M. Cohen and N. Pollock. Vancouver: Canadian Centre for Policy Alternatives – B.C. Office. Summary available from http://www.policyalternatives.ca/bc/withoutfoundation.html.

Rachlis, M.M., and C. Kushner (1994) *Strong Medicine: How to Save Canada's Health Care System.* Toronto: HarperCollins.

Rachlis, M.M., R.G. Evans, P. Lewis, and M.L. Barer (2001) 'Revitalizing Medicare: Shared Problems, Public Solutions.' Report. Tommy Douglas Research Institute. Vancouver. January. Available at http://www.tommydouglas.ca/reports/revitalizingmedicare.pdf

Redden, C.J. (1999) 'Rationing Care in the Community: Engaging Citizens in Health Care Decision Making.' *Journal of Health Politics, Policy and Law* 24, 136–8.

Relman, A.S. (1992) 'What Market Values Are Doing to Medicine.' *Atlantic Monthly*, March, 99–106.

Rhodes, P., and G.P. Murray Research (1994a) 'Media Guidelines.' Memo to Bill
173 Coalition, 25 October.
– (1994b) Memo to Lynn Moore: Revised – Visiting Queen's Park / Public Gal-
lery. 26 October.
Rice, T. (1998) *The Economics of Health Reconsidered.* Chicago: Health Administra-
tion Press.
Ross, N.A., M.C. Wolfson, J.R. Dunn, J.-M. Bertholet, G.A. Kaplan, and J.W.
Lynch (2000) 'Relation between Income Inequality and Mortality in Canada
and in the United States: Cross Sectional Assessment Using Census Data and
Vital Statistics.' *British Medical Journal* 320, 898–902.
Saint Elizabeth Visiting Nurses Association (1994a) 'Bill 173 Fact Sheet.'
– (1994b) 'Sample General Letter.'
Saltman, R.B. (1995) 'The Public-Private Mix in Financing and Producing
Health Services.' Mimeo report prepared for the World Bank. February.
Saltman, R.B., and C. von Otter (1992a) *Planned Markets and Public Competition:
Strategic Reform in Northern European Health Systems.* Philadelphia: Open Univer-
sity Press.
– (1992b) 'Reforming Swedish Health Care in the 1990s: The Emerging Role of
"Public Firms." ' *Health Policy* 21, 143–54.
– eds (1995) *State of Health. Implementing Planned Markets in Health Care: Balanc-
ing Social and Economic Responsibility.* Milton Keynes, U.K.: Open University
Press.
Saskatchewan Health Services Utilization and Research Commission (2000)
'The Impact of Preventive Home Care and Seniors Housing on Health Outcomes.' Summary Report No. 14. May. Available at http://www.hsurc.sk.ca/
reserch-studies/pdf.php3?id=2&section=l.
Schattschneider, E E. (1964) *The Semisovereign People: A Realist's View of Democracy
in America.* New York: Holt, Rinehart and Winston.
Schieber, G.J., and J.-P. Poullier (1991) 'International Health Spending: Issues
and Trends.' *Health Affairs* 10, 106–16.
Schlesinger, M. (1998) 'Mismeasuring the Consequences of Ownership: External Influences and the Comparative Performance of Public, For-Profit, and
Private Nonprofit Organizations.' In *Private Action and the Public Good.* Ed.
W.W. Powell and E.S. Clemens. New Haven, Conn.: Yale University Press.
Senior Citizens' Consumer Alliance for Long-Term Care Reform (SCCA) (1992)
'Consumer Report on Long-Term Care Reform.' Report prepared for the Pol-
icy Conference on Long-Term Care Reform. Old Mill, Toronto. 6 July.
– (1993) 'Consumer Response to the Government's Long-Term Care Reform
Policies.' A response prepared by the SCCA for Long-Term Care Reform.
October.

– (1994) 'A Consumer Response to Bill 173, An Act Respecting Long Term Care: An Urgent Plea to Reform Ontario's System of Long-Term Care Services.' Submission to the Standing Committee on Social Development. Government of Ontario. Toronto. 15 September.

Shamian, J., and E.Y. Lightstone (1997) 'Hospital Restructuring Initiatives in Canada.' *Medical Care* 35(10), Supplement, OS62–9.

Shapiro, E. (1992) 'There's No Place Like Home.' In *Restructuring Canada's Health Services System: How Do We Get There From Here?* Ed. R.B. Deber and G.G. Thompson. Toronto: University of Toronto Press.

– (1997) *The Cost of Privatization: A Case Study of Home Care in Manitoba.* Ottawa: Canadian Centre for Policy Alternatives.

Sheps, S.B., R.J. Reid, M.L. Barer, H. Krueger, K.M. McGrail, B. Green, R.G. Evans, and C. Hertzman (2000) 'Hospital Downsizing and Trends in Health Care Use among Elderly People in British Columbia.' *Canadian Medical Association Journal* 163, 397–401.

Simeon, R.E. (1976) 'Studying Public Policy.' *Canadian Journal of Political Science* 4, 548–80.

Spasoff, R.A. (1987) *Health For All Ontario – Report of the Panel on Health Goals for Ontario.* Toronto: Ontario Ministry of Health.

Standing Senate Committee on Social Affairs Science and Technology (2002) 'The Health of Canadians: The Federal Role.' Vol. 6. 'Recommendations for Reform.' Final report on the state of the health care system in Canada. October. Ottawa: Parliament of Canada. Available at http://www.parl.gc.ca/37/2/parlbus/commbus/senate/Com_e/SOCI_E/ repoct02vol6_e.htm.

Stapleton, D. (1994a) 'Memo to OCSA Board of Directors Re: Important Update Re Bill 173.' 16 November.

– (1994b) 'Memorandum to OCSA Board of Directors Re: Ad Hoc Group Concerned with Bill 173.' 19 October.

Starr, P. (1982) *The Social Transformation of American Medicine.* New York: Basic Books.

– (1989) 'The Meaning of Privatization.' In *Privatization and the Welfare State,* ed. S.B. Kamerman and A.J. Kahn. Princeton, N.J.: Princeton University Press.

Stevenson, H.M., and A.P. Williams (1985) 'Physicians and Medicare: Professional Ideology and Canadian Health Care Policy.' *Canadian Public Policy* 11, 504–21.

Stevenson, H.M., A.P. Williams, and E. Vayda (1988) 'Medical Politics and Canadian Medicare: Professional Response to the Canada Health Act.' *Milbank Quarterly* 66, 65–104.

Stewart, R., and M. Lund (1990) 'Home Care: The Ontario Experience.' *Pride Institute Journal of Long Term Home Health Care* 9, 15–25.

Stoddart, G.L., and R.J. Labelle (1985) *Privatization in the Canadian Health Care System: Assertions, Evidence, Ideology and Options.* Ottawa: Department of National Health and Welfare.

Stone, D.A. (1997) *Policy Paradox: The Art of Political Decision Making.* New York: W.W. Norton.

Sutherland, R. (2001) 'The Costs of Contracting Out Home Care: A Behind the Scenes Look at Home Care in Ontario.' CUPE Research. Ottawa. Available at http://www.cupe.ca/www/ContractingOut.

Sweeney, J. (1989) 'Long Term Care for the Elderly and People with Physical Disabilities.' Minister of Community and Social Services statement to the Ontario Legislature. 7 June.

Taft, K., and G. Steward (2000) *Clear Answers: The Economics and Politics of For-Profit Medicine.* Edmonton, Alta: Duval House Publishing / Parkland Institute / University of Alberta Press.

Taylor, M.G. (1987) *Health Insurance and Canadian Public Policy. The Seven Decisions that Created the Canadian Health Insurance System and their Outcomes.* 2d ed. Kingston, Ont.: McGill-Queen's University Press.

Thelen, K., and S. Steinmo (1992) 'Historical Institutionalism in Comparative Politics.' In *Structuring Politics: Historical Institutionalism in Comparative Analysis.* Ed. S. Steinmo, K. Thelen, and F. Longstreth. Cambridge: Cambridge University Press.

Tuohy, C.J. (1992) *Policy and Politics in Canada: Institutionalized Ambivalence.* Philadelphia, Pa.: Temple University Press.

– (1999a) *Accidental Logics: The Dynamics of Change in the Health Care Arena in the United States, Britain, and Canada.* New York: Oxford University Press.

– (1999b) 'Dynamics of a Changing Health Sphere: The United States, Britain, and Canada.' *Health Affairs* 18, 114–34.

Van Horne, R. (1986) *A New Agenda: Health and Social Service Strategies for Ontario's Seniors.* Toronto: Queen's Printer for Ontario.

Vogel, D. (2000) 'Unfulfilled Promise: How Health Care Reforms of the 1990s Are Failing Community and Continuing Care in B.C.' Part I in *Without Foundation: How Medicare Is Undermined by Gaps and Privatization in' Community and Continuing Care.* Ed. M. Cohen and N. Pollock. Vancouver: Canadian Centre for Policy Alternatives – B.C. Office. Summary available at http://www.policyalternatives.ca/bc/withoutfoundation.html.

Weir, M. (1992) *Politics and Jobs: The Boundaries of Employment Policy in the United States.* Princeton, N.J.: Princeton University Press.

Wessenger, P. (1994) *Hansard.* Legislative Assembly of Ontario. 15 June. Available at http://www.ontla.on.ca/hansard/house_debates/35_parl/session3/1144b.htm#P245_91559

Williams, A.P., P. Baranek, J. Lum, and R.B. Deber (2002) 'Mapping the Front Lines of Canadian Medicare: The Logics of Health Care Restructuring in Ontario.' Paper presented at the Congress of the Social Sciences and Humanities, Annual Meeting of the Canadian Political Science Association. 25 May–1 June.

Williams, A.P., J. Barnsley, S. Leggat, R.B. Deber, and P. Baranek (1999) 'Long Term Care Goes to Market: Managed Competition and Ontario's Reform of Community-Based Services.' *Canadian Journal on Aging* 18, 125–51.

Williams, A.P., R.B. Deber, P. Baranek, and A. Gildiner (2001) 'From Medicare to Home Care: Globalization, State Retrenchment and the Profitization of Canada's Health Care System.' In *Unhealthy Times: Political Economy Perspectives on Health and Care in Canada.* Ed. P. Armstrong, H. Armstrong, and D. Coburn. Toronto: Oxford University Press.

Williams, A.P., E. Vayda, M.L. Cohen, C.A. Woodward, and B.M. Ferrier (1995) 'Medicine and the Canadian State: From the Politics of Conflict to the Politics of Accommodation?' *Journal of Health and Social Behavior* 36, 303–21.

Wilson, J. (1995) 'Prescribing Solutions to Health Care.' Remarks by Jim Wilson, M.P.P. (Ontario), Progressive Conservative Health Critic, to the Lexium Conference. 31 May.

– (1996) 'Notes for Remarks by the Honourable Jim Wilson, Minister of Health, for Community Care Access Centres.' Toronto. 25 January.

World Health Organization (WHO) Regional Office for Europe (1978) 'Declaration of Alma-Ata.' International Conference on Primary Health Care. Alma-Ata, USSR. 6–12 September. Available at http://www.who.dk/AboutWHO/Policy/20010827_1.

– (1986) 'Ottawa Charter for Health Promotion.' First International Conference on Health Promotion. Ottawa, Canada. 17–21 November. Available at http://www.who.dk/AboutWHO/Policy/20010827_2.

Wright, T. (1997) 'A Special Report to the Legislative Assembly of Ontario on the Disclosure of Personal Information at the Ministry of Health.' From the World Wide Web site of the Information and Privacy Commissioner of Ontario. 20 February. Available at http://www.ipc.on.ca/english/pubpres/reports/health.htm.

Yin, R.K. (1989) *Case Study Research: Design and Methods.* London: Sage.

Zelder, M. (2001) 'How Private Hospital Competition Can Improve Canadian Health Care.' Public Policy Sources No. 35. Fraser Institute. Available at http://www.fraserinstitute.ca.

Index